Design and Implementation of the Modern Men's
Health Center

Joseph P. Alukal • Steven Lamm
Thomas J. Walsh
Editors

Design and Implementation of the Modern Men's Health Center

A Multidisciplinary Approach

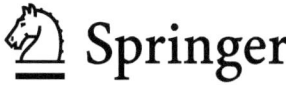 Springer

Editors
Joseph P. Alukal
Vagelos College of Physicians and Surgeons
Columbia University Irving Medical Center
New York, NY
USA

Steven Lamm
Preston Robert Tisch Center
New York University
New York, NY
USA

Thomas J. Walsh
University of Washington
Seattle, WA
USA

ISBN 978-3-030-54481-2   ISBN 978-3-030-54482-9   (eBook)
https://doi.org/10.1007/978-3-030-54482-9

This Springer imprint is published by the registered company Springer Nature Switzerland AG
The registered company address is: Gewerbestrasse 11, 6330 Cham, Switzerland

Preface

Over the past 2 years, while working on this book, there were numerous advances in medicine and men's health that helped shape our chosen content. But certainly no one event defined our experience in medicine—not just men's health—to a greater degree than the COVID-19 pandemic. Watching the sacrifice of our colleagues in healthcare, the suffering of our patients, the anxiety of the community as a whole—these experiences have shaped us tremendously (in particular given our practices in New York City and Seattle), and in turn have influenced our thinking about this book.

First and foremost, the pandemic made us even more appreciative of the tireless dedication of our authors, our partners, and our support staff in the clinics and hospitals. The willingness of healthcare providers and essential staff to do their best in the face of risk and suffering has been inspirational.

Second, the pandemic brought back to the forefront for both of us the humanism at the heart of medicine. Suffering, fear, illness, and death in patients stricken with COVID-19, quarantined at home, or hospitalized, these patients and their experiences evoke the desire to do everything in one's power to help. Research shows that men are disproportionately burdened by the negative impacts of COVID-19, including higher likelihoods of hospitalization and death due to the disease. It is unclear why this might be the case, and certain comorbidity may be the most important contributing factor, and in that light, this book became even more important. If something in here can make men become more healthy, and thereby impart them some resistance to the disease, then we've made a needed difference.

Third, we felt the pull to help the community we belong to—healthcare providers—in some meaningful way. Hopefully, this book can provide them a toolkit with which they can make their practices and men's health centers work better. If this makes their life any easier, and in turn helps them better navigate the demands of their healthcare system as the pandemic proceeds, we are happy to help. This is a difficult time, and we should all do what we can to help each other however we can, now more than ever.

We are thankful for the support of friends and family who helped us in the completion of this book, tolerating long nights spent reading and writing and shoehorning this additional bit of work into our already full professional and personal lives.

We are as well grateful for the support, patience, and knowhow of the editorial staff at Springer. Without this support, the finished product here would not have become a reality.

We hope within that product you will find a resource that can help you provide up-to-date and state-of-the-art care for your male patients. We hope that it will enable you to build or grow your own men's health center. And in that capacity, we hope you will be able to be the best doctor you can to your patients. Certainly, in this particular moment, no mission or calling is more important.

Best wishes for your own continued health and success.

New York, NY, USA	Joseph P. Alukal
New York, NY, USA	Steven Lamm
Seattle, WA, USA	Thomas J. Walsh

Contents

Contributors

Joseph P. Alukal, MD Department of Urology, Columbia University Irving Medical Center, New York, NY, USA

Denise Asafu-Adjei, MD, MPH Columbia University Irving Medical Center, Department of Urology, New York, NY, USA

Marc A. Bjurlin, DO, MSc Department of Urology, Lineberger Comprehensive Cancer Center, University of North Carolina at Chapel Hill, Chapel Hill, NC, USA

Kenneth Brill, MD Department of Medicine, NYU Grossman School of Medicine, New York, NY, USA

Benjamin Brucker, MD NYU, Department of Urology, New York, NY, USA

Joseph M. Caputo, MD Columbia University Irving Medical Center, Department of Urology, New York, NY, USA

Patricia Freitas Corradi, MD Rede Mater Dei de Saúde, Department of Endocrinology, Belo Horizonte, Minas Gerais, Brazil

Renato B. Corradi, MD Rede Mater Dei de Saúde, Department of Urology, Belo Horizonte, Minas Gerais, Brazil

Loren Wissner Greene, MD, MA (Bioethics) New York University School of Medicine, New York, NY, USA

Akash A. Kapadia, MD University of Washington, Department of Urology, Seattle, WA, USA

Matthew Katz, MD NYU, Department of Urology, New York, NY, USA

Cynthia W. Ko, MD, MS Department of Medicine, Division of Gastroenterology, University of Washington, Seattle, WA, USA

Rebecca Kosowicz, MD Department of Medicine, Division of Gastroenterology, University of Washington, Seattle, WA, USA

Steven Lamm, MD Preston Robert Tisch Center, New York University, New York, NY, USA

Vanessa L. Pascoe, MD Department of Dermatology, Beth Israel Deaconess Medical Center, Boston, MA, USA

Mike Pell Envisioneer, Woodinville, WA, USA

Benjamin H. Press, MD Department of Urology, Yale School of Medicine, New Haven, CT, USA

Susanne A. Quallich, PhD, ANP-BC, NP-C, CUNP, FAANP University of Michigan/Michigan Medicine, Department of Urology, Ann Arbor, MI, USA

Gundu H. R. Rao, PhD, MBBS Emeritus Professor, Laboratory Medicine and Pathology, Director, Thrombosis Research, Lillehei Heart Institute, University of Minnesota, Minneapolis, MN, USA

Maryam Safaee, MD Tibor Rubin Veteran's Administration Medical Center, Long Beach, CA, USA

Christopher I. Sayegh, MD Columbia University Irving Medical Center, Department of Urology, New York, NY, USA

Paul R. Shin, MD Reproductive Urology, Shady Grove Fertility and Reproductive Science Center, Rockville, MD, USA

Michi Shinohara, MD University of Washington, Division of Dermatology, Seattle, WA, USA

Molly M. Shores, MD VA Puget Sound Health Care System, University of Washington, Department of Psychiatry and Behavioral Sciences, Seattle, WA, USA

Michael Siev, MD NYU, Department of Urology, New York, NY, USA

Samir S. Taneja, MD Division of Urologic Oncology, Department of Urology, NYU Langone Health, New York, NY, USA

Thomas J. Walsh, MD, MBA University of Washington, Seattle, WA, USA

Vinson Wang, MD Columbia University Irving Medical Center, Department of Urology, New York, NY, USA

Hunter Wessells, MD, FACS Department of Urology, Harborview Injury Prevention and Research Center, Diabetes Research Center, University of Washington School of Medicine, Seattle, WA, USA

Alina Wong, MD Department of Medicine, Division of Gastroenterology, University of Washington, Seattle, WA, USA

Chapter 1
The Multidisciplinary Men's Health Center: A Modern-Day Necessity

Joseph P. Alukal and Thomas J. Walsh

Patient preference has driven a number of trends in the past 100 years of medicine including the rise of concierge practices, telemedicine, and same-day surgery among many other examples. In the end, convenience and access have driven all these trends; patients would like to more easily and completely access their doctor's expertise. They would like to do this without leaving their home or spending too much time in the doctor's waiting room, and given the busy constraints of modern life, this is entirely understandable.

As physicians, the drive to accommodate these demands can sometimes feel burdensome. Doctors feel that pressure to share their time and talent with their patients before you get to requests such as alternate schedules (nighttime and weekend hours), same-day appointments, and necessary phone call follow-ups that can't be billed for: all of these pressures conspire to create frustration, not to minimize it.

At first glance, the men's health center – multiple providers of all specialties but most notably urologists, primary care doctors, and cardiologists under one roof – seems to only cater to this pressure in the extreme. But in our own time spent at our home institutions in these centers, each of the practitioners involved in this book has noticed instead the opposite. The opportunity to work collaboratively with providers outside our specialty, the quality of the tailored care we can provide patients through our centers, and the opportunity to see our patients happy with the care they receive – each of these factors is tremendously rewarding, before you get to the necessity of the actual care and style of care being provided.

No demographic utilizes healthcare resources less than men between the ages of 18 and 45; this statistic is often cited, but it truly illuminates the crux of what we are

J. P. Alukal (✉)
Columbia University Irving Medical Center, New York, NY, USA
e-mail: jpa2148@cumc.columbia.edu

T. J. Walsh
University of Washington, Seattle, WA, USA
e-mail: walsht@uw.edu

© Springer Nature Switzerland AG 2021
J. P. Alukal et al. (eds.), *Design and Implementation of the Modern Men's Health Center*, https://doi.org/10.1007/978-3-030-54482-9_1

up against when we try to take care of men. Men simply do not want to go to the doctor. Whatever the predominant reason for this might be time constraints and busy professional lives (and yet somehow professional women find time to see their physicians) and sociologic programming asserting that men are tough and therefore shouldn't need help while ignoring the obvious observation that all men (all people, of course) get sick; whatever it may be, no matter what the reason, men benefit from seeing their doctor more than they currently do: for preventive care (smoking cessation, other cardiac prevention, screening for urologic and other cancers, suicide prevention, diet, exercise, and weight loss), for care of chronic issues (urinary issues, coronary artery disease, diabetes, hypertension, irritable bowel syndrome), and for acute care (orthopedic injury, post-even care for heart attack or stroke) – the list is almost endless. All of these topics have been covered by experts in this book. But most importantly, putting access to these types of care for patients in one setting ultimately makes it more likely that the patient will avail themselves of this resource and thereby stay healthier. The quality of the care and patient and physician satisfaction – yes all these things benefit in the multidisciplinary model, but you could be running the best multidisciplinary center in the world with high-quality care and an engaged and happy professional staff, and if you don't have any patients, your center isn't doing anybody any actual benefit.

Multidisciplinary care offers patients the opportunity to easily access their doctors through coordination of care, same-day add-on visits when needed, and streamlining of office logistics (easy sharing of charts, reports, results, etc.). This appeals to all patients, not just the busy professional. This appeal gets patients through the door. Of course, the quality of the care they receive is what will keep these patients coming back.

In this book, you will find expert opinion on cardiology, endocrinology, gastroenterology, dermatology, orthopedics, and urology. These expert authors can help you take steps toward the development of your own men's health center with a basis in the published data in terms of what conditions you can expect to treat and how best to treat them. Discussion of the role of the primary care provider as well as the nurse practitioner and physician assistant is found here as well. Algorithms for mental healthcare provided by the psychologist, psychiatrist, and other counselors are outlined. Finally, a discussion of the future of medicine and multidisciplinary care can be found within.

We hope this resource can help you in your men's health center to achieve the goal of providing the best care to your patients. It is through this effort that we aim to meet the public health challenge of making half of the population on the face of the earth live longer and healthier (in part by taking better care of themselves). We know you find this goal to be a valuable one as well; if you didn't, you wouldn't have picked up this book. Good luck! It is a worthy endeavor, and we are happy to help however we can.

Chapter 2
Urologic Disease in the Aging Male: A Look Across the Lifespan

Hunter Wessells

Introduction

Extending the longevity and quality of life of men is a primary function of a modern man's health center (MHC), through patient care, education, research, and outreach. While the most significant urological burden to a man's health comes in the years beyond 45, the importance of identifying health risks, and engaging men in their own health promotion, should begin decades earlier. The transition from parentally guided care under the supervision of a pediatrician to self-care poses an important initial point of exposure during adolescence and young adulthood. Others occur at predictable intervals based on the incidence and time to onset of a variety of conditions such as diabetes, obesity, heart disease, and various cancers. MHCs can be designed primarily to address *urological* problems or to provide men with broader services of health screening and/or health maintenance. Regardless of model, modern MHC's serve as platforms for *risk management* for men who, on their own, may manage risk poorly or well based on genetic, ethnic, racial, psychosocial, and environmental factors. Along with health risks, men's priorities evolve over the course of decades. The MHC can help men and their partner or families reduce the risks that men take in order to achieve better personal health outcomes.

It is instructional to review the CDC's Report ([1]; see Tables 2.1 and 2.2) outlining the leading causes of death across the age span. In younger patients, unintentional injuries and suicide predominate, whereas in older individuals other conditions come to the fore. Presenting urological symptoms of younger patients likely are not mechanistically linked to the most prevalent causes of death and disability. Thus, healthcare providers must actively engage younger men in an understanding of the

H. Wessells (✉)
Department of Urology, Harborview Injury Prevention and Research Center, Diabetes Research Center, University of Washington School of Medicine, Seattle, WA, USA
e-mail: wessells@uw.edu

© Springer Nature Switzerland AG 2021
J. P. Alukal et al. (eds.), *Design and Implementation of the Modern Men's Health Center*, https://doi.org/10.1007/978-3-030-54482-9_2

Table 2.1 Leading causes of death in males, 2015. A: Ages 10–44

Top five causes of death in males ages 10–44				
Rank	Age 10–14	Age 15–19	Age 20–24	Age 25–34	Age 35–44
1	Unintentional injuries 28.0%	Unintentional injuries 38.1%	Unintentional injuries 42.3%	Unintentional injuries 41.0%	Unintentional injuries 27.5%
2	Suicide 14.1%	Suicide 21.4%	Suicide 18.6%	Suicide 15.4%	Heart disease 15.5%
3	Cancer 12.8%	Homicide 19.1%	Homicide 18.2%	Homicide 11.5%	Suicide 11.4%
4	Homicide 6.1%	Cancer 4.8%	Cancer 3.5%	Heart disease 6.4%	Cancer 10.2%
5	Birth defects 5.0%	Heart disease 2.8%	Heart disease 3.1%	Cancer 5.1%	Homicide 5.1%

Source: CDC. https://www.cdc.gov/healthequity/lcod/men/2015/all-males/index.htm

Table 2.2 Leading causes of death in males, 2015. B: Ages 45–84

Top five causes of death in males, ages 45 and older				
Rank	Age 45–54	Age 55–64	Age 65+	Age 65–74	Age 75–84
1	Heart disease 22.6%	Cancer 29.5%	Heart disease 26.7%	Cancer 32.0%	Cancer 25.2%
2	Cancer 20.1%	Heart disease 24.4%	Cancer 23.8%	Heart disease 24.2%	Heart disease 25.2%
3	Unintentional injuries 13.6%	Unintentional injuries 6.2%	Chronic lower respiratory diseases 6.5%	Chronic lower respiratory diseases 6.8%	Chronic lower respiratory diseases 7.3%
4	Suicide 6.1%	Chronic liver disease 4.2%	Stroke 5.1%	Diabetes 4.0%	Stroke 5.2%
5	Chronic liver disease 5.5%	Chronic lower respiratory diseases 4.1%	Alzheimer's disease 3.6%	Stroke 3.9%	Alzheimer's disease 3.4%

Source: CDC. https://www.cdc.gov/healthequity/lcod/men/2015/all-males/index.htm

relationship between presenting symptoms and overall health, and their role in self-care. *Per contra*, in older patients, presenting urological symptoms often are directly linked to the most prevalent health conditions, such as genitourinary cancers and urological complications of diabetes, obesity, and cardiovascular disease.

Constellations of symptoms, signs, and related health maintenance and health screening can thus be stratified by age, and these strata guided construction of the American Urological Association *Men's Health Checklist* [2]. The broad age categories chosen reflect peak incidences of common urological diseases. The AUA Checklist can serve as a framework for designing services, referral guidelines, and capabilities of an MHC; thus, in this chapter we organized an evidence-based overview of men's health priorities by the same age categories.

General Considerations

Men's health centers provide urologic specific access and expertise in the care of urinary, sexual, and general medical conditions. Figure 2.1 represents graphically the range of problems that require urological expertise. Moving across the age spectrum, it is clear that medical knowledge and surgical expertise in congenitalism, reconstruction, andrology/infertility, urological oncology, and geriatric urology all contribute to optimal care of the aging male. At points along the lifespan, other determinants of health, including socioeconomic and biological factors, need to be considered. These may require specific infrastructure and resources, decisions on accessibility of care, advocacy for healthcare coverage for specific disorders such as ED and infertility, as well as depending on state and federal funding for the underserved which vary regionally within the United States.

Whether an MHC offers access to other specialists and resources within the center or accessed through other parts of a health system is beyond the scope of this chapter, and relates to financial models, space, collaborative environment, and other factors. Of paramount importance is that discoveries made in the MHC, whether they relate to congenital disorders, risk taking behavior, mental health, cancer, or

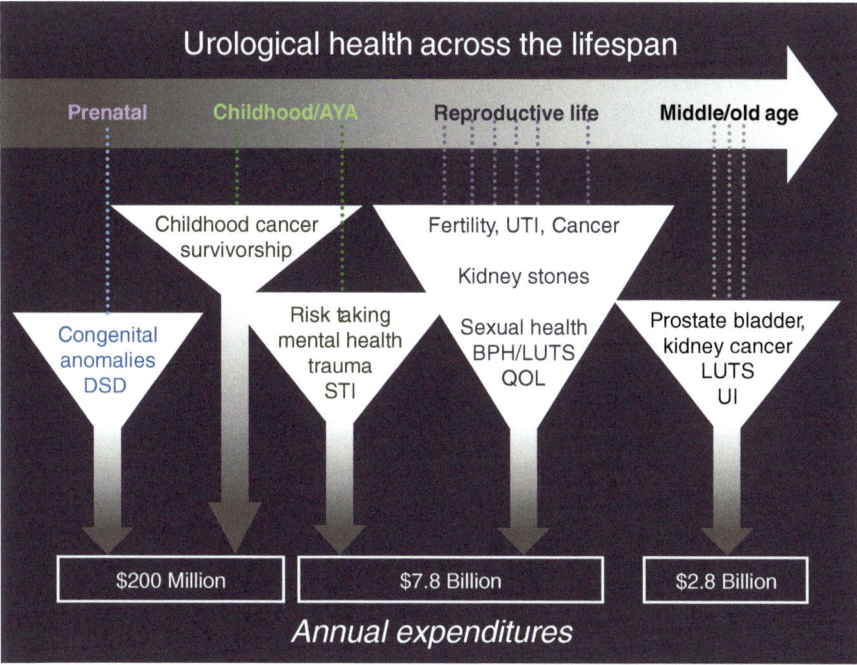

Fig. 2.1 Burden of urological diseases in men across the lifespan. (Adapted from data contained in NIH News Release May 1, 2007 https://www.nih.gov/news-events/news-releases/urologic-diseases-cost-americans-11-billion-year)

cardiovascular disease, are given thoughtful interface with other disciplines. The central role of a primary care provider for the patient cannot be overemphasized. Whether the men's health center will become a "medical home" or remain the domain of specialists will depend on many factors including the structure of health-care delivery and payment.

Adolescence and Young Adulthood (18–39 Years)

Urological disease management in younger men (18–39 years) has as an emphasis on the burden of inherited and congenital disorders; sexually transmitted infection; counseling regarding contraception; unintentional injury and its consequences; and urological disorders with peak incidence in young men (e.g., testis cancer). Drivers of unhealthy behaviors in this cohort include lack of health seeking behavior layered on top of poor decision making related to motor vehicle use, sexuality, sports, and recreational activities. Young men will typically use a MHC to seek care for a specific urological symptom or condition, which often stands in the way of goals related to relationships, family, and work. An example might be a man who presents with penile chordee or hypospadias as he considers marriage or starting a family. Any such visit should be leveraged to assess behaviors with long-term health consequences such as untreated mental health disorders; tobacco alcohol and substance use; and poor control of weight, diet, or exercise; and the resultant metabolic syndrome and obesity.

Injuries are the leading cause of death and disability in all men from adolescence through age 45. While rarely fatal, genitourinary trauma affects men twice as often as women and frequently represents a first interface with the healthcare system. The management of urotrauma has been codified in an AUA Guideline [3]. These individuals usually do not receive treatment in an MHC; nevertheless, several points bear noting. First, urologists can use these interactions as an opportunity to counsel about risk mitigation in motor vehicle driving (e.g., seatbelt and helmet use), extreme sports, and sexual activity which may result in a variety of injuries ranging from renal lacerations, bladder and urethral rupture, and penile fracture. Second, clinicians should anticipate the need for ancillary psychological, interpersonal, and/or reproductive counseling and therapy for patients with genital trauma when loss of sexual, urinary, and/or reproductive function is anticipated [4].

Sexually transmitted infections similarly provide an opportunity to asses associated bio-psychosocial determinants of the high-risk behavior. For specific literature on this topic, see Dariotis 2008 and Reidy 2008 [5, 6]. Symptoms leading to presentation with sexually tranmitted infection (STI) include lower urinary tract symptoms, hematuria, urinary tract infection, dysuria, urethral discharge, decrease force of stream, scrotal swelling, and the like.

Reproductive health concerns drive care-seeking behavior for a number of complaints, including male factor infertility, androgen deficiency, undescended testis, testis mass, scrotal disorders, phimosis, congenital chordee, Peyronie's disease, premature ejaculation, sexual dysfunction, and concerns about contraception, HIV infection, and sexually transmitted infection. Organic erectile dysfunction in this age range is rare, although increasingly it may be a consequence of obesity and metabolic disturbances. An emerging area of care improvement is the intersection of reproductive health and transgender care. Transgender patients seeking gender-affirming surgery from male to female and female to male each have specific needs including preservation of gametes, hormonal replacement, and gender-affirming surgery. An important resource is the World Professional Association for Transgender Health *Standards of Care for the Health of Transsexual, Transgender, and Gender Nonconforming People* [7].

Testicular cancer represents a unique diagnosis for which the modern MHC may serve as the best first point of contact. In addition to ready access to laboratory and radiology services needed prior to inguinal exploration, close association with a male fertility laboratory hard-wires timely assessment of semen quality, cryopreservation of sperm when indicated, and subsequent treatment of male factor infertility. Disparities in access to care across the United States reflect geographical, cultural, and fiscal barriers [8]. The services of an MHC thus align with the initial evaluation and management of testis mass as well as cancer survivorship needs, but may not be sufficient to address all the needs of complex cancer patients. A key responsibility of an MHC is to ensure availability of important downstream services, including urological, radiation, and medical oncology referral.

Middle Age (40–49 Years; 50–69 Years)

As men reach their 40s, the burden of disease related to unintentional injury and congenital conditions gives way to the impact of metabolic and cardiovascular disease and the rising prevalence of cancers. For an MHC-specific urological cancer detection and initial evaluation are added onto the cumulatively increasing rates of urolithiasis, infertility, organic erectile dysfunction, LUTS, and hypogonadism, which in this age range arise out of earlier periods of poor self-care, genetic predisposition, and concurrent diseases. Taken together, the greatest impact of a modern MHC may be in providing men the "No wrong door" point of entry into a healthcare system. In contrast to "Men's Clinics" focused on Testosterone Replacement Therapy [9] and costly ED treatments, the MHC committed to health equity and a wholistic approach to improving health for men will make sure that the underlying disorders driving urological disease and symptoms are addressed. In the critical 40–49 age range, secondary prevention and intervention strategies still have a chance to mitigate some of the risk of the many "benign" urological conditions listed above. In contrast, when these conditions present in older individuals, treatment of symptoms is.

Appropriate cancer screening, based on specialty society guidelines and US Public Health Task Force recommendations synthesize the best available evidence to inform high value decisions about healthcare. Table 2.3 links existing guidelines

Table 2.3 High-priority urological conditions affecting men and relevant American Urological Association Guidelines

Priority condition[a]	AUA guideline (date of guideline/update)
Developmental anomalies	Cryptorchidism 2014
Reproductive health and infertility	Testosterone Deficiency 2018; Vasectomy 2012/2015; Evaluation of the Infertile Male (BPS); Management of the Azoospermic Male (BPS)
Nephrolithiasis	Medical 2014; Surgical 2016
Urinary symptoms	BPH/LUTS 2018; Urethral Stricture 2016
Sexual dysfunction	Erectile dysfunction 2018; Peyronie's Disease 2015; Priapism 2003/2010; Premature Ejaculation 2004/2010
Renal cell cancer	Renal Mass and Localized RC 2017
CPPS/IC PBS	IC/PBS 2011/2014
Prostate cancer	Early Detection 2013/2018; Clinically Localized 2017
Bladder cancer	Asymptomatic Microhematuria 2012/2016

BPS best practice statement, *CPPS* chronic pelvic pain syndrome, *IC PBS* interstitial cystitis/painful bladder syndrome
[a]Priority areas as defined by the National Urology Research Agenda [15, 16]

created by the AUA to some high-priority men's urological conditions across the age spectrum. Interestingly, the subspecialization of urology into oncology-only surgical practices means that in integrated health systems and academic centers, counseling regarding PSA testing, evaluation of elevated PSA, and work-up of microhematuria will fall to urologists outside of cancer centers; the properly resourced MHC can easily incorporate these diagnoses into its workflow and use the opportunity to assess all aspects of a man's urological health.

MHCs contribute to improving outcomes for male urological cancer patients through the alleviation of side effects of treatment. Traditionally, urologists have managed the side effects of radiation therapy and radical pelvic surgery including urinary obstruction (e.g., stricture), ED, and urinary incontinence. An expanded role for the MHC can be to create pathways that include an initial visit prior to cancer treatment along with standardized intervention schedules early after.

Diabetes and the metabolic syndrome have long been linked to sexual and voiding dysfunctions. The identification of modifiable risk factors associated with ED and LUTS in men, such as glycemic control, blood pressure, smoking, diet, and exercise, represent the "tip of the iceberg" in terms of intervention opportunities. Another emerging area of overlap between the metabolic syndrome and urologic disease relates to urinary stone disease. Growing evidence supports the relationship between cardiovascular risk factors including body mass index, blood pressure, and overt cardiovascular disease with the risk of urolithiasis. For the time being, however, high-level evidence to support specific strategies is still lacking.

Another condition that crosses these age ranges is genitourinary pain syndromes including chronic prostatitis, chronic pelvic pain syndrome, and less commonly painful bladder syndrome/interstitial cystitis. The potential overlap and interplay of these chronic conditions with BPH/LUTS on the one hand, and other health conditions such as varicocele, hernia, and spermatocele make the MHC an appropriate environment for coordination of care and maximizing effectiveness of treatments for each symptom complex.

The relationship between urologic conditions such as infertility, erectile dysfunction, and hypogonadism with other significant health conditions including cardiovascular disease, urologic and other cancers, diabetes, and the metabolic syndrome point to the value in having a matrixed approach to men's health.

Older Age (70 Years and Over)

The accumulating burden of urological diseases seen as men exceed 70 years of age is significant: (ED 77%; LUTS 80%; prostate cancer 50%) and poses a challenge to the MHC [10–13]. Living with chronic diseases and mitigating bother and impact may take a front seat to definitive treatment or "cure" of symptoms accompany shifts of patient priorities and goals of health care. MHC can play an important role in maintaining quality of life, and physical functioning, in the face of cancer treatment, highly prevalent urological conditions, and the complications of diabetes and heart disease.

Individualized approach based on patient goals are critical to properly prioritize expectations around sexual function, urinary symptomatology, continued increasing burden of cancer diagnosis, and competing medical conditions. The benefits of screening against the side effects and cost of treatment must be balanced; for example, routine screening for androgen deficiency is no longer needed and may lead to unnecessary use of testosterone, similarly, the use of PSA screening for prostate cancer beyond age 70 must be balanced against life expectancy. Extensive evaluation of sexual dysfunction for reversible causes is no longer be relevant; goal-oriented approaches should be predominant for many of the men's health conditions including BPH, genital urinary pain, sexual dysfunction, and the like.

Infrastructure

A number of factors will determine the setting, equipment, and staffing needs of Men's Health Centers including target population, diagnoses, financial resources, and healthcare providers available to serve patients. The broad age spectrum defined in Fig. 2.1 and the AUA Checklist offers a model in which a MHC can serve as a resource to a larger more diverse male population in an integrated system, but will require significant investment in equipment and services to optimally serve patients, although these need not all be housed in the MHC.

Minimum necessary resources to assess common men's health conditions include a range of patient-reported measures of lower urinary tract and sexual symptoms;

clinical laboratory facilities for urinalysis and urine testing for STI; assays of total testosterone that meet CDC Hormone Standardization criteria [14]; semen analysis; and PSA testing. Equipment and facilities required to address cancer detection and diagnosis, care of male patients undergoing cytotoxic chemotherapy, and complex in-office assisted reproductive technology include high-resolution ultrasonography and relevant probes; prostate needle biopsy devices; flexible and/or rigid cysto-scopes; surgical instruments and procedure rooms suitable (covered extensively in other chapters). Equally important is the range of staff to address a range of issues including but not limited to: sexual therapists and other psychological counseling services to support men and couples; sperm cryopreservation facilities; genetic counseling for infertility and cancer risk assessment; and last but not least financial counselors to help patients navigate insurance coverage and planning for uncovered diagnoses.

Conclusions

The burden of disease from genitourinary disease changes significantly across the lifespan, and men's health care providers and MHC's need to develop a patient-oriented and personalized approach across all ages. Adolescent and young adults have different priorities and manage risk very differently. Often, the first point of contact is when the risk has already been taken, the problem already exists, and the opportunity is one to treat symptoms, educate, and mitigate risk. As men age, the risks and priorities change such that they are more likely to engage actively in health maintenance and health screening. This is the "sweet spot" for the modern Men's Health Center in terms of contributing to prevention, early detection and interven-tions to address a long list of highly prevalent conditions. At the end of the lifespan, there must be another transition away from expectations of cure and completely normal function. Instead, symptom improvement and maintenance of quality of life must be primarily sought.

References

1. Centers for Disease Control and Prevention. Leading cause of death in men. 2018. https://www.cdc.gov/healthequity/lcod/men/2015/all-males/index.htm.
2. American Urological Association. Men's health checklist. 2018. https://www.auanet.org/publications/mens-health-checklist.
3. Morey AF, Brandes S, Dugi DD 3rd, Armstrong JH, Breyer BN, Broghammer JA, Erickson BA, Holzbeierlein J, Hudak SJ, Pruitt JH, Reston JT, Santucci RA, Smith TG 3rd, Wessells H. Urotrauma: AUA guidelines. J Urol. 2014;192(2):327–35.
4. American Urological Association. Guidelines. 2018. https://www.auanet.org/guidelines.

5. Dariotis JK, Sonenstein FL, Gates GJ, Capps R, Astone NM, Pleck JH, Sifakis F, Zeger S. Changes in sexual risk behavior as young men transition to adulthood. Perspect Sex Reprod Health. 2008;40(4):218–25.
6. Reidy DE, Berke DS, Gentile B, Zeichner A. Masculine discrepancy stress, substance use, assault and injury in a survey of US men. Inj Prev. 2016;22(5):370–4.
7. World Professional Association for Transgender Health. Standards of care for the health of transsexual, transgender, and gender nonconforming people. 7th Version. https://www.wpath.org/publications/soc.
8. Mokdad AH, Dwyer-Lindgren L, Fitzmaurice C, Stubbs RW, Bertozzi-Villa A, Morozoff C, Charara R, Allen C, Naghavi M, Murray CJ. Trends and patterns of disparities in cancer mortality among US counties, 1980-2014. JAMA. 2017;317(4):388–406.
9. New York Times Editorial Board. Overselling testosterone, dangerously. Feb. 4, 2014.
10. Saigal C, Litwin M, editors. Urological diseases in America. Bethesda: NIDDK; 2006.
11. Saigal CS, Wessells H, Pace J, Schonlau M, Wilt T. Predictors and prevalence of erectile dysfunction in a racially diverse population. Arch Intern Med. 2006;166:207–12.
12. Parsons JK, Bergstrom J, Silberstein J, Barrett-Connor E. Prevalence and characteristics of lower urinary tract symptoms in men aged > or = 80 years. Urology. 2008;72:318–21.
13. Stangelberger A, Waldert M, Djavan B. Prostate cancer in elderly men. Rev Urol. 2008;10(2):111–9.
14. Centers for Disease Control and Prevention. Standardization of serum total testosterone measurements. CDC Laboratory/Manufacturer Hormone Standardization (HoSt) Program. 2013. https://www.cdc.gov/labstandards/pdf/hs/Testosterone_Protocol.pdf.
15. Miller DC, Saigal CS, Litwin MS, Urologic Diseases in America Project. The demographic burden of urologic diseases in America. Urol Clin North Am. 2009;36(1):11–27.
16. Schaeffer AJ, Freeman M, Giambarresi L. Introduction to the national urology research agenda: a roadmap for priorities in urological disease research. J Urol. 2010;184(3):823–4.

Chapter 3
Approach to Primary Care of the Male Patient

Steven Lamm and Kenneth Brill

Traditionally, primary care has been charged with several core tasks. These include the prevention, early diagnosis, and management of a wide variety of conditions. In the following chapter, a number of different topics will be covered. Each of these will be discussed in greater detail elsewhere in this book, but the focus of this chapter will be on prevention and screening from the primary care perspective. Over the years, the methods by which this has been accomplished has changed dramatically, but the tasks have not. The goal of these duties, together, is to improve our patients' quality of life, wellness, and longevity. It has long been thought that wellness was the absence of disease, but recently this attitude has been shifting. More considerations are being made for patients' quality of life and their personal, individualized goals as they progress through different stages of their life. In recent years, the field of primary care has undergone some of its most stark changes, bringing about a new area of primary care. Challenges that face the field today include engaging patients in shared decision-making processes. In the past, the physician would make recommendations to all of their patients with less regard for the individual situations, but now the attention has been turned to a patient-centered approach. Gone are the days of a "one size fits all" approach to medicine, and this landscape is set to change even more dramatically in the future.

A growing area of medicine is the role of genomics and big data. Our ability to collect and analyze a large amount of genetic data for our patients has expanded exponentially since the laborious days of the Human Genome Project, and now patients are even able to acquire their own genetic information through at-home kits

S. Lamm
Preston Robert Tisch Center, New York University Preston Robert Tisch Center, New York, NY, USA

K. Brill (✉)
Department of Medicine, NYU Grossman School of Medicine, New York, NY, USA
e-mail: kenneth.brill@nyulangone.org

© Springer Nature Switzerland AG 2021
J. P. Alukal et al. (eds.), *Design and Implementation of the Modern Men's Health Center*, https://doi.org/10.1007/978-3-030-54482-9_3

such as 23andMe and Ancestry. With the advent of these advanced genomic technologies, medicine will be thrust toward a focus on personalized medicine. Each patient will be able to have their specific genetic information analyzed and have prevention, screening, and treatment protocols designed specifically to suit them. As this ability expands, primary care physicians will be expected to keep up with the demands of their patients and will have to adapt to the rapidly changing landscape. Adding to the complexity of this new approach, medical management of patients will have to be personalized to consider more than a person's genes. Already there are some considerations being made with respect to a patient's socioeconomic status, but the relevance of this will be amplified as our ability to personalize our approach expands. Also, taking a patient's educational level into account and designing a management plan suited to them may help improve patient understanding, compliance, and satisfaction with their care, thus making the achievement of the goals of primary care that much simpler.

A common concern people have is how long they can expect to live and how long they can expect to live in good health. In fact, tremendous amounts of time, money, and effort are poured into attempting to answer these questions. Measures of the progress made in medicine are related as improvements in life expectancy, and that statistic is used as the water mark for how well or poorly a nation is doing at providing for their citizen's health. In recent news, the gaps between life expectancy in the United States and other developed nations have been reported as efforts to expand access in the United States gain popular support. Additionally, the disparity in life expectancy between the United States and other countries is being co-opted as proof of the effectiveness of socialized medical care. The longevity gap between people of different races and socioeconomic status within the United States has also received attention in the debate about improving healthcare in this country, with a large number of studies being conducted to attempt to explain these differences.

A longevity gap of another kind, however, has not received as much mainstream coverage as the previously mentioned disparities: life expectancy at birth between men and women. It is common knowledge that men tend to live shorter lives than women, though very little public attention has been aimed at questioning or understanding this gap in longevity. According to the National Vital Statistics Systems compiled by the National Center for Health Statistics in 2016, the average life expectancy at birth in 2016 was 78.6 years across all races, genders, and ethnicities [1]. However, when this is broken down by gender, the average life expectancy for men of all races and ethnicities is 76.1 years and 81.1 years for women, a difference of 5 years. If the life expectancy at 65 is considered, men still fall short of women: the same study reports a life expectancy of 18.0 years for men at age 65 and 20.6 years for women, more than 2 years sooner [1]. Clearly, this demonstrates that not only are there differences in the expected longevity of men and women but that at least some of these mortality risks persist throughout a man's life.

A review published in the *International Journal of Clinical Practice* in 2010 summarized many of the differences in disease prevalence and outcome in men and women. For the top 15 leading causes of death in 2010, men had a higher mortality rate in 12 out of 15, with five of these having a mortality risk more than twice as high for men. The largest gap in mortality was suicide, with men being four times as more likely to die by suicide than women [2]. When considering the prevalence of coronary heart disease, men have higher rates of disease than women at all ages over 60 and are significantly more likely to be diagnosed with a myocardial infarction for all ages before 75 [2]. Type 2 diabetes mellitus has become an increasingly important and common disease in recent years, with the rate of disease rising steadily since the early 1990s. However, the rates of disease among men have been rising more quickly than women, resulting in an ever-widening gap in the rates of DM2 between the genders [2]. Stepping away from cardiovascular health and risk factors, differences in mortality have been observed for cancer as well. Men have higher rates of lung cancer than women, which somewhat explains the differences in all cancer mortality. However, men have higher mortality rates for some of the most common causes of cancer death, including pancreatic cancer, leukemia, non-Hodgkin lymphoma, and liver and intrahepatic bile duct cancers [2].

This longevity gap, often, is taken for granted as a fact of life. It is likely that very few people would be surprised to know that men have a shorter life expectancy than women, but it is unlikely that most people understand how little is sure about the cause of this. The exact reasons for this gap are quite controversial. Arguments have been made that it is the Y chromosome itself that poses a threat to male mortality. Others have done experiments demonstrating negative physiologic effects of testosterone and numerous protective effects of estrogen, most notably with relation to cardiovascular health. Some studies have suggested that behavioral, environmental, and risk-taking differences between men and women account for a large portion of this decreased longevity. References to some such investigations can be found at the end of this chapter [3–7]. What is clear, however, is that being male makes a person inherently different and that whatever these differences are puts men at a high risk for early mortality. It could be argued that these increased risks together mark men as an endangered species, and attention must be turned to providing high-quality primary care to this enormous segment of the population.

From the above discussion, it is clear that the longevity gap between men and women is multifaceted, and no single factor can explain the difference between the sexes. In addition, more work must be done to fully understand the modifiable and unmodifiable factors that affect life expectancy and the sex difference in mortality. More attention should be turned to explaining and addressing this longevity gap between men and women, and primary care focused on issues related to men's health is a growing area of importance. As personalized and precision medicine rises to the forefront of healthcare, these issues will become more pressing as we search for ways to help male patients live longer, healthier lives. Wellness and primary prevention are also becoming more of a focus for primary care, and an increased understanding of the factors affecting men's health will be essential in providing care for male patients. Until personalized medicine becomes more robust, we have rigorously established guidelines for the prevention, screening, and diagnosis of some of our most common diseases, including cardiovascular disease and cancer (Table 3.1). In addition, more attention in recent years has been aimed at understanding and managing mental health in men, as well as sexually transmitted

Table 3.1 Screening recommendations by decade of life

Decade	Strong recommendations	Risk-based recommendations	Controversial recommendations	Discontinue screening
20–29	Blood lipids – *every 5 years, 3 years for abnormal* Blood pressure – *annually* Depression – *every visit* Alcohol/tobacco use – *every visit* HIV – *once, annually for high risk*			
30–39	Blood lipids – *every 5 years, 3 years for abnormal* Blood pressure – *annually* Depression – *every visit* Alcohol/tobacco use – *every visit* HIV – *once, annually for high risk*			
40–49	Blood lipids– *every 5 years, 3 years for abnormal* Blood pressure – *annually* Depression – *every visit* Alcohol/tobacco use – *every visit* HIV – *once, annually for high risk*	CAC score Colon cancer – *every 10 years*		
50–59	Blood lipids – *every 5 years, 3 years for abnormal* Blood pressure – *annually* Depression – *every visit* Alcohol/tobacco use – *every visit* HIV – *once, annually for high risk* Colon cancer – *every 10 years*	CAC score Lung cancer – *annually*	PSA – *every 2–4 years, at age 55*	
60–69	Blood lipids – *every 5 years, 3 years for abnormal* Blood pressure – *annually* Depression – *every visit* Alcohol/tobacco use – *every visit* HIV – *once, annually for high risk* Colon cancer – *every 10 years*	Lung cancer – *annually*	PSA – *every 2–4 years*	CAC score
70–79	Blood pressure – *annually* Depression – *every visit* Alcohol/tobacco use – *every visit* Colon cancer – *every 10 years*	Lung cancer – *annually*		Blood lipids, HIV (age 75), PSA
80–89	Blood pressure – *annually* Depression – *every visit* Alcohol/tobacco use – *every visit*			Colon cancer (age 85)

infections. The guidelines, as well as prevention and screening efforts, will remain to be the focus of this discussion. It should be noted, however, that these guidelines are not meant to be definitive rules for how to handle all patients and that individual choices must be made given each patient's individual risk profile and goals of care. These guidelines are also subject to change, as they often have in the past, but reflect our current best practices when approaching common diseases.

As of 2016, the leading cause of death in the United States was heart disease, and it was responsible for 165.5 deaths per 100,000 people [1]. There are some unmodifiable risk factors that lead to the development of heart disease. These include family history and genetic predisposition; however, these factors do not account for the entirety of a person's heart disease risk. There are a number of modifiable risk factors that can help protect patients from developing heart disease that can contribute to premature morbidity and mortality. Assessing cardiovascular risk is absolutely essential in evaluating the necessity of primary prevention and screening for both cardiovascular risk factors and early heart disease. One such method of risk assessment is the American College of Cardiology/American Heart Association Atherosclerotic Cardiovascular Disease (ASCVD) risk calculator. This allows clinicians to calculate lifetime risk of cardiovascular events for patients by taking blood pressure, lipid levels, smoking and diabetes status, and statin and aspirin therapy into account. This calculator also makes recommendations from the ACC/AHA for statin therapy based on a patient's lipid levels and the most up-to-date recommendations on LDL and HDL targets. Limitations of the calculator include the lack of a variable for family history and the inability to describe important factors about diabetes status, including the type of diabetes, length of disease course, and level of glycemic control. Another calculator for patients with type 2 diabetes is available from the UK Prospective Diabetes Study [8]. By better understanding our patient's cardiovascular risk, we can aim preventative efforts at the most at-risk populations and manipulate any modifiable risk factors that may explain a particular patient's risk.

Primary prevention is focused on identification and modification of risk factors for disease prior to the development of overt disease, and this should be the focus of a primary care physician. One possible target risk factor for the development of cardiovascular disease is the level of low-density lipoprotein cholesterol (LDL-C). LDL-C has been demonstrated to have a consistently positive relationship with the occurrence of cardiovascular events, and repeatedly it has been shown that modification of LDL-C levels adjusts the risk of future cardiovascular events. Notably, only lowering of LDL-C has been shown to provide benefit for patients without overt cardiovascular disease, while correction of HDL-C or triglycerides does not provide benefit in the absence of heart disease [9–12]. Initial trials of several cholesterol lowering statins including pravastatin, lovastatin, and rosuvastatin demonstrated a reduction in risk for first cardiovascular event and even all-cause mortality for both men and women [13–16]. Meta-analysis of studies of LDL-C reduction has shown that these drugs are associated with strong reductions in the risk for CVD events and mortality both in patients with established cardiovascular disease and patients without overt disease [17]. Clearly, early recognition and intervention for patients with demonstrated abnormalities in LDL-C are important for the primary prevention of cardiovascular events, and current consensus suggests that screening for and discussion of cardiovascular risk, including blood lipid monitoring, begin at the age of 20.

For patients with elevated LDL-C, current recommendations suggest moderate-intensity statin therapy as a primary preventative strategy for cardiovascular disease, along with diet and lifestyle modification. There have been no randomized trials comparing moderate- and high-intensity statin therapy for primary prevention, and the benefit in LDL-C reduction is not large when increasing intensity from moderate to high. In addition, side effect profile tends to be more tolerable on moderate-intensity therapy, further justifying the use of this approach in primary prevention. Current recommendations suggest that patients who are intolerant of statins with an LDL-C below 190 mg/dL should be managed conservatively with lifestyle and diet modifications in the absence of cardiovascular disease. In patients with a 10-year ASCVD risk of greater than 20%, ezetimibe and PCSK-9 inhibitors can be considered as primary prevention options in statin-intolerant patients, despite long-term safety and evidence for efficacy in primary prevention not being firmly established with randomized trials. Current goals of therapy have been established by the ACC/AHA. For adults with an LDL-C between 70 and 189 mg/dL, patients with a 10-year ASCVD risk of greater than or equal to 7.5% should be started on moderate- to high-intensity statin therapy, and patients with risk between 5% and 7.5% can be started on moderate-intensity therapy. In addition, patients with LDL-C at or above 190 mg/dL should be treated with high-intensity statin therapy, and additional non-statin cholesterol lowering therapy should be considered [18]. Recommendations from the US Preventative Task Force, the UK National Institute for Health and Clinical Excellence, and the 2016 European Society of Cardiology/European Atherosclerosis Society suggest a more conservative approach, with statin therapy being initiated in patients with a 10-year ASCVD risk of at least 10% [17, 19, 20]. Despite the difference in goals and initialization cutoffs, it is clear that control of LDL-C is an important and effective method of primary prevention for cardiovascular disease.

A noninvasive approach to assessing the atherosclerotic burden of a patient is coronary artery calcification (CAC) scoring. This evaluation involves the use of multidetector row CT scanners (MDCT) to assess for calcification of the coronary arteries. This test has been shown to be highly sensitive for stenosis of the coronary arteries of greater than or equal to 50%, but it is only moderately specific for coronary artery disease, especially in patients over the age of 60 where calcification can occur in the absence of CAD. A review of 16 studies found the sensitivity and specificity to be 91% and 49%, respectively [21]. The absence of CAC, in contrast, is highly predictive for the absence of coronary artery disease. In fact, patients with no CAC had a less than 1% chance of having atherosclerotic disease of the coronary arteries. In addition, higher CAC scores were associated with more specificity for coronary artery disease [22]. Therefore, it is important to consider CAC scoring for patients at high risk for coronary artery disease, and it is highly useful as a negative predictor in patients with concern for CAD. It is important to note that the approach to the diabetic patient with respect to CAC scoring is different, with studies suggesting that a score of zero may not predict long-term mortality in diabetic patients [23]. Overall, this screening test is useful in patients over the age of 40 without symptoms of CAD as a way to rule out subclinical atherosclerotic disease. It is an especially important tool in risk stratification and in patients who are at intermediate risk for CAD, as patients with low risk are not likely to have a positive score and high-risk patients will be treated aggressively. It can be helpful to have a CAC score in patients who may need treatment but are resistant to pharmacologic therapy, as a way to convince them of the importance of aggressive management. Even in high-risk patients who will be receiving therapy, a CAC score can help to confirm the presence of atherosclerotic disease without invasive testing, such as CT coronary angiography, and could help to lower our threshold for managing these patients aggressively.

As genetic testing becomes more robust, its application to primary prevention and screening will expand. There are two basic approaches to genetic testing: genomic screening and expression profiling. The first is what most people are familiar with, and it involves scanning a person's genome for genes that may predict the presence of a disease in the future. Expression profiling is a newer technique that allows us to assess which genes are overexpressed or underexpressed compared to what we expect. One such application of this technology is in heart disease, with the new Corus CAD Gene Expression Test. The test uses a sample of blood to assess for the expression of genes associated with cardiovascular disease. The aim of this new approach is to accurately assess for the presence of atherosclerotic heart disease without patients having to undergo invasive coronary angiography, which is often negative for patients who meet the criteria for ICA. This new test has not been extensively studied in a diverse patient population, but early findings suggest that this test performs well and could be a highly useful tool in CAD screening [24]. Currently, Corus is most useful in patients who present with atypical chest pain, with a low suspicion for CAD, and is best seen as a reassurance for patients rather than a positive marker of disease. In addition, lipoprotein(a) has received more attention as a predictive tool for cardiovascular disease risk. It has been shown that this protein has a near-linear relationship with the risk of a cardiovascular event, and the levels of this protein are not affected by statin therapy. While Lp(a) has clear value as a risk marker, thus far there has not been substantial evidence that drugs used to lower Lp(a), such as nicotinic acid and PCSK9 antibodies, have a clinically significant impact on CVD risk [25, 26]. Regardless, the possible utility of Lp(a) as a risk factor for cardiovascular disease should not be overlooked.

The most important modifiable risk factor for the development of heart disease is hypertension [27]. The American College of Cardiology and the American Heart Association updated their definitions of hypertension in 2017 to reflect the most recent developments in our understanding of the impact of high blood pressure. According to their definitions, normal blood pressure is defined as a systolic reading below 120 mmHg and a diastolic reading below 80 mmHg. Elevated blood pressure is between 120 and 129 mmHg systolic and below 80 mmHg diastolic. Hypertension is classified into two stages. Stage 1 hypertension is a systolic pressure between 130 and 139 mmHg or a diastolic pressure between 80 and 89 mmHg. Stage 2 hypertension is defined as a systolic pressure of at least 140 mmHg or a diastolic pressure of at least 90 mmHg [28]. This reflects a broader definition of hypertension than in the past, lowering our cutoffs for considering treatment of patients with abnormal blood pressures.

There are many factors that can contribute to a person's risk of developing primary, or essential, hypertension. Some of these include advanced age, obesity, family history, race, kidney disease, high-sodium diet, alcohol consumption, and physical inactivity [29–33]. Screening for hypertension is recommended by a number of societies, including the ACC/AHA, on an annual basis for all patients above 18 years of age without a previous history of hypertension. In patients with identified risk factors, such as those previously mentioned, or for patients with observed elevated blood pressure, screening should be done at least semiannually or more frequently for patients at the highest risk. For patients with elevated blood pressure or stage 1 hypertension, the ACC/AHA has recommendations for several non-pharmacologic interventions. These include dietary salt restriction, weight loss, exercise, potassium supplementation, DASH diet, and limited alcohol intake [28]. The PREMIER trial demonstrated that comprehensive lifestyle modifications both reduced the rate of hypertension and the use of antihypertensive pharmacologic therapy, although the reduction was not statistically significant. Nevertheless, these findings motivate the push for DASH diet and exercise recommendations for patients with elevated blood pressure or stage 1 hypertension [34].

For patients with stage 2 hypertension or stage 1 hypertension with other factors such as age over 65, type 2 diabetes, established cardiovascular disease, chronic kidney disease, or a 10-year ASCVD risk above 10%, the ACC/AHA recommends pharmacologic management of their hypertension [28]. Appropriate pharmacologic management of hypertension has been shown to reduce the relative risk for heart failure, stroke, and myocardial infarction when compared to placebo [35]. In addition, it has been shown that 100 patients need to be treated for 4 or 5 years to prevent cardiovascular events in two patients, although the short duration of the study may underestimate the total benefit of pharmacologic antihypertensive therapy [36]. The appropriate management of hypertension is important for avoiding many of the cardiovascular and extra-cardiac complications of uncontrolled high blood pressure, including left ventricular hypertrophy, systolic and diastolic heart failure, ischemic stroke, intracranial hemorrhage, ischemic heart disease, and chronic kidney disease [27, 37–43].

Another important cardiovascular risk factor that has been gaining increasing attention is obesity. Obesity is defined using set definitions based on body mass index (BMI) established by the National Institutes of Health and World Health Organization, as well as prediction of a patient's cardiovascular risk. Normal weight is between 18.5 and 24.9 kg/m^2, and overweight is between 25 and 29.9 kg/m^2. Obesity is divided into three classes. Class I is between 30 and 34.9 kg/m^2, Class II is between 35 and 39.9 kg/m^2, and Class III is greater than 40 kg/m^2 [44–46]. Obesity has been increasing in prevalence among adult men for several years in the United States. From 2007 to 2008, 32.2% of American men were obese (BMI over 30 kg/m^2), and 4.2% of men were severely obese (BMI over 40 kg/m^2). By

2015–2016, 37.9% of men were obese and 5.6% were severely obese, representing the increasing trends in unhealthy lifestyle and weight gain in the United States [47].

When screening obese patients, it is important to consider several factors in addition to a calculation of BMI. Weight history has been shown to be important in evaluating the potential impact of obesity on a patient's future health. For men, even a small weight gain of greater than or equal to 5 kg after the age of 20 has been shown to increase the risk of coronary heart disease and type 2 diabetes regardless of initial BMI [48]. Comorbid cardiovascular risk factors are important to consider when counseling patients about weight loss. These include hypertension, dyslipidemia, elevated triglycerides, impaired fasting glucose, obstructive sleep apnea, and tobacco use [45]. Other noncardiac comorbidities may be present, such as osteoarthritis, cholelithiasis, NAFLD, depression, and a general reduction in the quality of life, and screening for these important complications of obesity is important in addition to the recognized cardiovascular risks and comorbidities.

The approach to the management of patients who are overweight or obese depends in part on their weight and any present comorbidities. In general, it is important to consider weight loss intervention in patients with a BMI greater than 25 kg/m^2 with the goal of preventing, treating, and reversing any complications related to increased weight. There is no evidence-based goal for weight targets, but the guidelines discussed below are based on current consensus. Patients with a BMI between 24.9 and 30 kg/m^2 without comorbid cardiovascular disease or other risk factors should be counseled on dietary changes and exercise programs with the aim of preventing further weight gain. In patients with BMI over 30 kg/m^2 or between 24.9 and 30 kg/m^2 with cardiovascular disease or risk factors, sleep apnea, or osteoarthritis, it should be the goal to achieve weight loss through behavioral modification, diet, exercise, or more aggressive intervention in patients at highest risk of complications [49].

Second to cardiovascular disease in all-cause mortality is cancer. In 2016, cancer was responsible for 155.8 deaths per 100,000 people, a slight decline from the 2015 figure of 158.5 deaths [1]. In fact, for patients under the age of 85, cancer outranks cardiovascular disease as the leading cause of mortality [50]. It is estimated that, worldwide, there are 14 million cases of cancer and 8 million cancer deaths each year. Importantly, the large amount of morbidity and mortality is occurring in spite of increasing evidence that many malignancies are preventable [51, 52]. It has been demonstrated that there are many modifiable cancer risk factors and that these account for the lion's share of malignancies. One study showed that two-thirds of malignancies could be attributed to tobacco use, excess weight, inactivity, and poor diet [53]. As discussed earlier, the role of personalized and precision medicine is perhaps most obvious in the prevention and treatment of cancer. As our ability to perform genetic testing and tailor treatments to specific mutations improves, we will become more efficient and effective at reducing the burden of morbidity and mortality from malignancy. Here, we will discuss current methods of prevention and screening for some of the most common and deadly malignancies in men: colorectal, lung, and prostate cancer.

Colorectal cancer is among the most common malignancies in the United States. It is the third most common malignancy diagnosed in men, and it accounts for 694,000 deaths annually, which is approximately 8.3% of cancer deaths overall [54]. The lifetime incidence of colorectal cancer is 4.4%, with 90% of the cases occurring after the age of 50 and nearly one-third of patients diagnosed with CRC eventually dying [55].

There are several identified risk factors for the development of colorectal cancer. Among the most prominent is family history of CRC. In fact, the increase in life-time risk for colorectal cancer in patients with a positive family history has been estimated to be between a two- and sixfold increase in the absence of familial malig-nancy syndromes [56]. Age is another firmly established risk factor, with the rates of colorectal cancer increasing with advanced age. A recent rise in the rate of colorectal cancer in younger populations may change the current understanding of CRC epidemiology, but we still consider those of advanced age to be at the highest risk. Race has also been shown to be an important risk factor for colorectal cancer, with black patients being both more likely to be diagnosed with CRC and more likely to die from it [57]. In addition, black patients are more likely to have large polyps (greater than 9 mm) during screening colonoscopies than white patients [58]. These risks may be explained by a combination of healthcare utilization, screening rates, and environmental and genetic risk factors that differ between black and non-black patients. Most relevantly to the issue of men's health, gender is a recognized risk factor for colorectal cancer. The rates of advanced adenomas found during screening colonoscopies were 8% in men and 4.3% in women, and the rates of colorectal cancer on screening colonoscopies were 1.4% for men and 0.6% for women. In addition, these adenomas and carcinomas were found at younger ages in men than in women [59–62]. Two studies compared the risk of finding advanced adenoma during a screening colonoscopy between men and women, and both found that men were at higher risk, with a relative risk of 1.83 and 1.91, making men nearly twice as likely as women to have advanced adenoma [63, 64]. Even in patients with traditionally low risk factors such as a negative family history and negative guaiac test, men have nearly twice the risk of women for having an advance neoplasm on screening colonoscopy, at 8.6% of men compared to 4.5% of women [64]. The risk factors described above must be carefully concerned when approach-ing preventative efforts, and the burden of disease emphasizes the important role primary prevention can play.

There are a number of screening guidelines that have been laid down for patients of average risk, but the two most often used will be discussed here. The US Preventive Services Task Force makes a strong recommendation that screening begins at age 50 for patients at average risk for colorectal cancer. Unlike previous recommendations, the USPSTF does not state a preference for any particular screening modality, emphasizing the importance of patient preference and the superiority of any screening method above a lack of screening. Screening options suggested include colonoscopy, fecal immunochemical testing (FIT) for occult blood, sigmoidoscopy plus FIT, computed tomography colonography (CTC), FIT-DNA multitargeted stool DNA testing, guaiac-based fecal occult blood testing (gFOBT), or sigmoidoscopy alone. They show through modeled life expectancy that efficacy is roughly equivalent across most of these modalities, with FIT-DNA being slightly lower and gFOBT or sigmoidoscopy alone being less efficacious. Screening should be discontinued when a patient's life expectancy is less than 10 years [65]. In contrast to the USPSTF, the American Cancer Society updated their guidelines in 2018 to recommend screening for patients over 45 and to strongly recommend for screening of patients over 50, which was aimed to reflect the rising prevalence of colorectal cancer in younger adults [66]. The ACS recommends six different screening options with varying frequency of repetition. They recommend colonoscopy every 10 years, CTC every 5 years, sigmoidoscopy every 5 years, take-home high-sensitivity gFOBT every year, take-home FIT every year, and multitargeted stool DNA test every 3 years. If any of these non-colonoscopy screening tests are found to be positive, they should be followed by prompt colonoscopy. Like the USPSTF, the ACS recommends any screening modality the patient will adhere to as superior to a lack of screening, despite their preference for colonoscopy as the gold standard screening modality. The ACS recommends screening for patients up to age 75 with a life expectancy of more than 10 years, individualized screening for patients between age 76 and 84, and discontinuation of screening for all patients over age 85 [67]. Due to the relatively slow progression of most sporadic cases of colorectal cancer and the ease of removal of precancerous lesions, primary prevention and screening are essential in caring for patients in the primary care setting.

Another common malignancy in men is lung cancer. In fact, lung cancer is the leading cause of cancer death in both men and women, with the most recent American Cancer Society report stating that there are over 234,000 new cases of lung cancer and over 154,000 lung cancer-related deaths each year in the United States [68, 69]. Prevention is absolutely essential for addressing lung cancer. The majority of lung cancer is associated with smoking, and even lung cancer in non-smokers has been connected to smoke exposure. It is thought that cigarette smoking is the causal agent in 85–90% of all lung cancer. As a result, the most important primary prevention strategy for lung cancer is aggressive screening for and counseling on smoking and early initiation of smoking cessation programs [70, 71]. Screening for asymptomatic lung cancer through several modalities has been analyzed with mixed results. In the Prostate, Lung, Colorectal, and Ovarian Cancer Screening Trial, screening for each of these malignancies was compared to no screening to determine the impact on incidence and mortality for different cancers [72]. For lung cancer, chest radiographs were used to screen the trial population for asymptomatic lung cancer over a period of 13 years. The participants were not identified as high risk and were intended to be representative of the general population. By the end of the trial, there was no significant difference in lung cancer incidence or mortality between the screening and control groups. Even when looking at only current or former smokers, no mortality difference was detected in those that were screened compared to those that were not. In addition, only 20% of diagnosed cases of lung cancer were diagnosed during screening [73]. This demonstrates that chest radiograph is not an effective screening method for lung cancer.

The National Lung Screening Trial analyzed the benefit of low-dose helical computed tomography (LDCT) as a screening tool for asymptomatic lung cancer. This was not the only trial of LDCT but was the only trial with a large enough sample or long enough trial period to demonstrate clear results. The NLST was stopped early after findings indicated a relative mortality reduction of 20% and an absolute mortality reduction of 62 lung cancer deaths per 100,000, demonstrating clear mortality benefit for screening with LDCT. However, the false-positive cumulative rate in the LDCT group was 96.4%, and many patients needed to undergo further evaluation when a positive finding was indicated on LDCT [74]. Taken together, this trial supports lung cancer screening by LDCT when a patient is considered at high risk where the risk of false positive is outweighed by the possibility of covert lung cancer. In addition, it is known that regular screening has a positive effect on smoking cessation risk, representing another positive outcome for screening of high-risk patient populations with LDCT.

For men, prostate cancer is a common cause of both malignancy and death in the United States. It is the most commonly diagnosed visceral cancer, responsible for an expected 165,000 diagnoses and 29,000 deaths by the end of 2018 [69]. It is second only to nonmelanoma skin cancer and lung cancer as the leading cause of cancer and cancer death in American men, and it is the most commonly diagnosed and seventh deadliest cancer in men around the world [75]. There are a small number of well-established risk factors for the development of prostate cancer. The primary risk factor is age. The development of prostate cancer in men before the age of 40 is rare, but the risk increases exponentially with advanced age [76]. In fact, the risk of prostate cancer ranges from 5% to 46% for men between ages 51 and 60 up to 40–73% for men ages 81–90 [77]. Another significant risk factor is ethnicity, with African American men being more likely to be diagnosed with prostate cancer and more likely to be diagnosed at a young age [76]. This is thought to be a combination between socioeconomic, environmental, and genetic factors that all combine to play a role in the increase risk for early prostate cancer in African American men [78, 79]. Certain genetic factors have been identified as increasing the risk for prostate cancer, including mutations in DNA repair pathways such as *BRCA2* and *ATM*. There have been some studies evaluating the role of a number of factors including diet, smoking, hormone levels, and drug or environmental exposures in the development of prostate cancer, but none of these have shown more than a minimal effect on risk.

The current wisdom for the screening of prostate cancer has changed recently, in contrast to the previous efforts at early detection. Specifically, the US Preventive Services Task Force has made new recommendations for screening in 2018. They recommend that men are involved in the decision-making process for whether screening is appropriate from the ages of 55 to 69. Men should be informed of the potential benefits of screening as well as the risks, such as false positives and over-diagnosis, and the utility of screening should be evaluated on an individualized basis. Men above the age of 70 should not be screened, and they find no sufficient evidence to make different screening recommendations for high-risk men, including African American men and men with a family history of prostate cancer [80]. The current recommendation if screening is warranted or requested is measurement of prostate-specific antigen (PSA). There are a number of different methods for measuring PSA, but it has been shown that elevations in PSA can precede clinical disease by at least 5 years and perhaps much longer [81–83]. The American Cancer Society currently suggests an abnormal cutoff for PSA levels of 4.0 ng/dL, which yields a 21% sensitivity for any prostate cancer and 51% for high-grade cancer. The specificity of this cutoff is 91% [84]. There are a number of different nonmalignant conditions that can result in an elevated PSA level, including prostatitis and benign prostatic hypertrophy, among others. Due to how common it is, the effectiveness of PSA screening in men with BPH was evaluated and was found to be a poor discriminator in men with symptomatic disease [85]. A common screening method for prostate cancer was digital rectal exam (DRE). It can detect abnormalities in the prostate on the posterior or lateral aspects, which are the most common origins for prostate neoplasms. However, DRE cannot detect cancer in other parts of the prostate, and malignancies discovered by DRE alone are clinically or pathologically advanced. Early prostate cancers are undetectable by DRE definitionally [86, 87]. As a result of this, DRE alone is not recommended as a screening modality for prostate cancer.

As is clear from the above discussions, our ability to screen for and, more importantly, prevent these cancers in men is limited in important ways. For some malignancies like lung cancer, the root causes are clear and our efforts at effective primary prevention are improving dramatically and already causing notable shifts in the morbidity and mortality associated with lung cancer. However, many malignancies such as colorectal and prostate cancer are genetic diseases at heart, either through familial association or mutation accumulation with aging. As a result, these diseases offer exciting opportunities for the application of ever-improving technology in genetic analysis. As personalized and precision medicine becomes more robust, we may be able to recognize more modifiable genetic risk factors and intervene before the formation of early malignant transformation. Until such day arrives, the above guidelines have been demonstrated to be our best practices in the prevention and early detection of colorectal, lung, and prostate cancers.

Our society has recently begun to look at mental health as a topic that should be discussed openly rather than act as a source of shame, but despite this shift in public opinion, many men still are not discussing their mental health openly, especially in a primary care setting. The most common mental health diagnosis in a primary care setting is depression, and the perception is that women are affected more often than men. However, it is often the case that men experience different symptoms than the classic depressive symptoms. Men are more likely to experience anger, agitation, and irritability as the primary mood disturbance rather than sadness, which can make it difficult for the family, physician, and patient to recognize the major depressive episode. Men are also more likely to engage in high-risk activity or have comorbid substance abuse issues [88]. As discussed before, the most worrying fact about depression in men is that they are almost four times as likely as women to attempt or complete suicide, making this an absolutely essential issue to screen for in all patients [2]. The primary care physician faces both the opportunity to diagnosis and intervene in these mental health issues, but they also face the challenge of appropriately screening patients. Effective screening is dependent on the ability of the primary care physician to form a trusting relationship with the patient and to encourage honest and open discussion of issues related to mental health, thus subverting expectations of masculinity that may prevent a conversion about depressive symptoms.

Alcohol use is widespread in the population, with 51.7% of Americans over the age of 12 reporting at least one drink within the last 30 days, 24.9% reporting binge drinking, and 6.5% reporting heavy drinking [89, 90]. The rates of alcohol abuse disorder among men and women differ, with men being much more likely to fit criteria. In 2007, the rate of alcohol abuse disorder as defined by the DSM-IV was 12.4% for men and 4.9% for women [91]. This has several important health consequences for men. In fact, alcohol abuse is the third leading cause of preventable death in the United States, and it is responsible for more than 85,000 deaths per year directly [92]. A recent analysis showed a dose-dependent relationship between alcohol consumption and non-MI cardiovascular disease, and this was associated with a lower life expectancy. In addition, they recommend lowering the threshold for alcohol consumption from 14 drinks per week for men to 7 drinks per week, as this was associated with the lowest mortality [93]. Aside from the cardiovascular risk, alcohol abuse increases the risk of suicide. A meta-analysis of over 400,000 patients showed that alcohol abuse was associated with an increased risk of suicidal ideation, suicide attempts, and suicide completion, with odds ratios of 1.86, 3.13, and 2.59, respectively [94]. The lifetime rate of suicide attempts is much higher in those that abuse alcohol compared to the general population, with 7% of alcohol abusers attempting suicide at some point in their life versus 1% of the general population [95–97]. Clearly, the risks associated with excessive alcohol consumption are enormous, and the associated effects exacerbate some of the gravest threats to life expectancy for men. It is essential that primary care doctors screen for alcohol abuse and discuss safe alcohol consumption with their male patients, as intervention is essential to curb the impact of alcohol on men's health.

Often an uncomfortable topic for providers and patients, sexual health is an important aspect of wellness that should receive attention during primary care visits. Worldwide, there are 2 million new HIV infections each year. With no effective vaccines against the virus, behavioral interventions remain the primary method by which we can reduce our patient's risk of infection [98]. Primary care physicians should discuss their patient's sexual activity and assess for their risk of HIV and other sexually transmitted infections. High-risk patients, especially men who have sex with men (MSM), should be screened aggressively, and discussions about HIV prevention should be initiated. Recently, it has been shown that the primary method by which HIV transmission can be prevented is through viral suppression. In fact, in patients who have achieved full viral suppression, the risk of transmission through intimate contact is negligible, and these patients can be considered noninfectious from this perspective. This makes antiretroviral therapy the mainstay in HIV prevention [99–101]. For HIV-negative patients, there are new approaches to protecting them from contracting the virus. The CDC has issued guidelines for offering pre-exposure prophylaxis, or PrEP, to patients who engage in high-risk sexual activity or are in a serodifferent relationship. The most extensively studied PrEP regimen is once-daily tenofovir disoproxil fumarate-emtricitabine (TDF-FTC), sold in the United States under the brand name Truvada. Truvada can be given in 90-day supplies and renewed after a negative HIV test [102]. Adherence to the regimen is absolutely essential for effective protection, so primary care physicians prescribing PrEP regimens should discuss this with patients and assess for a patient's ability to comply when deciding whether to initiate PrEP. Because of the disproportionate HIV prevalence in the MSM community, physicians caring for gay men in the primary care should be proactive in discussing sexual health and infection prevention.

A growing issue for adults has been insufficient sleep, and many patients are not aware of the broad health impacts of chronic sleep insufficiency. The amount of scientific evidence for a specific amount of sleep is actually quite sparse, even in children and adolescents where the importance of sufficient sleep has received more attention. Our best recommendations are from the American Academy of Sleep Medicine, which recommends at minimum of 7 hours of sleep per night for adults [103]. However, it is extremely common that people do not get this amount of sleep, with nearly one-third of adults reporting less than 7 hours of sleep on workday nights [104]. The importance of healthy sleep cannot be overstated, with sleep insufficiency resulting in an increase in the rates of motor vehicle and workplace accidents, as well as being associated with increased cardiovascular risk, immunosuppression, and obesity [105–110]. There have been a number of studies looking at the impact of sleep on all-cause mortality, with some suggesting that both sleep insufficiency and oversleeping are associated with an increase in mortality. Meta-analysis of the available research on the topic has yielded mixed results [111–113]. A special note should be made with regard to the prevalence of sleep apnea syndrome in men. Obstructive sleep apnea is two to three times more likely in men than women, with male gender being an important risk factor for OSA [114, 115]. In North America, between 20% and 30% of men have obstructive sleep apnea, making it one of the most common causes for disturbances in sleep [116, 117]. The most common presentations of sleep apnea are snoring and wake-time sleepiness, but many men will not have daytime sleepiness. As a result, choking or gasping during sleep is seen as the most useful sign, and careful sleep history taking is essential for catching this syndrome before it negatively impacts the patient's overall health [118]. It is clear that sleep insufficiency has important implications for overall well-being, and it is absolutely critical that primary care providers discuss their patients' sleep habits and emphasize the vital role that healthy sleep behavior has on a patient's general health.

The above discussion is intended to demonstrate the current best practices with respect to some of the most common issues in the primary care of the male patient. Of course, there are a number of other preventative and screening considerations that must be made, but these represent the most important health issues facing men, and thus they must form the core of our approach to primary prevention and screening. A summary of the recommendations discussed here can be found in the accompanying table. The guidelines covered are ever-changing based on our newest understanding of these diseases, and individual modifications can be made based on each patient's individual risk profile. Times are also changing dramatically in the field of primary care, with genomics and big data becoming more widespread, and patients are demanding more openness and communication in their relationship with their physicians. Primary care providers must be prepared to apply this individualistic approach to medicine and become more flexible in their approach to each patient. Men's health is a growing field of interest, and it's important that primary care prepares to fill this need and provide for the specific situations facing the male patient.

References

1. Xu J, Murphy SL, Kochanek KD, Arias E. Mortality in the United States, 2015. NCHS Data Brief. 2016;(267):1–8. https://doi.org/10.1056/NEJM184002260220306.
2. Pinkhasov RM, Shteynshlyuger A, Hakimian P, Lindsay GK, Samadi DB, Shabsigh R. Are men shortchanged on health? Perspective on life expectancy, morbidity, and mortality in men and women in the United States. Int J Clin Pract. 2010;64(4):465–74. https://doi.org/10.1111/j.1742-1241.2009.02289.x.
3. Newman AB, Brach JS. Gender gap in longevity and disability in older persons. Epidemiol Rev. 2001;23(2):343–55. https://doi.org/10.1093/oxfordjournals.epirev.a000810.
4. Bonhomme JJ. The gender longevity gap: is it really biology? J Mens Health. 2009;6(3):151–4. https://doi.org/10.1016/j.jomh.2009.06.004.
5. Schünemann J, Strulik H, Trimborn T. The gender gap in mortality: how much is explained by behavior? J Health Econ. 2017;54:79–90. https://doi.org/10.1016/j.jhealeco.2017.04.002.
6. Regan JC, Partridge L. Gender and longevity: why do men die earlier than women? Comparative and experimental evidence. Best Pract Res Clin Endocrinol Metab. 2013;27(4):467–79. https://doi.org/10.1016/j.beem.2013.05.016.
7. Marais GAB, Gaillard JM, Vieira C, et al. Sex gap in aging and longevity: can sex chromosomes play a role? Biol Sex Differ. 2018;9(1):1–14. https://doi.org/10.1186/s13293-018-0181-y.
8. King P, Peacock I, Donnelly R. The UK Prospective Diabetes Study (UKPDS): clinical and therapeutic implications for type 2 diabetes. Br J Clin Pharmacol. 1999;48:643–8. https://doi.org/10.1046/j.1365-2125.1999.00092.x.
9. Wallis EJ, Ramsay LE, Haq IU, et al. Coronary and cardiovascular risk estimation for primary prevention: validation of a new Sheffield table in the 1995 Scottish health survey population. BMJ. 2000;320(7236):671–6. https://doi.org/10.1136/bmj.320.7236.671.
10. Ballantyne CM, Grundy SM, Oberman A, et al. Hyperlipidemia : diagnostic and therapeutic perspectives primary prevention of coronary heart disease. J Clin Endocrinol Metab. 2015;85(6):2089–112. https://doi.org/10.1210/jcem.85.6.6642-1.
11. Grundy SM, Bilheimer D, Chait A, Clark LT, Denke M, Havel RJ, Hazzard WR, Hulley SB, Hunninghake DB, Kreisberg RA, Etherton PK. Summary of the second report of the National Cholesterol Education Program (NCEP) Expert Panel on detection, evaluation, and treatment of high blood cholesterol in adults (adult treatment panel II). J Am Med Assoc. 1993;269(23):3015–23.
12. Jeremiah Stamler MD, Deborah Wentworth MPH, Neaton JD. Is relationship between serum cholesterol and risk of premature death from coronary heart disease continuous and graded? Findings in 356 222 primary screenees of the multiple risk factor intervention trial (MRFIT). J Am Med Assoc. 1986;256(20):2823–8.
13. Shepherd J, Cobbe S, Ford I, et al. Prevention of coronary heart disease with pravastatin in men with hypercholesterolemia. West of Scotland Coronary Prevention Study Group. N Engl J Med. 1995;333(20):1301.
14. Downs JR, Clearfield M, Weis S, Whitney E, Shapiro DR, Beere PA, Langendorfer A, Stein EA, Kruyer W, Gotto AM Jr. Primary prevention of acute coronary events with lovastatin in men and women with average cholesterol levels. J Am Med Assoc. 1998;279(20):1615–22.

15. Jamerson K, Weber MA, Bakris GL, Dahlöf B, Pitt B, Shi V, Hester A, Gupte J, Gatlin M, Velazquez EJ, for the A trial investigators*. Abstract. Rosuvastatin to prevent vascular events in men and women with elevated C-reactive protein paul. N Engl J Med. 2017;359:1315–23. https://doi.org/10.1056/NEJMoa1706198.
16. Yusuf S, Bosch J, Dagenais G, et al. Cholesterol lowering in intermediate-risk persons without cardiovascular disease. N Engl J Med. 2016;374(21):2021–31. https://doi.org/10.1056/NEJMoa1600176.
17. Roger Chou MD, Tracy Dana MLS, Ian Blazina MPH, Monica Daeges BA, Jeanne TL. Statins for prevention of cardiovascular disease in adults. J Am Med Assoc. 2016;316(19):2008–24.
18. Stone NJ, Robinson JG, Lichtenstein AH, et al. 2013 ACC/AHA guideline on the treatment of blood cholesterol to reduce atherosclerotic cardiovascular risk in adults. Circulation. 2014;129(25 suppl 2):S1–S45. https://doi.org/10.1161/01.cir.0000437738.63853.7a.
19. Guideline development group. Cardiovascular disease: risk assessment and reduction including lipid modification. 2014;(August 2015):1–50. http://www.nice.org.uk/guidance/cg181/chapter/Introduction.
20. Catapano AL, Graham I, De Backer G, et al. ESC/EAS guidelines for the management of dyslipidaemias. Eur Heart J. 2016;37(39):2999–3058l. https://doi.org/10.1093/eurheartj/ehw272.
21. O'Rourke RA, Brundage BH, Froelicher VF, Greenland P, Grundy SM, Hachamovitch R, Pohost GM, Shaw LJ, Weintraub WS, Winters WL Jr, Forrester JS, Douglas PS, Faxon DP, Fisher JD, Gregoratos G, Hochman JS, Hutter AM Jr, Kaul SWM. American College of Cardiology/American Heart Association Expert Consensus document on electron-beam computed tomography for the diagnosis and prognosis of coronary artery disease. Circulation. 2000;102(1):126–40.
22. Haberl R, Becker A, Leber A, et al. Correlation of coronary calcification and angiographically documented stenoses in patients with suspected coronary artery disease: results of 1,764 patients. J Am Coll Cardiol. 2001;37(2):451–7. https://doi.org/10.1016/S0735-1097(00)01119-0.
23. Valenti V, Hartaigh BÓ, Cho I, Schulman-Marcus J, Gransar H, Heo R, Truong QA, Shaw LJ, Knapper J, Kelkar AA, Sciarretta S, Chang H-J, Callister TQ, Min JK. Absence of coronary artery calcium identifies asymptomatic diabetic individuals at low near-term but not long-term risk of mortality: a 15-year follow-up study of 9715 patients. Circ Cardiovasc Imaging. 2016;9(2):1–18. https://doi.org/10.1161/CIRCIMAGING.115.003528.Absence.
24. Vargas J, Lima JAC, Kraus WE, Douglas PS, Rosenberg S. Use of the Corus® CAD gene expression test for assessment of obstructive coronary artery disease likelihood in symptomatic non-diabetic patients. PLoS Curr. 2013;5.
25. Guyton JR, Blazing MA, Hagar J, et al. Extended-release niacin vs gemfibrozil for the treatment of low levels of high-density lipoprotein cholesterol. Niaspan-Gemfibrozil Study Group. Arch Intern Med. 2000;160:1177–84. https://doi.org/10.1001/archinte.160.8.1177.
26. CARLSON LA, HAMSTEN A, ASPLUND A. Pronounced lowering of serum levels of lipoprotein Lp(a) in hyperlipidaemic subjects treated with nicotinic acid. J Intern Med. 1989;226(4):271–6. https://doi.org/10.1111/j.1365-2796.1989.tb01393.x.
27. Wilson P. Established risk factors and coronary artery disease: the Framingham Study. Am J Hypertens. 1994;7:7S.
28. Whelton PK, Carey RM, Aronow WS, et al. 2017 ACC/AHA/AAPA/ABC/ACPM/AGS/APhA/ASH/ASPC/NMA/PCNA Guideline for the Prevention, Detection, Evaluation, and Management of High Blood Pressure in adults: a report of the American College of Cardiology/American Heart Association Task Force. Hypertension. 2018;71(6):140–4.
29. Sonne-Holm S, Sørensen TI, Jensen G, Schnohr P. Independent effects of weight change and attained body weight on prevalence of arterial hypertension in obese and non-obese men. BMJ Br Med. 1989;299(September):299–302. https://doi.org/10.1136/bmj.299.6702.767.
30. Suzanne O. Hypertension in women. Vasc Biol Hypertens Program, Div Cardiovasc Dis Univ Alabama Birmingham, 35294, USA. 2010;302(4):401–11. https://doi.org/10.1001/jama.2009.1060.Diet.
31. Staessen JA, Wang J, Bianchi G. Essential hypertension. In: xPharm: the comprehensive pharmacology reference, vol. 361; 2003. https://doi.org/10.1016/B978-008055232-3.60057-1.

32. Wang N-Y, Young JH, Meoni LA, Ford DE, Erlinger TP, Klag MJ. Blood pressure change and risk of hypertension associated with parental hypertension. Arch Intern Med. 2008;168(6):643–8.
33. Carnethon MR, Evans NS, Church TS, et al. Joint Associations of Physical Activity and Aerobic Fitness on the Development of Incident Hypertension: Coronary Artery Risk Development in Young Adults (CARDIA). Hypertension. 2011;56(1):49–55. https://doi.org/10.1161/HYPERTENSIONAHA.109.147603.Joint.
34. Elmer PJ, Obarzanek E, Vollmer WM, Simons-Morton D, Stevens VJ, Young DR, Lin P-H, Champagne C, Harsha DW, Svetkey LP, Ard J, Phil M. Effects of comprehensive lifestyle modification on diet, weight, physical fitness, and blood pressure control: 18-month results of a randomized trial. Ann Intern Med. 2006;144(7):485–95.
35. Turnbull F. Effects of different regimens to lower blood pressure on major cardiovascular events in older and younger people: meta-analysis of randomised trials. BMJ. 2008;336(7653):1121–3. https://doi.org/10.1136/bmj.39548.738368.BE.
36. Hebert PR, Moser M, Mayer J, Glynn RJ, Hennekens CH. Recent evidence on drug therapy of mild to moderate hypertension and decreased risk of coronary heart disease. Arch Intern Med. 1993;153(5):578–81.
37. Lorell BH, Carabello B. Left ventricular hypertrophy: pathogenesis, detection, and prognosis. Circulation. 2000;102(4):470–9.
38. Vakili BA, Okin PM, Devereux RB. Prognostic implications of left ventricular hypertrophy. Am Heart J. 2001;141(3):334–41. https://doi.org/10.1067/mhj.2001.113218.
39. Levy D, Larson MG, Vasan RS, Kannel WB, Ho KKL. The progression from hypertension to congestive heart failure. J Am Med Assoc. 1996;275(20):1557–62.
40. Staessen JA, Fagard R, Thijs L, et al. Randomised double-blind comparison of placebo and active treatment for older patients with isolated systolic hypertension. Lancet. 1997;350:757–64.
41. Thrift AG, McNeil JJ, Forbes ADG. Risk factors for cerebral hemorrhage in the era of well-controlled hypertension. Melbourne Risk Factor Study (MERFS) Group. Stroke. 1996;27(11):2020–5.
42. Coresh J, Wei GL, McQuillan G, Brancati FL, Levey AS, Jones C, Klag MJ. Prevalence of high blood pressure and elevated serum creatinine level in the United States. Arch Intern Med. 2001;161(9):1207–16.
43. Hsu C-Y, McCulloch CE, Darbinian J, Go AS, Iribarren C. Elevated blood pressure and risk of end-stage renal disease in subjects without baseline kidney disease. Arch Intern Med. 2005;165(8):923–8.
44. MacMahon S, Baigent C, Duffy S, et al. Body-mass index and cause-specific mortality in 900 000 adults: collaborative analyses of 57 prospective studies. Lancet. 2009;373(9669):1083–96. https://doi.org/10.1016/S0140-6736(09)60318-4.
45. Clinical Guidelines on the identification, evaluation, and treatment of overweight and obesity in adults--The Evidence Report. National Institutes of Health. Obes Res Clin Pract. 1998;6(6):464.
46. Obesity: preventing and managing the global epidemic. Report of a WHO consultation. World Health Organ Tech Rep Ser. 2000;894:1–253.
47. Hales CM, Fryar CD, Carroll MD, Freedman DS, Ogden CL. Trends in obesity and severe obesity prevalence in US youth and adults by sex and age, 2007-2008 to 2015-2016. J Am Med Assoc. 2018;319(16):1723–5.
48. Willett WC, Dietz WH, Colditz GA. Guidelines for healthy weight. N Engl J Med. 1999;341:427–34.
49. Apovian M, Ard JD, Comuzzie AG, et al. 2013 AHA/ACC/TOS guideline for the management of overweight and obesity in adults: HHS public access preamble and transition to ACC/AHA guidelines to reduce cardiovascular risk. Circulation. 2014;129(25):102–38. https://doi.org/10.1161/01.cir.
50. Siegel R, Ward E, Brawley O, Jemal A. Cancer statistics, 2011 the impact of eliminating socioeconomic and racial disparities on premature cancer deaths. CA Cancer J Clin. 2011;61:212–36. https://doi.org/10.3322/caac.20121.Available.

51. Torre LA, Bray F, Siegel RL, Ferlay J. Global cancer statistics, 2012. CA Cancer J Clin. 2015;65(2):87–108. https://doi.org/10.3322/caac.21262.
52. Brawley OW. Avoidable cancer deaths globally. CA Cancer J Clin. 2011;61(2):67–8. https://doi.org/10.3322/caac.20108.
53. Colditz GA, DeJong W, Emmons K, Hunter DJ, et al. Harvard report on cancer prevention volume 2: prevention of human Cancer. Cancer Causes Control. 1997;8(S1):S1–3.
54. Siegel R, Miller K, Jemal A. Cancer statistics, 2015. Cancer J Clin. 2015;65(1):29. https://doi.org/10.3322/caac.21254.
55. International Agency for Research on Cancer. Colorectal cancer. Lancet. 2018;876:49–50. https://doi.org/10.1016/S0140-6736(13)61649-9.
56. Johns LE, Houlston RS. A systematic review and meta-analysis of familial colorectal cancer risk. Am J Gastroenterol. 2001;96:2992–3003.
57. Jemal A, Siegel R, Ward E, Hao Y, Xu J, Thun MJ. Cancer statistics, 2010. CA Cancer J Clin. 2009;59(4):1–25. https://doi.org/10.1002/caac.20073.Available.
58. Lee B, Holub J, Peters D, Lieberman D. Prevalence of colon polyps detected by colonoscopy screening of asymptomatic Hispanic patients. Dig Dis Sci. 2012;57(2):481–8. https://doi.org/10.1007/s10620-011-1898-1.
59. Ferlitsch M, Reinhart K, Pramhas S, Wiener C, Gal O, Bannert C, Hassler M, Kozbial K, Dunkler D, Trauner M, Weiss W. Sex-specific prevalence of adenomas, advanced adenomas, and colorectal cancer in individuals undergoing screening colonoscopy. J Am Med Assoc. 2011;306(12):1352–8.
60. Brenner H, Hoffmeister M, Stegmaier C, Brenner G, Altenhofen L, Haug U. Risk of progression of advanced adenomas to colorectal cancer by age and sex: estimates based on 840 149 screening colonoscopies. Gut. 2007;56(11):1585–9. https://doi.org/10.1136/gut.2007.122739.
61. Nowacki MP, Butruk E. Colonoscopy screening for detection of advanced neoplasia. N Engl J Med. 2007;356(6):632–4. https://doi.org/10.1056/NEJMc063405.
62. Rundle AG, Lebwohl B, Vogel R, Levine S, Neugut AI. Colonoscopic screening in average risk individuals ages 40 to 49 versus 50 to 59 years. Gastroenterology. 2013;134(5):1311–5. https://doi.org/10.1053/j.gastro.2008.02.032.COLONOSCOPIC.
63. Nguyen SP, Bent S, Chen YH, Terdiman JP. Gender as a risk factor for advanced neoplasia and colorectal cancer: a systematic review and meta-analysis. Clin Gastroenterol Hepatol. 2009;7(6):676–681.e3. https://doi.org/10.1016/j.cgh.2009.01.008.
64. Schoenfeld P, Cash B, Flood A, et al. Colonoscopic screening of average-risk women for colorectal neoplasia. N Engl J Med. 2005;353(8):844–6; author reply 844–846. https://doi.org/10.1056/NEJMc051651.
65. Force UPST. Screening for colorectal cancer. J Am Med Assoc. 2016;315(23):2564–75.
66. Peterse EFP, Meester RGS, Siegel RL, et al. The impact of the rising colorectal cancer incidence in young adults on the optimal age to start screening: microsimulation analysis I to inform the American Cancer Society colorectal cancer screening guideline. Cancer. 2018;124(14):2964–73. https://doi.org/10.1002/cncr.31543.
67. Wolf AMD, Fontham ETH, Church TR, et al. Colorectal cancer screening for average-risk adults: 2018 guideline update from the American Cancer Society. CA Cancer J Clin. 2018;68(4):250–81. https://doi.org/10.3322/caac.21457.
68. Siegel RL, Miller KD, Jemal A. Cancer statistics, 2017. CA Cancer J Clin. 2017;67:7–30. https://doi.org/10.3322/caac.21387.
69. Siegel RL, Miller KD, Jemal A. Cancer statistics, 2018. CA Cancer J Clin. 2018;68:7–30. https://doi.org/10.3322/caac.21387.
70. Alberg AJ, Samet JM. Epidemiology of lung cancer. Chest. 2003;123:21S–49S. https://doi.org/10.1378/chest.123.1.
71. Fontham ETH, Correa P, Reynolds P, Wu-Williams A, Buffler PA, Greenberg RS, Chen VW, Alterman T, Boyd P, Austin DF, Liff J. Environmental tobacco smoke and lung cancer in non-smoking women. J Am Med Assoc. 1994;271(22):1752–9.

72. Hasson MA, Fagerstrom RM, Kahane DC, et al. Design of the prostate, lung, colorectal and ovarian (PLCO) cancer screening trial. Control Clin Trials. 2000;21(6):329S–48S. https://doi.org/10.1016/S0197-2456(00)00100-8.

73. Oken MM, Hocking WG, Kvale PA, et al. Screening by chest radiograph and lung cancer mortality: the prostate, lung, colorectal, and ovarian (PLCO) randomized trial. J Am Med Assoc. 2011;306(17):1865–73. https://doi.org/10.1001/jama.2011.1591.

74. Team TNLSTR. Reduced lung-cancer mortality with low-dose computed tomographic screening. N Engl J Med. 2011;365(5):395–409. https://doi.org/10.1056/NEJMoa1511939.

75. Collaboration GB of DC. Global, regional, and national cancer incidence, mortality, years of life lost, years lived with disability, and disability-adjusted life-years for 32 cancer groups, 1990 to 2015: a systematic analysis for the global burden of disease study. JAMA Oncol. 2017;3(4):524–48. https://doi.org/10.1001/jamaoncol.2016.5688.Global.

76. Hankey BF, Feuer EJ, Clegg LX, Hayes RB, Legler JM, Prorok PC, Ries LA, Merrill RMKR. Cancer surveillance series: interpreting trends in prostate cancer--part I: evidence of the effects of screening in recent prostate cancer incidence, mortality, and survival rates. J Natl Cancer Inst. 1999;91(12):1017–24.

77. Delongchamps NB, Singh A, Haas GP. The role of prevalence in the diagnosis of prostate cancer. Cancer Control. 2006;13(3):158–68. https://doi.org/10.1177/107327480601300302.

78. Baquet CR, Horm JW, Gibbs TGP. Socioeconomic factors and cancer incidence among blacks and whites. J Natl Cancer Inst. 1991;83(8):551–7.

79. Ingles SA, Coetzee GA, Ross RK, et al. Association of prostate cancer with vitamin D receptor haplotypes in African-Americans. Cancer Res. 1998;58(8):1620–3. https://doi.org/10.1016/0013-4686(90)87055-7.

80. Grossman DC, Curry SJ, Owens DK, et al. Screening for prostate cancer. J Am Med Assoc. 2018;319(18):1901–13. https://doi.org/10.1001/jama.2018.3710.

81. Gann PH, Hennekens CH, Stampfer MJ. A prospective evaluation of plasma prostate-specific antigen for detection of prostatic cancer. J Am Med Assoc. 1995;273(4):289–94. https://doi.org/10.1001/jama.1995.03520280035036.

82. Draisma G, Boer R, Otto SJ, van der Cruijsen IW, Damhuis RA, Schröder FH de KH. Lead times and overdetection due to prostate-specific antigen screening: estimates from the European randomized study of screening for prostate cancer. J Natl Cancer Inst. 2003;95(12):868–78.

83. Whittemore AS, Cirillo PM, Feldman D, Cohn BA. Prostate specific antigen levels in young adulthood predict prostate cancer risk: results from a cohort of black and white Americans. J Urol. 2005;174(3):872–6. https://doi.org/10.1097/01.ju.0000169262.18000.8a.

84. Wolf AMD, Wender RC, Etzioni RB, Thompson IM, D'Amico AV, et al. American Cancer Society Guideline for the early detection of prostate cancer. CA Cancer J Clin. 2010;60:70–98. https://doi.org/10.3322/caac.20066.Available.

85. Meigs JB, Barry MJ, Oesterling JEJS. Interpreting results of prostate-specific antigen testing for early detection of prostate cancer. J Gen Intern Med. 1996;11(9):505–12.

86. Tricoli JV, Schoenfeldt M, Conley BA. Detection of prostate cancer and predicting progression current and future diagnostic markers. Clin Cancer Res. 2004;10(301):3943–53. https://doi.org/10.1002/(SICI)1096-8644(199705)103:1<119::AID-AJPA8>3.0.CO;2-R.

87. Mitchell TS. Screening for prostate cancer. Urol Nurs. 1994;14(1):9–11. https://doi.org/10.1002/14651858.CD004720.pub3.

88. Road D, Terrace E. Men & depression. National Institute of Mental Health, 2008.

89. Park-lee E, Porter JD, Pemberton MR, Tice P. Key substance use and mental health indicators in the United States: results from the 2015 National Survey on Drug Use and Health. 2015. https://doi.org/10.1016/j.drugalcdep.2016.10.042.

90. Services H, Institutes N, Abuse A. Helping patients who drink too much: a clinician's guide. National Institute on Alcohol and Alcoholism. 2005;7(3769).

91. Hasin DS, Stinson FS, Ogburn E, Grant BF. Prevalence, correlates, disability, and comorbidity of DSM-IV alcohol Abuse and dependence in the United States. Arch Gen Psychiatry. 2008;64(7):830–42. https://doi.org/10.1001/archpsyc.64.7.830.

92. Harwood H. Updating estimates of the economic costs of alcohol abuse in the United States: estimates, update methods, and data. Natl Inst Alcohol Abus Alcohol. 2000;69(3):1–17. https://doi.org/10.1016/j.amepre.2011.06.045.

93. Wood AM, Kaptoge S, Butterworth AS, et al. Risk thresholds for alcohol consumption: combined analysis of individual-participant data for 599 912 current drinkers in 83 prospective studies. Lancet. 2018;391(10129):1513–23. https://doi.org/10.1016/S0140-6736(18)30134-X.

94. Darvishi N, Farhadi M, Haghtalab T, Poorolajal J. Alcohol-related risk of suicidal ideation, suicide attempt, and completed suicide: a meta-analysis. PLoS One. 2015;10(5):1–14. https://doi.org/10.1371/journal.pone.0126870.

95. Ohberg A, Vuori E, Ojanperä I, Lonnqvist J. Alcohol and drugs in suicides. Br J Psychiatry. 1996;169(1):75–80. https://doi.org/10.1192/bjp.169.1.75.

96. Yaldizli Ö, Kuhl HC, Graf M, Wiesbeck GA, Wurst FM. Risk factors for suicide attempts in patients with alcohol dependence or abuse and a history of depressive symptoms: a subgroup analysis from the WHO/ISBRA study. Drug Alcohol Rev. 2010;29(1):64–74. https://doi.org/10.1111/j.1465-3362.2009.00089.x.

97. Hingson R, Heeren T, Winter M, Wechsler H. Magnitude of alcohol-related mortality and morbidity among U.S. college students ages 18–24: changes from 1998 to 2001. Annu Rev Public Health. 2005;26(1):259–79. https://doi.org/10.1146/annurev.publhealth.26.021304.144652.

98. Maartens G, Celum C, Lewin SR. HIV infection: epidemiology, pathogenesis, treatment, and prevention. Lancet. 2014;384(9939):258–71. https://doi.org/10.1016/S0140-6736(14)60164-1.

99. Rodger AJ, Cambiano V, Bruun T, et al. Sexual activity without condoms and risk of HIV transmission in serodifferent couples when the HIV-positive partner is using suppressive antiretroviral therapy. J Am Med Assoc. 2016;316(2):171–81. https://doi.org/10.1001/jama.2016.5148.

100. Muessig KE, Cohen MS. Advances in HIV prevention for Serodiscordant couples. Curr HIV/AIDS Rep. 2014;11(4):434–46. https://doi.org/10.1007/s11904-014-0225-9.

101. Cohen MS, Chen YQ, McCauley M, Gamble T, Hosseinipour MC, Kumarasamy N, Hakim JG, Kumwenda J, Grinsztejn B, Pilotto JHS, Godbole SV, Mehendale S, Chariyalertsak S, Santos BR, Mayer KH, Hoffman IF, Eshleman SH, Eron J, Gallant J, Havlir D, Swindells S, Ribaudo H, Elharrar V, Burns D, Taha TE, Nielsen-Saines K, Celentano D, Fleming TR, for the H 052 ST. Prevention of HIV-1 infection with early antiretroviral therapy. N Engl J Med. 2011;365(6):493–505. https://doi.org/10.1056/NEJMoa1603827.

102. Preexposure prophylaxis for the prevention of HIV infection in the United States-2017 update clinical providers' supplement. 2017. https://www.cdc.gov/hiv/pdf/risk/prep/cdc-hiv-prep-provider-supplement-2017.pdf.

103. Watson NF, Badr MS, Belenk G, Bliwise DL. Recommended amount of sleep for a healthy adult. Sleep. 2015;38(6):843–4. https://doi.org/10.5665/sleep.4716.

104. Liu Y, Wheaton AG, Chapman DP, Cunningham TJ, Lu HCJ. Prevalence of healthy sleep duration among adults — United States, 2014. Morb Mortal Wkly Rep. 2016;65:137–41.

105. Besedovsky L, Lange T, Born J. Sleep and immune function. Pflugers Arch. 2012;463(1):121–37. https://doi.org/10.1007/s00424-011-1044-0.

106. St-Onge MP, Grandner MA, Brown D, et al. Sleep duration and quality: impact on lifestyle behaviors and cardiometabolic health: a scientific statement from the American Heart Association. Circulation. 2016;134(18):e367–86. https://doi.org/10.1161/CIR.0000000000000444.

107. Rajaratnam SMW, Barger LK, Lockley SW, Shea SA, Wang W, Landrigan CP, O'Brien CS, Qadri S, Sullivan JP, Cade BE, Epstein LJ, Wh DP. Sleep disorders, health, and safety in police officers. J Am Med Assoc. 2011;306(23):2567–78. http://www.ncbi.nlm.nih.gov/pubmed/22187276

108. Gottlieb DJ, Ellenbogen JM, Bianchi MT, Czeisler CA. Sleep deficiency and motor vehicle crash risk in the general population: a prospective cohort study. BMC Med. 2018;16(1):1–10. https://doi.org/10.1186/s12916-018-1025-7.

109. Ayas NT, Barger LK, Cade BE, et al. Extended work duration and the risk of self-reported percutaneous injuries in interns. J Am Med Assoc. 2006;296(9):1055–62. https://doi.org/10.1001/jama.296.9.1055.

110. Barger LK, Ayas NT, Cade BE, et al. Impact of extended-duration shifts on medical errors, adverse events, and attentional failures. PLoS Med. 2006;3(12):2440–8. https://doi.org/10.1371/journal.pmed.0030487.

111. Kurina LM, McClintock MK, Chen JH, Waite LJ, Thisted RA, Lauderdale DS. Sleep duration and all-cause mortality: a critical review of measurement and associations. Ann Epidemiol. 2013;23(6):361–70. https://doi.org/10.1016/j.annepidem.2013.03.015.

112. Cappuccio FP, D'Elia L, Strazzullo P, Miller MA. Sleep duration and all-cause mortality: a systematic review and meta-analysis of prospective studies. Sleep. 2010;33(5):585–92. https://doi.org/10.1093/sleep/33.5.585.

113. Manoharan S, Jothipriya A. Sleep duration and mortality - a systematic review. J Pharm Sci Res. 2016;8(8):867–8. https://doi.org/10.1111/j.1365-2869.2008.00732.x.

114. Quintana-gallego E, Carmona-bernal C, Capote F, Botebol-benhamou G, Polo J. Gender differences in obstructive sleep apnea syndrome : a clinical study of 1166 patients. Respir Med. 2004;98:984–9. https://doi.org/10.1016/j.rmed.2004.03.002.

115. Young T, Skatrud J, Peppard PE. Risk factors for obstructive sleep apnea in adults. J Am Med Assoc. 2004;291(16):2013–6.

116. Young T, Palta M, Dempsey J, Peppard P, Nieto FJ, Hla KM. Burden of sleep apnea: rationale, design, and major findings of the Wisconsin Sleep Cohort Study Terry. WMJ. 2009;108(5):246–9.

117. Peppard PE, Young T, Barnet JH, Palta M, Hagen EW, Hla KM. Increased prevalence of sleep-disordered breathing in adults. Am J Epidemiol. 2013;177(9):1006–14. https://doi.org/10.1093/aje/kws342.

118. Myers KA, Mrkobrada M, Simel DL. Does this patient have obstructive sleep apnea? The rational clinical examination systematic review. J Am Med Assoc. 2013;310(7):731–41. https://doi.org/10.1001/jama.2013.276185.

Chapter 4
Cardiometabolic Diseases in the Adolescents, Young Adults, and the Elderly

Gundu H. R. Rao

Introduction

"The ultimate public health goal is not just to control disease, or just to reduce high risk, but to prevent the development of high risk in the first place, amongst individuals and entire populations," wrote Professor Henry Blackburn, pioneer cardiovascular epidemiologist of the University of Minnesota, in his introduction to our first book on coronary artery disease, some two decades ago [1]. He further elaborated his thoughts on the essentials of preventive cardiology, – "Applications to cardiovascular health include the prevention of both individual risk and overall population risk, that is dealing with 'sick population as well as sick individuals'. The future for prevention of individual high risk lies in targeting these individuals, promoting individual and family health, education and motivation of health professionals in preventive practice, along with wider provision of preventive services." According to public health experts, modern medicine has failed to stop, reduce, reverse, or prevent the increase in the incidence and prevalence of metabolic diseases, such as hypertension, excess weight, obesity, type-2 diabetes, and vascular diseases. This observation is supported by numerous recent publications indicating the increase in the incidence of metabolic diseases to epidemic proportions worldwide [2–20].

The first observations among population cohorts were oriented toward individual risks in the North American culture in Minnesota in 1947, and Framingham, MA in 1948. Another approach led by the well-known pioneering epidemiologist and researcher Professor Ancel Keys focused on the factors that determined cardiovascular (CVD) risk differences among entire populations, as in the Seven Countries Study. Ancel Keys gave the study its scope, design, and direction and coordinated the program from Minnesota, with field surveys beginning in 1957 in the United States, Italy, Greece, Yugoslavia, the Netherlands, Finland, and Japan. The main

G. H. R. Rao (✉)
Emeritus Professor, Laboratory Medicine and Pathology, Director, Thrombosis Research, Lillehei Heart Institute, University of Minnesota, Minneapolis, MN, USA

© Springer Nature Switzerland AG 2021   35
J. P. Alukal et al. (eds.), *Design and Implementation of the Modern Men's Health Center*, https://doi.org/10.1007/978-3-030-54482-9_4

conclusions of the Seven Countries Study were that the mass burden and epidemic of atherosclerotic diseases: (1) has cultural origins, (2) is preventable, (3) can change rapidly, and (4) is strongly influenced by the fatty composition of the habitual diet [21]. It showed that serum cholesterol, blood pressure, diabetes, and smoking were universal risk factors for CVD. Continuation of these studies in the North Karelia province, Finland, with the specific aims to reverse the excess incidence of CVD by changing the population life styles, was successfully accomplished [22].

The Framingham Heart Study (FHS), with congruent findings from other studies in the United States and abroad, provides a sound basis for successful medical action and health promotion policy to reduce the death rate from these diseases [23]. The FHS was a landmark monograph on the predictive power of blood pressure, blood cholesterol level, and smoking habit for heart and blood vessel diseases. Roy Dawber, the first director of the FHS, states, "The characteristics of persons who already have the disease are not necessarily the same as those that predispose to the disease. Observations of population characteristics must be made well before disease becomes overt, if the relationship of these characteristics to the development of the disease, is to be established with reasonable certainty." The Office of the Science Policy of the National Institutes of Health (NIH), USA, claims, "The Framingham Heart Study contributed significantly in laying down the foundation for preventive health care. FHS changed the way we study and approach chronic disease in the medical and public health spheres. We now go beyond treating disease once it occurs, by emphasizing disease prevention and addressing modifiable risk factors." In fact, large clinical studies have indeed demonstrated the benefits of robust management of modifiable risk factors on clinical outcomes of premature mortality [24–26].

In view of the galloping rate the CMDs are increasing worldwide, Millennium Development Goals (MDGs) and the commitments made on the NCDs at the United Nations General Assembly in 2011 and 2014, and in the 2030, 'Agenda for Sustainable Development', recommend NCD targets for halt in the rise of the twin epidemics of obesity and type-2 diabetes by 2025. Without any positive action, 1.9 million people worldwide will remain at risk from the poor health outcomes associated with overweight, obesity, and diabetes. Syndemic of cardiometabolic diseases is a complex topic, and we will not be able to cover all aspects of these lifestyle disorders. We will briefly discuss some salient findings, comment on global economic impact, and present our viewpoints about some cost-effective prevention strategies. As we have mentioned in the introduction, the future for prevention of individual high risk lies in targeting these individuals, promoting individual and family health, education, and motivation of health professionals in preventive practice, along with wider provision of preventive services.

Discussion

Childhood and Adolescent Obesity

More than one-third of adults and 17% of the youth in the United States are obese [27]. Weight and height were measured in 9120 participants as a part of the National

Health and Nutrition Examination Survey (NHANES). In children and adolescents aged 2–19 years, obesity was defined as a body mass index (BMI) at or above 95th percentile of the CDC growth charts. Obesity and childhood obesity in particular are the focus of many public health efforts worldwide. In the United States, new regulations have been implemented by the US Department of Agriculture for food packages, and the CDC has funded state- and community-level interventions [28]. There have been numerous reports, recommendations, and guidelines by the Institutes of Medicine, the US Surgeon General, and the White House. In spite of all these, the prevalence of childhood obesity in the United States is at an all-time high, with nearly one-third of all children and adolescents considered overweight [29]. The causes of weight problems in children may include busy families cooking less and eating out more, easy access to cheap, high-calorie fast food and junk food, bigger food portions both in restaurants and at home, kids consuming huge amounts of sugar in sweetened drinks, kids spending less time actively outside, more time watching TV, playing video games, junk food in schools, and elimination of physical education programs.

Gordon-Larsen and associates of the University of North Carolina, Population Center, examined obesity incidence in a nationally representative cohort of US teens, followed into their early 30s, using measured height, weight data, in individuals enrolled in Wave 11(1996;12-21 years), wave 111 (2001;17–26 years), and wave 1 V (2008-early release data) of the National Longitudinal Study of Adolescent Health. Authors concluded, "Obesity prevalence doubled from adolescence to the early 20s and doubled again from the early to late 20s or early 30s, with strong tracking from adolescence into adulthood. This trend is likely to continue owing to high rates of pediatric obesity [29]. Childhood obesity is a global problem, not just the problem in the United States. In England, UK, more than a third of children leave primary school overweight or obese. Being obese in childhood increases the chance of being obese as adult and doubles the risk of dying prematurely. Evidence suggests that the prevalence of childhood obesity is strongly correlated with socioeconomic status and is highest among children living in the most deprived areas [30]. As a part of the UK Government's childhood obesity plan, a national sugar reduction program has been launched to reduce 20% of calories from everyday foods over a 5-year period. Children and adolescents are more susceptible to food marketing than adults, which makes reducing children's exposure to obesogenic foods necessary to protect them from harm [9].

NCD Risk Factor Collaborators report (2016), "If post-2000 trends in the increase of these diseases continue, the probability of meeting the global obesity target is virtually zero. If these trends continue, by 2025, global obesity will reach 18% in men and surpass 22% in women; severe obesity will surpass 6% in men and 9% in women. Nonetheless, underweight remains in the world's poorest regions, especially in South Asia [10]." Is obesity the same "monster" we are discussing worldwide? Does it have the same clinical manifestation in all the obese individuals? The largest increase in men's mean BMI occurred in high-income English-speaking countries and in women in Central America. These increases were also more pronounced in Melanesia, Polynesia, and Micronesia. The NCD Risk Factor Collaborators defined obesity using body-mass index (BMI) in adults and

BMI-for-age in children and adolescents. Systematic reviews of a large amount of high-quality and consistent evidence show that the use of BMI to define obesity is highly specific but has low-to-moderate sensitivity [8]. As a result, BMI-based estimates of obesity prevalence are highly conservative for all ages and both sexes. South Asians have a very high incidence of type-2 diabetes and coronary artery disease, despite a low prevalence of obesity as defined by the BMI. Based on a collaborative study done at the Madras Diabetes Research Foundation (MDRF), Chennai, India, and the staff of the University of Minnesota, a hypothesis was developed to explain the increased burden of diabetes in this population. They hypothesized that increased risk might be due to high propensity to accumulate abdominal fat or visceral fat. Furthermore, this hypothesis was tested by comparing the characteristics between young adults of the NHANES (111) and to young adults of the Chennai Urban Rural Epidemiology Study (CURES). Compared to the US adults, the waist–weight ratio was significantly higher in men and women from Chennai, India, in spite of their lower BMI [31].

Prediabetes and Early-Onset Diabetes

Excess weight can greatly affect one's health in many ways, with type-2 diabetes (T2D) being one of the most serious implications. When an individual predisposed to diabetes has excess weight, the cells in the body become less sensitive to the insulin. There is some evidence that fat cells are more resistant to insulin than muscle cells. Prime examples include Barker's observations of fetal origin of adult disease (FOAD), the role of protein kinase C-epsilon in fat cell metabolism, and observations related to adiposity-related disorders [32–34]. Population-based data suggest that pediatric obesity is being followed by an increase in type-2 diabetes, particularly in adolescents and minority groups. Change in the BMI during and after adolescence is the most important predictive variable of adult obesity. Furthermore, oxidative stress, chronic inflammation, endothelial dysfunction, and subclinical atherosclerosis may be some of the pathophysiological mechanisms explaining the increased risk of atherosclerotic CVD and diabetes associated with obesity. Obesity has been spreading rapidly throughout the world. Following in its wake is type-2 diabetes, which will affect half a billion people worldwide by 2030 [35]. Swedish researchers, considering over 62,000 Danish individuals, have demonstrated that childhood overweight is associated with an increased risk for type-2 diabetes in adulthood [36].

According to recent report by the CDC, USA, 50% of the adults in the United States are prediabetic (84 million). Prediabetes is a high-risk state and prevalence of prediabetes is increasing worldwide in an alarming rate and will reach half a billion by 2030 [37]. For prediabetic individuals, lifestyle modification seems to be the cornerstone of diabetes prevention, with evidence of a 40–70% relative-risk reduction. In view of the fact both the genetic and environmental factors contribute to T2D progression, it has been proposed that Asian ethnicities have been unable to adapt to food and lifestyle related to Western diet pattern. This increased risk for T2D has been reported for both northern (Chinese) and southern (Indian) Asians [37]. The number of people with diabetes has risen from 108 million in 1980 to 422 million in 2014. The global prevalence of diabetes among young adults over 18 years of age has risen from 4.7% in 1980 to 8.5% in 2014. Diabetes prevalence has been rising more rapidly in middle- and low-income countries. The age of onset of type-2 diabetes is falling, not uncommon in those aged less than 30 years, including children, adolescents, and young adults, and has been reported with different ethnic and cultural backgrounds. Available evidence suggests that early-onset T2D is a more aggressive disease phenotype than later-onset cohort and develops CVD complications with more adverse CVD risk profile and relatively higher risk of myocardial infarction and death [38].

Metabolic diseases such as hypertension, overweight, obesity, diabetes, and vascular diseases have rapidly increased worldwide. In the last three decades, the number of people with obesity has increased two-fold and the number of people with diabetes by four-fold worldwide. Increase in the incidence of diabetes, particularly in the developing countries, has been greater; and more than 80% of the people with diabetes live in these resource poor countries [39]. The authors of this article bring about a very important component of this regional, ethnic problem: adverse intrauterine environment and epigenetic changes, which was the basis of now famous, 'Barker's Hypothesis' of fetal origin of adult diseases [32, 33]. They attribute recent increase in diabetes prevalence to changes in dietary pattern, sedentary behavior, and obesity superimposed on a background of genetic/epigenetic susceptibilities.

Cardiometabolic Diseases in Adolescents, Young Adults, and the Elderly

If one does an Internet search on metabolic disease, one gets lots of articles on metabolic syndrome. What we refer to in this article as metabolic diseases are hypertension, overweight, obesity, diabetes, and vascular complications, which promote heart attack and stroke [40–43]. On the other hand, if we have to consider the risks that promote the development of metabolic diseases, then we will have to pay attention to metabolic alterations that lead to oxidative stress, chronic inflammation, elevated levels of blood glucose and lipids, altered flow dynamics, endothelial dysfunction, hardening of the arteries, subclinical atherosclerosis, and various vascular dysfunctions. Although these risk factors have been associated with diabetes, hypertension, and cardiovascular disease, most of the clinical studies of such association have focused on adults 40 years or older. A prospective study, by CDC, of participants in the third NHANES (1988–1994), age 12–39 years at the time of survey monitored adiposity, glycated hemoglobin, cholesterol levels, blood pressure, and self-reported smoking. After adjusting for age, gender, and race/ethnicity, results showed that smokers were at 86% greater risk for early death; those with a waist-to-height ratio of >0.65 were at 139% greater risk, and those with HBA1c level <6.5% were at 281% greater risk than normal subjects [44].

Coronary artery disease has remained as the number one killer, followed by stroke, worldwide [45]. Having said that, it is important to understand that there exist regional, ethnic/racial, and age-related variations in various regions and countries of the world. Global burden of diseases group, in a recent report, discussed regional variations of the CVD among the US States [46, 47]. The authors of this seminal study found that it took 25 years for states with the largest burden of CVD to achieve levels observed among the healthiest states in 1990. States with the highest burden of CVD in 1990 were Kentucky, West Virginia, Alabama, Arkansas, Louisiana, Tennessee, and Oklahoma, while Mississippi still continues to lag as the state with the largest CVD burden. An important finding was that socioeconomic status did not fully explain the variation in CVD burden between the states. The lowest rate of CVD burden was in Minnesota, Colorado, and areas of New England and the Pacific Northwest, including Massachusetts, New Hampshire, Washington, Connecticut, Vermont, and Oregon. In the early 1990s, we initiated our studies in India to determine the causes of excess burden of diabetes and CAD in South Asians. We published our first book on this topic in 2001 [1]. In the introduction to this book, I wrote, "Studies done in Africa, New Zealand, Singapore, Malaysia, Fiji, United Kingdom, and the USA have revealed a high incidence of CAD in men and women of South Asian origin compared to other ethnic groups." Recent Scientific Statements by the prestigious American Heart Association confirms our earlier findings on excess burden of CVD in this ethnic population, calls for action as well as focuses on risk factors that affect this population, in order to develop clinical strategies, to reduce the CVD burden, and provides future directions to reduce or reverse CVD in this population [48, 49]. The all-age prevalence of most leading NCDs increased substantially in India from 1990–2016, but the age-standardized prevalence increased for diabetes, cerebrovascular disease, and ischemic heart disease [50–52]. The highest rates in 2015 were in Andhra Pradesh, Punjab, and Tamil Nadu. The mortality rate rose to more than double those of the United Kingdom or the United States [53]. When considered best health indicators, the State of Kerala was ranked very high. However, the burden of CVD deaths in this community now exceeds that of industrialized nations [54, 55].

Irrespective of the age, adolescents, young adults, and adults, by and large, seem to have a high risk for developing cardiometabolic diseases such as obesity, diabetes type-2, and vascular diseases. For instance, results from the NHANES, conducted by the National Center for Health Statistics indicates that an estimated 40% of adults aged 20 and over have obesity, including 7.6% with severe obesity. These surveys did not include persons over the age of 74. National Health Examination Survey (NHES) was conducted in the 1960s (NHES1-1960-62, NHES 11-1963-65, NHES111-1966-70) and included 7, 500 individuals. Beginning 1970, a new survey was initiated, with larger cohorts, National Health and Nutrition Examination Survey (NHANES: 1971–75, 1976–80, 1982–84, 1988–94, 1999-present). In a short overview like this, it is not possible to cover all aspects of the cardiometabolic diseases in the young adults and the elderly. We urge readers to refer to the reviews and original articles on this topic [9–11, 41–43, 56]. Older adults with diabetes are a large heterogenous population, who are at risk for adverse cardiovascular events [57]. On the other hand, if we look at all-cause mortality statistics in a state (Florida; 2017), where elderly individuals live, then cancer is the number one killer (23%), not CVD (17%).

Preventive Strategies for Cardiometabolic Diseases

Global economic burden of preventable diseases is huge. According to a summary report published in the Harvard Gazette [58], "eight million largely preventable deaths from various diseases costed 6 trillion dollars in lost economic welfare in low-and middle-income countries." Since metabolic diseases are lifestyle diseases, it is possible to stop, reduce, reverse, or prevent these diseases. Researchers at the University of Newcastle, UK, have demonstrated that just low-calorie diet alone will reverse diabetic conditions [59]. Halting obesity is possible and requires the willingness, cooperation, commitment of all the stakeholders and policy makers. Halting the twin epidemics of obesity and diabetes requires dynamic approach; effective interventions, development of healthy diets, recommendation of healthy lifestyles and encouragement of physical activity. At the population level, it requires commitment by multiple stakeholders and national-level interventions similar to Tobacco Initiatives. Encourage and recommend provision of healthy food in public institutions, initiate public campaigns and social marketing on healthy practices and physical activity. Reduce the content of free sugars and fat (Trans) in foods and beverages. Increase availability, affordability of healthy foods, including fruits and vegetables (Harvard Food Plate?). Restrict marketing of foods high in sugars, fat and salt to children and adolescents.

In a seminal study in 52 countries, representing every inhabited continent, Yusuf and associates from McMaster University, Canada, demonstrated the potential benefits of managing modifiable risk factors in reducing premature mortality [24]. Similar to the JAMA Network report, INTERHEART study showed that abnormal lipids, smoking, hypertension, diabetes, abdominal obesity, psychosocial factors, consumption of fruits, vegetables, alcohol, and regular physical activity account for most of the risk of myocardial infarction worldwide in both sexes at all ages and all regions [24]. The investigators from the Departments of Nutrition and Epidemiology, Harvard T. H. Chan School of Public Health, Boston, MA, defined the following five low-risk lifestyle factors as the modifiable risk factors for improving longevity: (1) never smoking; (2) body mass index of 18.5–24.9 kg/m^2; (3) 30 min/day of moderate-to-vigorous physical activity; (4) moderate alcohol intake (5–30 g/day for men and 5–15 g/day for women); (5) and a high-quality diet. Based on the data from 34 years follow-up, the authors concluded, "Adopting a healthy lifestyle could substantially reduce premature mortality and prolong life expectancy in the US adults. One of the major take home message from this seminal study is that prevention should be a top priority for national health policy, and preventive care should be an indispensable part of the US healthcare system [26, 60, 61].

It is of great interest that a collaborative study by prestigious US and international institutions such as the Center for Human Genetic Research and Cardiology Division, Mass. Gen. Hospital; Division of Preventive Medicine and others, concluded, "Across four studies involving 55,685 participants, lifestyle factors were independently associated with susceptibility to coronary artery disease" [26]. Among participants at high genetic risk, a favorable lifestyle was associated with nearly 50% lower relative risk of coronary disease than was an unfavorable lifestyle. These observations from large clinical studies and their conclusion fit very well with the observations of Professor Frank Hu, of Harvard TH Chan School of Public Health, indicating that a healthy diet pattern, moderate alcohol consumption, non-smoking status, a normal weight, and regular physical activity were each associated with a low risk of premature mortality. In spite of the fact that it has been fairly well established by large clinical studies, that robust management of modifiable risks or adherence to a low-risk lifestyle could prevent premature mortality and prolong life expectancy, these observations and recommendations seem to have not made any significant impact in stopping, reversing, reducing, or preventing cardiometabolic diseases worldwide.

It is important to understand that the majority of clinical studies, which have demonstrated the benefits of a healthy lifestyle, healthy diet, and exercise on the reduction of premature mortality, have not contributed to the reduction in the increase of metabolic diseases. In view of this observation, we need to concentrate on the primary prevention strategies both at the level of the individual and at the level of the populations. As we have noted earlier, there is still a great need for the development of interventions to prevent FOADs in the developing countries. If at all possible, we need to develop intervention for the prevention of metabolic risks at the early stages of life. Now that it is well established that childhood and adolescent overweight will continue to plague the adult life, we need to concentrate on interventions for overweight reduction and weight management. For instance, a recent study examined the role of leisure-time physical activity during adolescence (15–18 years), or early (19–29), middle (35–39), and later (40–61) adulthood and all-cause mortality [62]. This study with over 300,000 participants found that maintaining physical activity into later adulthood was associated with 29–36% lower risk for all-cause mortality.

Currently diagnostic tools are available for monitoring various metabolic risks. We are already using continuous glucose monitors of Abbott Diabetes Care and Dexcom G6 to monitor interstitial glucose and empower the patients to take care of their glycemic load (Fig. 4.1). Similarly, clinicians can use non-invasive risk assessment platforms developed by LD Technologies (www.ldteck.com) to monitor metabolic risks and cluster of risks (Fig. 4.2). Using such technologies will help them not only to identify the risks, but also to follow the benefits or otherwise of diet, lifestyle, and treatment interventions. Using the revised version of such platforms, which provide a composite of cardiometabolic risk score, autonomic nervous

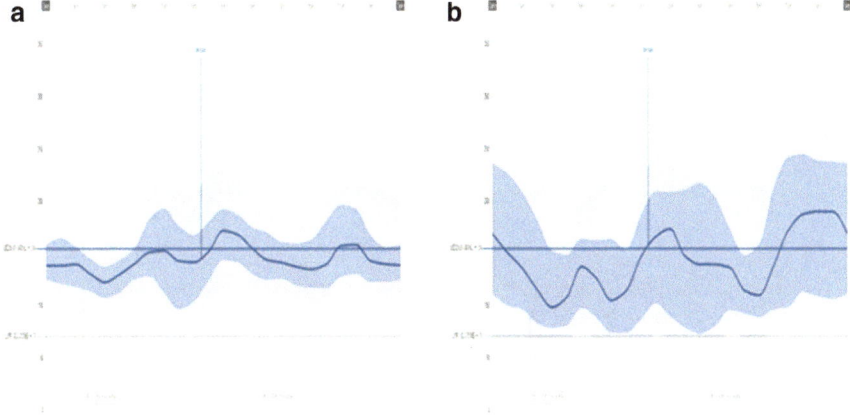

Fig. 4.1 Continuous glucose monitoring. (Courtesy: Abbott Diabetes Care)

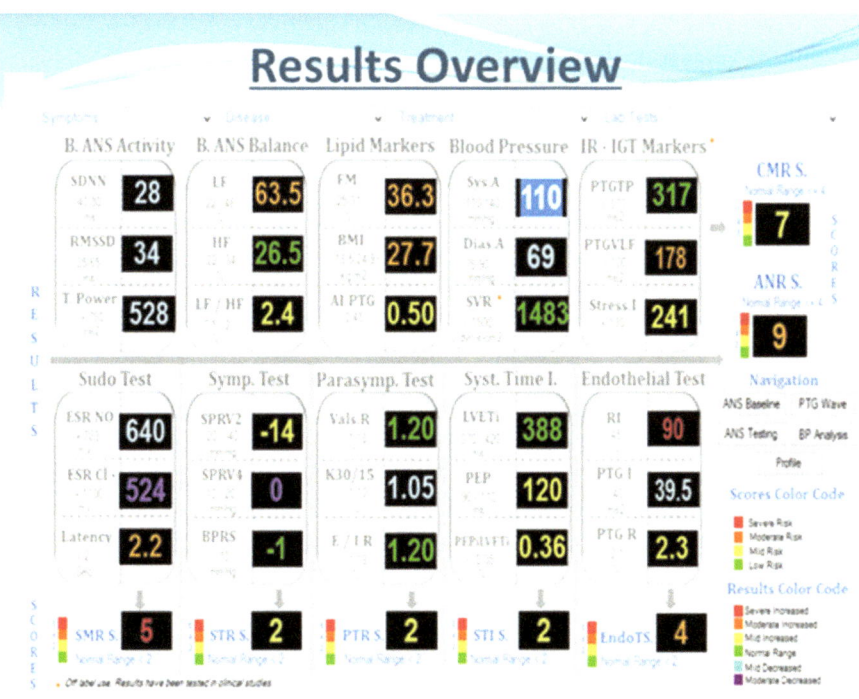

Fig. 4.2 Monitoring metabolic risks. (Courtesy: LD-Technologies)

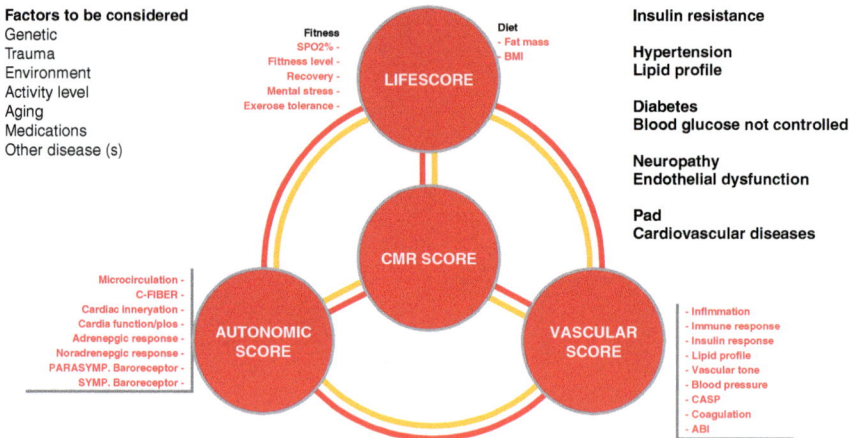

Fig. 4.3 Factors to be considered for stratification of physiological and metabolic fitness. (Courtesy: Dr Albert Maarek, LD-Technologies, Miami, Florida)

system risk score, and vascular risk score, one could develop a life score and state of wellness (Fig. 4.3). Having said that, all of these newly developed technologies need clinical validation [63–67].

Conclusions

Metabolic diseases, such as hypertension, overweight, obesity, diabetes, and vascular diseases, have rapidly increased to epidemic proportions worldwide. No country has stopped, reduced, or prevented the increase in the incidence of these diseases. Clinical studies have demonstrated the beneficial effects of healthy diet, healthy lifestyle, and exercise in preventing premature mortality in industrialized nations. Global economic burden of these preventable diseases is very high (several trillions of dollars). It is high time we call for collective action. If the increase in the incidence of these diseases is not checked, many of the developing nations, which share the greater economic burden, will face unprecedented economic disaster in the near future. Just writing reports, or signing agreements, or passing resolutions will not reduce the global burden of metabolic diseases. The recent GBD 2015 study estimates demonstrated that none of the 188 participating countries currently meets all of the UNs health-related sustainable development goals. At the level of the individual, creating awareness, early diagnosis of the risks, and robust management of identified risks will significantly reduce premature mortality. At the population level, it is the collective responsibility of the individuals and the various stakeholders to develop appropriate preventive strategies.

Primary prevention of cardiometabolic diseases through population-wide motivational strategies has been discussed by many research groups including National Institute of Stroke, New Zealand, Department of clinical sciences Lund University,

Center for Translational Research, National Heart, Lung, and Blood Institute, USA. According to these researchers, in 2007, there was a 'Head to Head' debate in the British Medical Journal [68] between researchers, who argued that screening individuals at high risk of CVD would be effective as well as cost-effective. They also argued that whole population approaches would be more cost-effective. On the other hand, the North Karelia project, an ongoing CVD prevention project for over three decades, has demonstrated a population-wide strategy for stroke/CVD prevention. We are of the opinion that for primary metabolic disease prevention, the emphasis should be to prevent at any level of the metabolic risk. Having said that, who is responsible for developing such a strategy? Global Health Partners should initiate moves to develop preventive strategies, similar to Tobacco Initiative or HIV/AIDS initiatives. We have been advocating an affordable healthcare program in India, which is population wide as well as individual approach integrated, at the primary care for CMD prevention. We also have advocated integration of emerging technologies to facilitate such integrated care (RIBURST study for prevention of Global Stroke is a fine example).

Worldwide, 23% of the adult population is insufficiently active, defined as not achieving at least 150 minutes of moderate or 75 minutes of high-intensity activity per week. A recent report by the CDC [69], states that only about 23% of US adults actually manage to work out during their leisure hours. The percentage of people who get enough exercise varies greatly by state, from a low of 13.5% of adults in Mississippi to a high of 32.5% in Colorado. Physical activity, healthy diet, and healthy lifestyle are simple cost-effective interventions. We need to find ways and means to encourage individuals of all age groups to follow these three prevention strategies. "No strenuous exercise, just being more active in daily life prolongs life," asserts a new study presented at the *EuroPrevnt 2019 by the European Society of Cardiology*. A study conducted on cardiorespiratory fitness, by Ekblom-Bak, included 316,137 adults aged 18–74 years, who had their first occupational health screening between 1995 and 2015 in Sweden. A "one size fits all" approach will not hold good in our approach for the early diagnosis, risk stratification, risk prediction, and the management of cardiometabolic diseases. While designing population-based prevention strategies, one should keep in mind the variations in the CMD disease burden as it relates to geographic, socioeconomic, and ethnic/racial differences. We mentioned early on that management of lifestyle disease should be the responsibility of individuals. Having said that, we need to create this knowledge of health science (Arogya-Jnana; Ayur-Jnana) in every individual, with an emphasis on healthy diet, healthy lifestyle, desire to live with life-time of fitness, and a supreme feeling of wellness.

References

1. Rao GHR, Kakkar VV. Coronary artery disease in south Asians: epidemiology, risk factors, and prevention. New Delhi: JP Medical Publishers; 2001.ISBN 81-7179-811-X.
2. NCD Risk Factor Collaboration (NCD-RisC). Worldwide trends in blood pressure from 1975 to 2015: a pooled analysis of 1479 population-based measurement studies with 19.1 million participants. Lancet. 2017;389:P37–55.

 3. Global Burden of Metabolic Risk Factors for Chronic Disease Collaboration. Cardiovascular disease, chronic kidney disease, and diabetes mortality burden of cardiometabolic risk factors from 1980 to 2010: a comparative risk assessment. Lancet Diabetes Endocrinol. 2014;2:634–47.
 4. NCD Risk Factor Collaboration. Worldwide trends in diabetes since 1980: a pooled analysis of 751 population-based studies with 4.4 million participants. Lancet. 2016;387:1513–30.
 5. Kearnery PM, Whelton M, Reynolds K, et al. Global burden of hypertension: analysis of worldwide data. Lancet. 2005;365:217–23.
 6. Evans A, Tolonen H, Hense HW, et al. Trends in coronary artery disease risk factors in the WHO MONICA project. Int J Epidemiol. 2001;30:S35–40.
 7. Juonala M, Vikari JS, Hurti-Kahonen B, et al. The 21-year follow up of the cardiovascular risk in young Finns Study: risk factor levels, secular trends and east-west difference. J Intern Med. 2004;255:457–68.
 8. Reilly JJ, El-Hamdouchi A, Diouf A, et al. Determining the worldwide prevalence of obesity. Lancet. 2018;391:1773–4.
 9. NCD Risk Factor Collaboration (NCD-RisC). Worldwide trends in body mass-index, underweight, overweight, and obesity from 1975 to 2016: a pooled analysis of 2416 population-based measurement studies in 128.9 million children, adolescents, and adults. Lancet. 2017;390:2627–42.
10. NCD Risk Factor Collaboration (NCD-RisC). Trends in adult body-mass index in 200 countries from 1975 to 2014: a pooled analysis of 1968 population-based measurement studies with 19.2 million participants. Lancet. 2016;387:1377–96.
11. The Global Burden of Metabolic Risk Factors for Chronic Diseases Collaboration (BMI Mediate Effects). Metabolic mediators of the effects of body-mass index, overweight, and obesity on coronary artery disease and stroke: a pooled analysis of 97 prospective cohorts with 1.8 million participants. Lancet. 2014;383:970–83.
12. WHO. Global action plan for the prevention and control of non-communicable diseases 2013-2020? Geneva: World Health Organization; 2013.
13. Kontis V, Mathers CD, Rehm J, et al. Contribution of six risk factors to achieving the 25 x25 non-communicable disease mortality reduction target: a modeling study. Lancet. 2014;384:427–37.
14. Ng M, Fleming T, Robinson M, et al. Global, regional and national prevalence of overweight and obesity in children and adults during 1980–2013: a systematic analysis for the Global Burden of Disease Study 2013. Lancet. 2014;384:766–81.
15. NCD Risk Factor Collaboration (NCD-RisC). Worldwide trends in diabetes since 1980: a pooled analysis of 751 population-based studies with 4.4 million participants. Lancet. 2016;387:P1513–30.
16. Seuring T, Archangelidi O, Suhrcke M. The economic costs of type-2 diabetes: a global systematic review. PharmacoEconomics. 2015;33:811–31.
17. Danaei G, Finucane MM, Lu Y, et al. National, regional, and global trends in fasting glucose and diabetes prevalence since 1980: systematic analysis of health examination surveys and epidemiological studies with 370 country-years and 2.7 million participants. Lancet. 2011;378:31–40.
18. Beagley J, Guariguata L, Weil C, et al. Global estimates of undiagnosed diabetes in adults. Diabetes Res Clin Pract. 2014;103:150–60.
19. Gakidou E, Mallinger L, Abott-Klafter J, et al. Management of diabetes and associated cardiovascular risk factors in seven countries: a comparison of data from national health surveys. Bull World Health Organ. 2011;89:172–83.
20. Shen X, Vaidya A, Wu S, et al. The diabetes epidemic in China: an integrated review of national surveys. Endocr Pract. 2016;22(9):1119–29. https://doi.org/10.4158/EP161199.RA.
21. Keys A, Aravanis C, Blackburn H, et al. Seven countries. A multivariate analysis of death and coronary artery disease. Cambridge: Harvard University Press; 1980.
22. Puska P. Successful prevention of non-communicable diseases: 25 year experiences with North Karelia Project in Finland. Public Health Med. 2002;4(1):5–7.

23. Framingham Heart Study. Reduction of mortality rate in coronary artery atherosclerosis by a low cholesterol Low-fat diet. Am Heart J. 1951;42:538–45.
24. Yusuf S, Hawken S, Ounpuu S, et al. Effect of modifiable risk factors associated with myocardial infraction in 52 countries (the INTEHEART study): case-control study. Lancet. 2004;364(9438):937–52.
25. Di Cesare M, Bennet JE, Best N, et al. The contributions of risk factors trends to cardiometabolic mortality decline in 26 industrialized countries. Int J Epidemiol. 2013;42:838–48.
26. Khera AV, Emdin CA, Drake I, et al. Genetic risk, adherence to a healthy lifestyle, and coronary artery disease. N Engl J Med. 2016;375:2349–58.
27. Ogden CL, Carroll MD, Kit BK, et al. Prevalence of childhood and adult obesity in the United States. JAMA. 2014;311(8):806–14.
28. Kahn LK, Sobush K, Keener D, et al. Center for Disease Control and Prevention. Recommended community strategies and measurements to prevent obesity in the United States. MMWR Recomm Rep. 2009;58(RR-7):1–26.
29. Datar A, Nicosia N. Junk food in schools and childhood obesity. J Policy Anal Manage. 2012;31(2):312–37. PMID 23729952.
30. Perkins C, DeSouza E. Trends in childhood height and weight, and socioeconomic equalities. Lancet. 2018;3(4):PE160–1.
31. Bajaj HS, Pereira MA, Mohan RA, et al. Comparison of relative waist circumference between Asian Indian and US adults. J Obes. 2014;2014:461956.
32. Dover GJ. The barker hypothesis: how pediatricians will diagnose and prevent common adult-onset diseases. Trans Am Clin Climatol Assoc. 2009;120:199–207.
33. Yajnik CS, Fall CH, Coyaji KJ, et al. Neonatal anthropometry: the thin-fat Indian baby. The Pune Maternal Nutrition Study. Int J Obes Relat Metab Disord. 2003;27(2):173–80.
34. Brandon AE, Liao BM, Diakanastasis B, et al. Protein Kinase C epsilon in adipose tissue, but not liver improves glucose tolerance. Cell Metab. 2019;29:183. https://doi.org/10.1016/j.cmet.2018.09.013.
35. Bjerregaard LG, Jensen BW, Angquist L, et al. Change in overweight from childhood to early adulthood and risk for type-diabetes. N Engl J Med. 2018;378:1302–12.
36. Tabak AG, Herder C, Ratmann W, et al. Prediabetes: a high-risk state for diabetes development. Lancet. 2012;379:2279–90.
37. Yip WCY, Sequeira IR, Plank LD, et al. Prevalence of prediabetes across ethnicities: a review of impaired fasting glucose (IFG) and Impaired Glucose tolerance (IGT) for classification of Dysglycemia. Nutrients. 2017;9:1273.
38. Song SH, Hardisty CA. Early-onset type-diabetes mellitus: an increasing phenomenon of elevated cardiovascular risk. Expert Rev Cardiovasc Ther. 2014;6(3):315–22.
39. Nanditha A, Ma RCW, Ramachandran A, et al. Diabetes in Asia and Pacific: implications for the global epidemic. Diabetes Care. 2016;39(3):472–85.
40. Rao GHR. Handbook of coronary artery disease. New Delhi: Nature/Springer Healthcare; 2017. ISBN 978-93-80780-96-2.
41. Rao GHR. Prevention or reversal of cardiometabolic diseases. J Clin Prevent Cardiol. 2018;7(1):22–8.
42. Rao GHR. Cardiometabolic disease: a global perspective. J Cardiol Cardiovasc Ther. 2018;12:JOCCT.MSID.555834.
43. Rao GHR. Cardiometabolic risk in India. J Clin Prevent Cardiol. 2019;8:25–33.
44. Saydah S, Bullard KM, Imperatore G, et al. Cardiometabolic risk factors among US adolescents and young adults and risk of early mortality. Pediatrics. 2013;131(3):e679–86.
45. Rao GHR. The tsunami of cardiometabolic diseases: an overview. J Diabetes Obes Metab Syndr. 2019;1(1):01–9.
46. Global Burden of Cardiovascualr Disease Collaboration. The burden of cardiovascular disease among US States, 1990-2016. JAMA. 2018;3:375. https://doi.org/10.1001/jamacardio.2018.0385.
47. GBD 2016 Causes of Death Collaborators. Global, regional, and national age-sex specific mortality for 264 causes of death, 1980–2016: a systematic analysis for the Global Burden of Disease Study 2016. Lancet. 2017;390(10100):1151–210.

48. Volgman AS, Palaniappan LS, Aggarwal NT, et al. Atherosclerotic cardiovascular disease in South Asians: epidemiology, risk factors, and treatments: as Scientific statement of the American Heart Association. Circulation. 2018;138:e1–e34.
49. Palaniappan LP, Araneta MRG, Assimes TL, et al. Call to action: cardiovascular disease in South Asians. A science advisory from the American Heart Association. Circulation. 2010;122(12):1242–52.
50. Prabhakaran D, Jeemon P, Roy A. The global burden of disease study: cardiovascular disease in India: current epidemiology and future directions. Circulation. 2016;133:1605–20.
51. India State-level Disease Burden Initiative Collaborators. Nations within a nation: variations in epidemiological transition across the states of India, 1990-2016 in the Global Burden of Disease Study. Lancet. 2017;390:2437–60.
52. India State-level Disease Burden Initiative CVD Collaborators. The changing patterns of cardiovascular disease and their risk factors in the states of India: the Global Burden of Disease Study 1990-2016. Lancet. 2018;6:PE1339–51. https://doi.org/10.1016/S2214-109X(18)30407-8.
53. Prabhakaran D, Jeemon P, Roy A. Cardiovascular disease in India: current epidemiology and future directions. Circulation. 2016;133:1605–20.
54. Ke C, Gupta R, Xavier D, et al. Divergent trends in ischemic heart disease and stroke mortality in India from 2005 to 2015: a nationally representative mortality study. Lancet. 2018;6(8):PE914–23.
55. Soman CR, Kutty VR, Safraj S, et al. All-cause mortality in Kerala state of India results from a 5-year follow-up of 161, 942 rural community dwellings. Asia Pac J Public Health. 2011;23:896–903.
56. Norheim OF, Jha P, Admasu K, et al. Avoiding 40% of the premature deaths in each country, 2010-2030: review of national mortality trends to help quantify the UN Sustainable Development Goal for health. Lancet. 2015;385:239–52.
57. Wilcox T, Blaum C, Newman JD. Diabetes management in older adults with cardiovascular disease. Am Coll Cardiol Expert Analysis 2018. https://www.acc.org/latest-in-cardiology/articles/2018/02/28/12/19/diabetes-management-in-older-adults-with-cvd.
58. Harvard Medical School. Preventable deaths from lack of high-quality medical care cost trillions. ScienceDaily. 4 June 2018. www.sciencedaily.com/releases/2018/06/180604160447.htm.
59. Taylor R. Type-2 diabetes: etiology and reversibility. Diabetes Care. 2013;36(4):1047–55.
60. Li Y, Pan A, Wang DD, et al. Impact of healthy lifestyle factors on life expectancies in the US population. Circulation. 2018;138:345–55. https://doi.org/10.1161/CIRCULATIONAHA.117.032047.
61. Brett AS, Arnett DK, et al. Primary prevention of cardiovascular disease: new guideline. Am Coll Cardiol/Am Heart Assoc. NEJM JW Gen Med Feb 1 2019 (e-pub).
62. Saint-Maurice PF, Coughlan D, Kelly SP. Association of leisure-time physical activity across adult life course with all-cause and cause-specific mortality. JAMA. 2019;2(3):e190355. https://doi.org/10.1001/jamanetworkopen.2019.0355.
63. Rao GHR. Integration of novel emerging technologies for the management of type-2 diabetes. Arch Diabetes Obes. 2018;1(1):ADO.MS.ID.000102. https://doi.org/10.3274/ADO.2018.
64. Rao GHR. Integrative approaches to the management of cardiometabolic diseases. J Cardiol Cardiovasc Sci. 2018;2(3):37–42.
65. Rao GHR. Integration of emerging technologies: cardiometabolic diseases. Indian J Cardio Biol Clin Sci. 2018;5(1):111.
66. Rao GHR. Novel approaches for the management of cardiometabolic risks. Int J Diabetes Endocrinol. 2019;1(1):102.
67. Rao GHR. Global syndemic of metabolic diseases. Editorial. Acta Sci Nutr Health. 2019;33:53–7.
68. Jackson R, Wells S, Rodgers A. Will screening individuals at high risk of cardiovascular events deliver large benefits? Yes. BMJ. 2008;337:a1371. Published 28 Aug 2008. https://doi.org/10.1136/bmj.a1371.
69. Blackwell DL, Clarke TC. State variation in meeting the 2008 Federal Guidelines for both aerobic and muscle-strengthening activities through leisure-time physical activity among adults aged 18-64: United States, 2010-2015. National Health Statistics Reports Number 112, June 28, 2018.

Chapter 5
Male Infertility

Akash A. Kapadia and Thomas J. Walsh

Introduction

Infertility affects nearly 15% of couples worldwide and is defined as failure to conceive a natural pregnancy after 1 year of regular unprotected intercourse [1]. Despite gender biases in evaluation, 20% of infertile couples are found to have male factor as the sole cause, while another 30% of couples will be infertile in part due to male factor, resulting in approximately equal contribution of both genders to the cause [2]. Semen analysis is the most widely accepted screening tool to evaluate for male factor infertility. If abnormalities are identified, formal evaluation by a urologist is paramount.

It must also be emphasized that while some causes of male infertility may be treated with medical or surgical therapy, other causes may be diagnosed but may not be amenable to treatment. Finally, in some instances, the *idiopathic* causes of male infertility may neither be identified nor treated. In difficult cases, the expertise of a reproductive urologist should be recruited in guiding couples in the right direction toward parenthood.

This chapter will outline the reproductive anatomy and physiology that play a critical role in defining pathology. Furthermore, the chapter will guide a complete evaluation of the male, outlining causes of male fertility. Additional testing will be highlighted along the way. Finally, both medical and surgical treatments will be discussed specific to the pathology.

A. A. Kapadia (✉)
University of Washington, Department of Urology, Seattle, WA, USA
e-mail: kapadiaa@uw.edu

T. J. Walsh
University of Washington, Seattle, WA, USA

© Springer Nature Switzerland AG 2021
J. P. Alukal et al. (eds.), *Design and Implementation of the Modern Men's Health Center*, https://doi.org/10.1007/978-3-030-54482-9_5

Reproductive Anatomy and Physiology

In order to adequately evaluate men for infertility, one must understand the functioning of the hypothalamic-pituitary-gonadal (HPG) axis. The HPG axis is critical in the development and maturation of the phenotypic male and plays a pivotal role in the endocrine (testosterone production) and exocrine (sperm production) functions of the testes.

Anatomy of the Hypothalamic-Pituitary-Gonadal Axis (Fig. 5.1)

Hypothalamus

As the name suggests, the hypothalamus is located below the thalamus and is also in close proximity to the pituitary gland. It is linked to the anterior pituitary gland via both a portal vascular system and neuronal pathways. It is directly responsible for secretion of gonadotropin-releasing hormone (GnRH), a 10-amino acid peptide with a half-life of approximately 5–7 minutes. GnRH results in cyclical secretion of both follicle-stimulating hormone (FSH) and luteinizing hormone (LH) from the anterior pituitary gland, after which it is almost entirely removed from circulation on the first pass.

GnRH secretion is highly sensitive to a variety of factors including stress, exercise, diet, hormones, and medications. Modulators of GnRH secretions are outlined below (Table 5.1). Pulsatile release of GnRH occurs every 60–120 minutes, but its release can vary temporally as well as seasonally. The role of GnRH agonists (e.g., leuprolide acetate) in disrupting pulsatile GnRH release as a means of androgen deprivation (suppression of testosterone production) is well understood.

Anterior Pituitary

The pituitary gland is a pea-sized structure composed of anterior and posterior halves and located in the sella turcica of the skull. The anterior pituitary gland secretes a series of peptide hormones, including the gonadotropins. Pulsatile release of GnRH from the hypothalamus stimulates both production and release of LH and FSH by a calcium flux-dependent mechanism. The sensitivity of the pituitary gonadotrophs for GnRH can vary with the patient's age and hormonal status.

LH and FSH are known to function solely in the gonads and are the main pituitary hormones that regulate testis function. Both are glycoproteins composed of alpha and beta polypeptide subunits, coded by separate genes. The alpha subunits are identical in both hormones and share high fidelity to all other pituitary hormones. The beta subunits confer the hormones their unique immunologic and biologic identities. LH secretion is pulsatile and varies from 8 to 16 pulses per day. The

Fig. 5.1 Major components of the HPG axis and recognized hormone feedback pathways. GnRH gonadotropin-releasing hormone, PRL prolactin, T testosterone, FSH follicle-stimulating hormone, LH luteinizing hormone, + positive feedback, − negative feedback. (Turek [3])

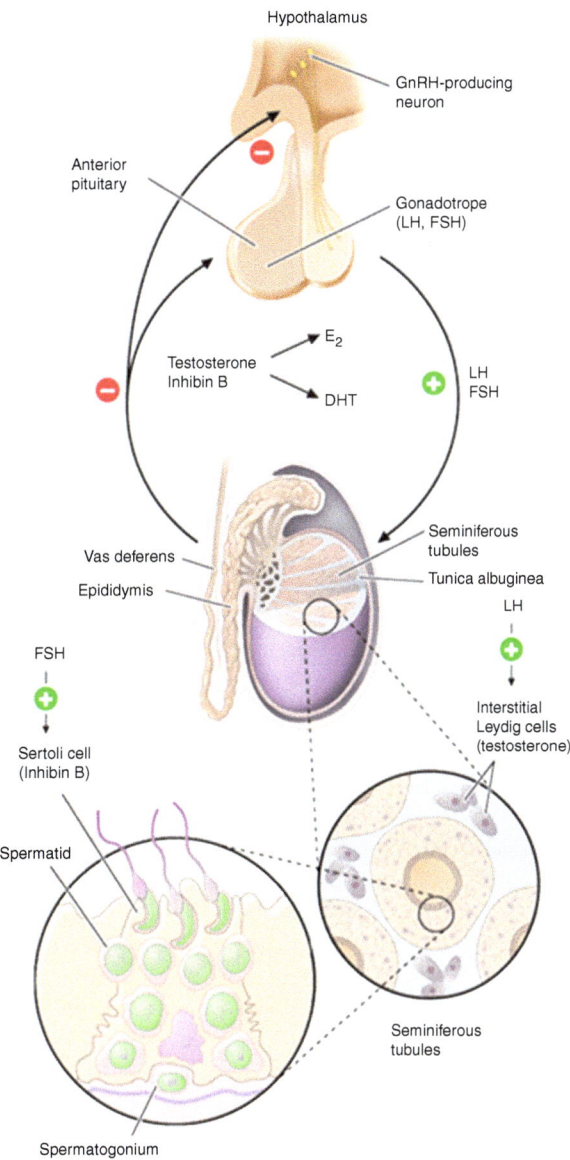

Table 5.1 GnRH modulators

GnRH modulator	Type of feedback	Examples
Prostaglandins	Positive/stimulatory	PGE2
Peptide hormones	Negative/inhibitory	FSH, LH
Sex steroids	Negative/inhibitory	Testosterone
Catecholamines	Variable	Dopamine

PGE2 prostaglandin E2

pulse patterns reflect GnRH release and are regulated by androgens and estrogens through negative feedback. FSH secretion is also pulsatile, occurring every 1.5 hours. Both hormones also demonstrate a degree of amplitude variation reflected by GnRH secretion, though the responsiveness of FSH to GnRH is not as well measured due to its longer serum half-life and its smaller amplitude response. Additionally, FSH is also influenced by gonadal proteins inhibin and activin independent of GnRH secretion.

Both LH and FSH act by way of increasing intracellular cyclic adenosine monophosphate (cAMP). LH induces steroidogenesis within Leydig cells by conversion of cholesterol to pregnenolone and testosterone within the mitochondria. FSH acts upon Sertoli cells and spermatogonial membranes. In the developing male, it induces seminiferous tubule growth, and in adults it maintains normal spermatogenesis.

Another anterior pituitary hormone, prolactin, can also impact fertility due to its influence on the HPG axis. In the pregnant female, prolactin (a large globular protein) facilitates milk production and lactation; however, its role in men is poorly understood. It is theorized to increase the concentration of LH receptors on Leydig cells, thereby sustaining high intratesticular testosterone levels. Normal prolactin levels may be critical in maintaining libido, though elevated prolactin levels interfere with pulsatile GnRH release. Marked elevation of prolactin levels during workup of the male may be a sign of pituitary microadenoma (prolactinoma) and should be further evaluated.

Testis

The testis is comprised of two compartments: seminiferous tubules and interstitium. The seminiferous tubules, which make up approximately 80% of testicular volume, produce spermatozoa with the aid of Sertoli cells. The interstitium, primarily composed of Leydig cells, is the site of steroidogenesis. Together, the two compartments control the endocrine and exocrine function of the testis. Not surprisingly, testicular atrophy or hypotrophy is known to correlate with semen parameters.

Endocrine Testis

In the normal male, 5 g of testosterone is produced per day and secreted in an irregular pulsatile fashion. It is metabolized into dihydrotestosterone (DHT) via 5-alpha reductase and into estradiol via aromatases in target tissues. DHT is a more potent androgen than testosterone, and conversion of testosterone to DHT is required for androgen action in many target tissues. While aromatase is present in many tissues, adipocytes play an important role in the aromatization of testosterone to estradiol. Estradiol is an important regulator of the HPG axis via negative feedback. As such, testosterone itself indirectly regulates its own production.

Only 2% of testosterone circulates as "free testosterone," which is considered the biologically active fraction. The remaining circulating testosterone is either tightly bound to sex hormone-binding globulin (SHBG) or loosely bound to albumin. Many conditions can alter circulating SHBG levels, thereby altering the amount of free or bioavailable testosterone levels, for example, chronic corticosteroid use, diabetes, and obesity lead to decreased production of SHBG and therefore a decrease in total testosterone in spite of a normal free fraction. Conversely, conditions such as cirrhosis of the liver and hypothyroidism as well as aging lead to increased SHBG production and therefore an elevation of total testosterone level.

Exocrine Testis

Sertoli cells, in response to FSH, produce a number of proteins essential for seminiferous tubule growth during development and spermatogenesis during adulthood. These proteins include androgen-binding protein, transferrin, ceruloplasmin, lactate, clusterin, prostaglandins, plasminogen activator, and other growth factors. FSH stimulates the testis to produce the hormone inhibin, which provides inhibitory feedback at the pituitary and hypothalamus. By contrast, activin, another hormone produced by the testis, leads to stimulatory effect on FSH secretion.

Spermatogenesis (Fig. 5.2)

Spermatogenesis is a specialized process of multipotent stem cell regeneration (mitosis), differentiation into haploid spermatids (meiosis), and spermiogenesis, resulting in transformation of spermatids to mature spermatozoa. This process occurs exclusively within the seminiferous tubules of the testis and involves a complex interaction between Sertoli cells and germ cells.

Sertoli Cells

The seminiferous tubules are lined with Sertoli cells, which are linked to each other via tight junctions. These junctional complexes separate the basement membrane from the adluminal compartment and form the blood-testis barrier. As such, spermatogenesis occurs unperturbed in an immunologically privileged site. Immunologic sanctuary is a critical feature of spermatogenesis as immune recognition develops within the first year of life, while spermatozoa are not produced until a male reaches puberty. Therefore, disruption of the blood-testis barrier due to postpubertal testicular insult can be an important cause of infertility to consider from development of antisperm antibodies.

Sequential stages in human spermatogenesis

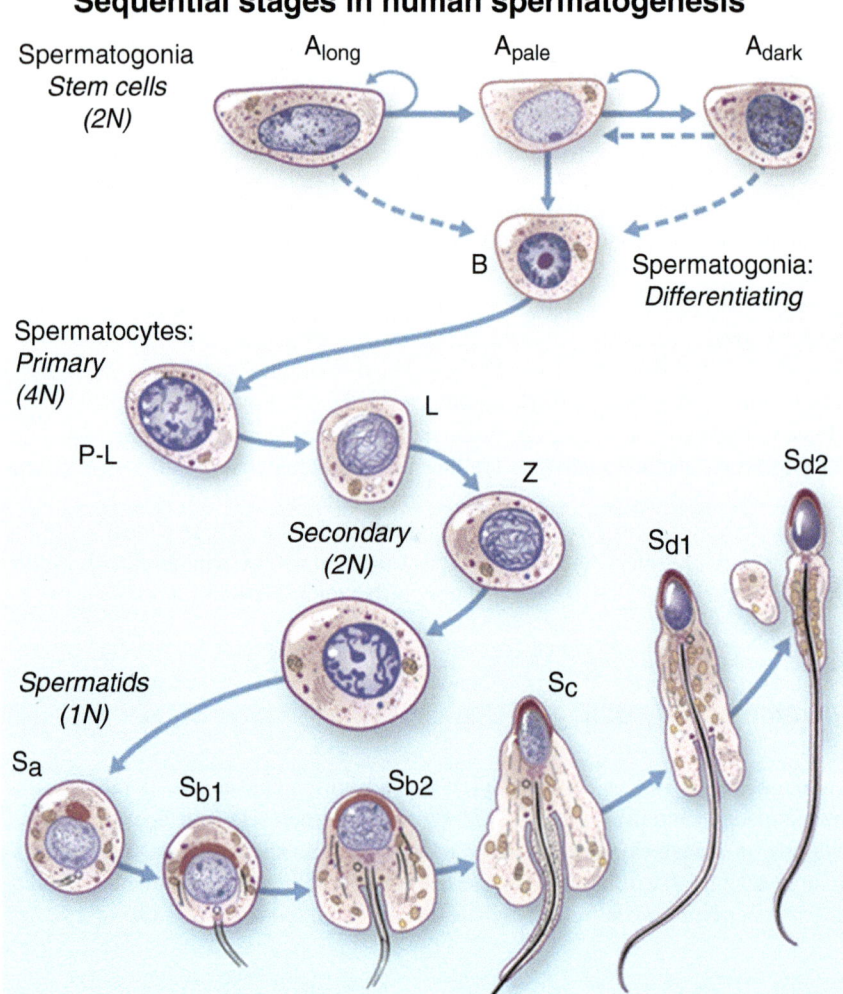

Fig. 5.2 Representation of the tree-shaped Sertoli cell with a thickened central portion, or "trunk," and more delicate processes, or "limbs". (Russell [4])

Germ Cells

Germ cells, or spermatogonia, line the basement membrane of the seminiferous tubules, which are arranged in a highly ordered, structural fashion. Spermatogenesis occurs in the direction of the luminal compartment in the following order: spermatogonia → primary spermatocytes → secondary spermatocytes → spermatids → spermatozoa. In total, 13 stages of germ cell differentiation have been identified in humans with the latter stages of germ cell development occurring within the luminal compartment. Germ cells are staged in order of development based on their histologic morphology: dark type A (Ad) spermatogonia; pale type A (Ap) spermatogonia; type B spermatogonia; preleptotene, leptotene, zygotene, and pachytene primary spermatocytes; secondary spermatocytes; and Sa, Sb, Sc, Sd1, and Sd2 spermatids.

Stages of Spermatogenesis

Spermatogenesis is a continuous process of division of spermatogonial stem cells into elongated spermatids. As such, the germinal epithelium is abundant with spermatogonia at different stages of spermatogenesis taking approximately 60–80 days for an individual cycle. Starting from puberty, a unique process of rapid and organized cell division ensues, resulting in large quantities—up to 300 sperm per gram of testis tissue per second. Type B spermatogonia undergo mitosis to produce diploid primary spermatocytes (2n), which then duplicate their DNA during interphase. After the first meiotic division, each daughter cell contains a single partner of the homologous chromosome pair and is termed a secondary spermatocyte (2n). During the second meiotic division, the chromatids separate at the centromere, yielding haploid spermatids (n).

Spermiogenesis

Spermiogenesis signifies the development of elongated spermatozoa from immature spermatids (n). This process occurs in the basilar compartment of the seminiferous tubules and requires several weeks. It entails an elaborate process of (1) development of the acrosome, (2) formation of the flagellum, (3) organization of the mitochondria around the midpiece, (4) compaction of nuclear material, and (5) elimination of residual cytoplasm. At completion, the mature spermatozoa have remarkably little cytoplasm.

Maturation

It is worth emphasizing that testicular spermatozoa have limited to no motility and, hence, lack the capability of naturally fertilizing an egg. They undergo maturation and gain motility only after traversing the epididymis. The steps of spermatozoa maturation that take place within the epididymis include alterations in cell membrane polarity, membrane protein composition, immunoreactivity, phospholipid and fatty acid content, and adenylate cyclase activity. This process of maturation takes approximately 10–15 days, as sperm travels through the length of the epididymis.

Fertilization

Ovulation takes place in the middle of the female menstrual cycle and can be predicted by changes in body temperature or cervical mucus, by luteinizing hormone surge, or simply by timing. Favorable cervical mucus changes facilitate entry of sperm into the uterus and protect the integrity of sperm against the inherently acidic vaginal environment. Once sperm enters the reproductive tract, they undergo physiologic changes termed *capacitation*. Fertilization normally takes place in the ampulla of the fallopian tubes. Once contact is made with an egg, sperm undergo *hyperactivation*, resulting in profound changes in motility (prominent lashing motions of the sperm tail). The acrosome then releases lytic enzymes that allow penetration of the outer surface of the egg. The acrosomal reaction results in ligand-receptor-mediated contact between the surfaces of the sperm and the egg. Once a single sperm enters the zona pellucida of the ovum, further penetration by additional sperm is disallowed. The egg then resumes meiosis and undergoes metaphase II. The sperm centriole, located in the midpiece, is critical in the formation of the metaphase spindle and ongoing embryogenesis [5–14].

Evaluation of the Male

The goal of an infertility evaluation is to (1) identify and rectify reversible causes of male infertility such that a couple can conceive naturally or with minimal technological assistance, (2) identify irreversible conditions that allow use of assisted reproductive technology (ART) using the male partner's sperm, (3) distinguish irreversible conditions in which the male partner's sperm may be either absent or unobtainable, (4) diagnose medical conditions that may require further workup and treatment, and (5) identify specific genetic conditions that may be transmitted to and impact the offspring. It must be emphasized that both partners should undergo evaluation in parallel due to equal contribution of both males and females in 50% of cases. A complete urologic evaluation of the male includes history, physical exam, and laboratory testing. It may also include adjunctive testing, imaging studies, and diagnostic procedures.

History

A comprehensive medical, surgical, sexual, and reproductive history is the first step to the evaluation of a male. Specific components of the evaluation include (1) childhood and adolescent conditions or illnesses; (2) sexual health and coital practices as well as duration of infertility; (3) prior paternity or treatments for infertility; (4) current or prior medical illnesses and medications; (5) prior surgeries or treatments;

(6) exposures to gonadal toxins such as radiation, chemotherapy, heat, chemical solvents, and pesticides; and (7) environmental toxins such as tobacco, marijuana, alcohol, and recreational drugs.

A common question that arises during discussion of sexual history is how a couple should time intercourse in order to achieve a pregnancy. In general, semen parameters are optimal after 1–2 days of abstinence, and therefore a frequency of intercourse every 1–2 days is ideal, although intercourse every day around the time of female ovulation is still considered the best strategy for increasing the probability of a pregnancy. The use of products during intercourse should also be addressed, as water-based lubricants like K-Y Jelly, skin lotions, and saliva can reduce sperm motility. Alternative lubricants include egg whites or vegetable, peanut, or safflower oils.

A general medical history should also include recent illnesses or acute infections, as spermatogenesis can be transiently impacted. As spermatogenesis takes at least 60 days, the impact of such illnesses may not be evident for 2 months. Surgeries of the bladder, pelvis, and retroperitoneum may lead to ejaculatory dysfunction from damage to the bladder neck and sympathetic or pelvic nerve plexus. Surgeries of the pelvis (hernia) or scrotum can cause damage or obstruction of the vas deferens.

Many childhood diseases can lead to chronic and permanent infertility. Postpubertal viral (mumps) orchitis can affect unilateral (30%) and bilateral (10%) testes. Pressure necrosis from severe tissue edema can lead to testis atrophy. Cryptorchidism is a well-known cause of subfertility, resulting in abnormal sperm counts in 30% of men with unilateral and 50% of men with bilateral disease.

Medications, both prescription and over the counter, can severely impact semen parameters. Pesticides have also been shown to decrease sperm counts by altering the normal testosterone/estrogen homeostasis. Ionizing radiation can result in decreased sperm production with as little as 10 cGy with more permanent damage resulting from higher doses. Several medications listed in Table 5.2 as well as social and recreational drugs such as tobacco and marijuana are implicated in aberrant spermatogenesis.

Physical Examination

The goal of a complete examination in the male is to identify any general health conditions that may contribute to infertility. A general overview should assess body habitus and signs of virilization, as decreased body hair or gynecomastia may be a sign of androgen deficiency (e.g., Klinefelter syndrome) or estrogen excess.

A thorough scrotal exam should be performed with the patient standing. The contents should be evaluated carefully and efficiently to avoid undue discomfort in young men. Examination of the testes includes assessment of size, consistency, asymmetry, and any associated anomalies. Size may be assessed by measuring along the long and wide axis; alternatively, volume may be assessed with the use of an orchidometer (Fig. 5.3). Mean testis length and width in normal men has been

Table 5.2 Components of history

Development history
Cryptorchidism
Hypospadias or other genitourinary congenital abnormalities
Childhood malignancies and treatments
Mumps orchitis
Pubertal development

Medical history
Recent fevers or illnesses
Chronic conditions—diabetes, hypertension, coronary disease, cancer
Genetic conditions—cystic fibrosis, Klinefelter syndrome (family history)

Surgical history
Orchidopexy or orchiectomy
Herniorrhaphy
Pelvic, perineal, or scrotal trauma
Pelvic, bladder, retroperitoneal surgery
Transurethral surgeries (TURP)

Sexual history
Timing and frequency of intercourse
Libido
Erections and ejaculation
Use of lubricants

Fertility history
Duration of infertility
Previous fertility treatments
Previous pregnancies (both partners)
Female evaluation

Medications	
SSRIs	Testosterone
Antipsychotics	DHEA
Imipramine	5-alpha reductase inhibitors
Amitriptyline	Alpha blockers
Nitrofurantoin	Opioids
Cimetidine	Sulfasalazine
Spironolactone	

Social history
Alcohol
Tobacco or marijuana
Cocaine
Anabolic steroids
Chronic heat exposure (hot tubs/saunas)

Occupational history
Ionizing radiation
Aniline dyes
Pesticides
Heavy metals (lead)

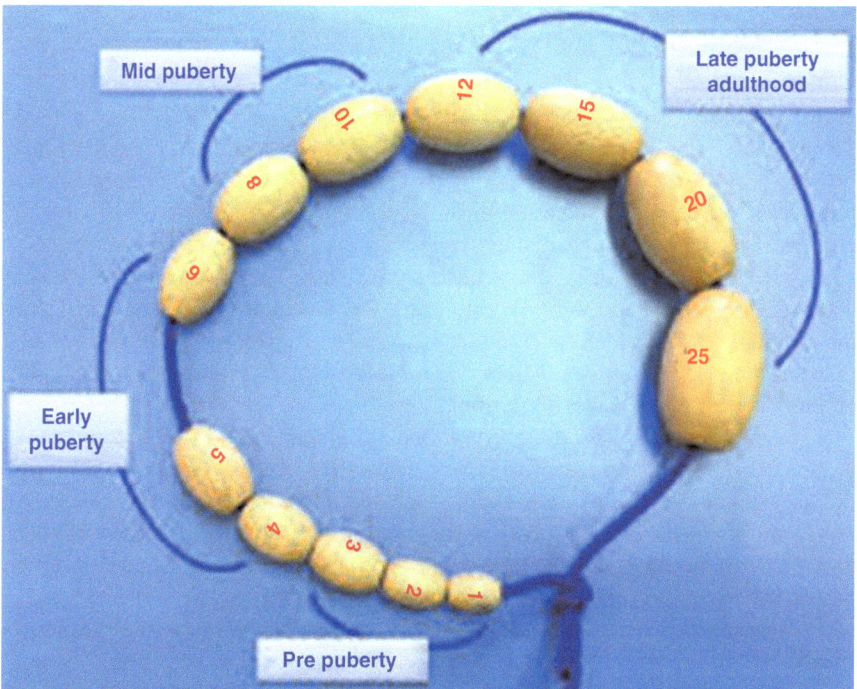

Fig. 5.3 Prader orchidometer for measuring testicular volume. (Lombardo [15])

determined to be 4.6 cm (range 3.6–5.5 cm) and 2.6 cm (range 2.1–3.2 cm). Mean volume, likewise, has been determined to be 18.6 ml (±4.6 ml). In terms of consistency, normal testes are typically firm and uniform, while abnormal testes are soft. Small testes with normal consistency are considered hypotrophic, while soft testes are considered atrophic. Masses or lesions found on exam should prompt an evaluation for testicular cancer.

Evaluation of the peritesticular area should note irregularities of the epididymis, such as induration, tenderness, or cysts. Evaluation of the spermatic cord should note presence or absence as well as characteristics of the scrotal vas deferens. Of infertile men, 2% may present with congenital absence of the vas deferens (CAVD) not previously diagnosed. Visual inspection of the scrotum may suggest a high-grade varicocele. Palpable engorgement of the pampiniform plexus similar to a "bag of worms" is indicative of a varicocele with or without a Valsalva maneuver that induces retrograde blood flow. Approximately 90% of varicoceles are found on the left side and may be associated with testis hypotrophy and asymmetry.

Examination of the penis should look for abnormalities such as phimosis, hypospadias, or curvature that may result in difficulty with intercourse and delivery of semen to the upper vaginal vault. A prostate exam should evaluate for size, consistency, and abnormal masses that may indicate infections, prostate cancer, or seminal vesicle enlargement due to ejaculatory duct obstruction [16–21].

Laboratory Testing

Semen Analysis

Semen analysis is the cornerstone of evaluation for male infertility. While it does provide critical information on sperm production and patency of the reproductive tract, it is not a complete measure of fertility. It merely suggests the likelihood of decreased fertility, although studies suggest that there are parameters of adequacy below which it may be difficult to achieve a pregnancy. The semen parameters were most recently validated by the World Health Organization (2010) and considered the minimum values of "normal" determined by semen parameters of men deemed to be fertile and with proven paternity. Of all the semen parameters, sperm count and motility correlate best with fertility.

Semen parameters can be highly variable, often depending on collection technique. Period of abstinence prior to testing can introduce significant variability. Semen volume can rise by up to 0.4 ml, and sperm concentration can increase by 10–15 million/ml with each day of abstinence up to 1 week. After 5 days of abstinence, sperm motility seems to decrease. Therefore, it is recommended that semen be collected after 48–72 hours of abstinence.

Semen can be obtained via masturbation (preferred), *coitus interruptus* (less ideal), or with the use of special non-spermicidal condom. The specimen should be analyzed within 1 hour of procurement due to impact on motility with prolonged duration. Of note, the specimen should also be kept at body temperature during transport. It is recommended that two semen analyses be obtained for a baseline evaluation.

Semen Characteristics and Measured Variables

Semen is typically a coagulum and liquefies 15–30 minutes after ejaculation. Normal ejaculate volume is considered to be at least 1.5 ml. Low ejaculate volume may be a sign of incomplete collection, ejaculatory duct obstruction, retrograde ejaculation, or androgen deficiency. Sperm concentration > 15 million/ml is deemed to be normal. Sperm motility is assessed by the percent and quality of movement (rapid and linear movement). Sperm morphology assesses the characteristics of the sperm head, midpiece, and tail. By the strictest classification (Kruger morphology), only 4% of sperm in the ejaculate are considered normal in appearance. See Tables 5.3 and 5.4 for critical parameters of semen analysis and the frequency of semen analysis findings in infertile men.

Table 5.3 Semen analysis (critical parameters)

Ejaculate volume	$\geq$1.5 ml
Sperm concentration	$>15 \times 10^6$ sperm/ml
Motility	>39%
Morphology	$\geq$4% normal forms

Table 5.4 Frequency of semen analysis findings in infertile men

All normal	55%
Isolated abnormal	37%
Low motility	26%
Low count	8%
Low volume	2%
Poor morphology	1%
No sperm	8%

Computer-Assisted Semen Analysis

In order to eliminate subjectivity in manual analysis, computer-assisted semen analysis (CASA) utilizes video digitalization and microchip processing to evaluate sperm characteristics. The future of technology utilization is promising, yet accuracy remains to be seen as CASA can overestimate sperm counts by 30% due to cross-contamination from immature sperm or leukocytes. On the contrary, high sperm concentration leads to underestimation in sperm motility. CASA does have an important value in the research setting at this time.

Semen Leukocyte Analysis

Leukocytes (white blood cells) are present in the ejaculate in relatively small numbers and play an important role in immune surveillance and eradication of abnormal sperm. Increase in leukocytes in the ejaculate, termed leukocytospermia or pyospermia, is defined as $>1 \times 10^6$ leukocytes/ml. Leukocytospermia is present in 2.8–23% of infertile men. Its impact on subfertility is not clearly elucidated and remains a matter of debate. It is suspected, however, that leukocytospermia can be a sign of presence of antisperm antibodies (ASA), which is of clinical relevance.

Antisperm Antibody (ASA) Test

The blood-testis barrier, described in the previous section, creates an immunologic sanctuary; however, when this barrier is broken, autoimmune infertility can occur from exposure to sperm antigens. Causes of autoimmune infertility include prior vasectomy, trauma, or surgery of the testis, which may lead to sperm antigen exposure and production of ASA. It is believed that ASA affects sperm transport through the reproductive tract or egg fertilization. Testing for ASA should be considered when (1) repeated semen analysis shows sperm agglutination or clumping, (2) idiopathic persistent leukocytospermia, (3) low sperm motility with history of testis injury or surgery, or (4) unexplained infertility. It is worth noting that testing for ASA in the modern era of fertility treatment is of decreasing utility, as no direct treatments exist.

Seminal Fructose and Post-ejaculate Urinalysis

In men with semen analyses demonstrating low ejaculate volumes and abnormal sperm concentration, the first steps should be noninvasive evaluations for a seminal vesicle abnormality or retrograde ejaculation.

Seminal vesicles contribute nearly 80% of the volume to the ejaculate, and seminal fluid is typically acidic (pH < 7.2) and rich in fructose. Therefore, testing for seminal fructose is indicated in men with low ejaculate volumes and no sperm. Positive testing suggests seminal vesicle agenesis or ejaculatory duct obstruction. A post-ejaculate urinalysis should also be considered in order to evaluate for retrograde ejaculation. This study inspects the first voided volume after ejaculation for the presence of sperm. If sperm is identified in the urine, a diagnosis of retrograde ejaculation is confirmed.

Hypoosmotic Swelling Test

When semen analyses suggest complete absence of sperm motility, it is prudent to evaluate sperm viability. Indeed, there are conditions, such as immotile cilia syndrome, in which sperm are perfectly viable but lack motility. Cell viability can be evaluated by testing for hypoosmotic swelling. When introduced to a hypoosmotic environment, viable cells with functional membrane and transporters swell in order to attain equilibrium with the environment. In the viable sperm, one can observe tail coiling and head swelling. Identifying immotile but viable sperm may allow couples to achieve healthy embryos via intracytoplasmic sperm injection (ICSI); therefore, this test should be considered when faced with absent sperm motility.

Sperm Penetration Assay

The sperm penetration assay (SPA) is utilized in order to test the ability of sperm to undergo "capacitation" as well as penetration and fertilization of the egg. The study is conducted with specially prepared hamster egg in the laboratory setting. The hamster egg is capable of interspecies fertilization but incapable of further development. SPA can be considered in couples with unexplained infertility. Furthermore, in specific situations, it may help decide whether a couple should elect for intrauterine insemination (IUI) with a good SPA result or in vitro fertilization and intracytoplasmic sperm injection (IVF-ICSI) with a poor SPA result.

Sperm DNA Fragmentation Assay

It is believed that fragmentation or disturbances in the sperm DNA (single- or double-stranded breaks) can lead to aberrant sperm function and resultant infertility. It is rare to encounter abnormally fragmented sperm in fertile men but occurs in a larger percentage of infertile men. When conventional semen studies cannot detect apparent sperm abnormalities, testing for sperm DNA integrity may be utilized. In general, there are two forms of DNA fragmentation testing: direct DNA fragmentation assays and denatured sperm DNA assays. Direct DNA fragmentation assays (TUNEL and Comet) are generally preferred by andrology laboratories due to a more effective correlation with clinical outcomes. As the name implies, denatured sperm DNA assays (SCD and SCSA) perform structural analysis on sperm following DNA denaturation by using either gel dispersion or flow cytometry. As a whole, these tests can detect infertility that is not apparent on conventional semen analyses.

Some known reversible causes of DNA fragmentation include tobacco use, excessive heat, infections, varicoceles, and certain medical conditions. The current role of DNA fragmentation testing is reserved for a select group of men in whom testing may determine treatment choices [22–35].

Hormonal Assessment

Assessment of the hypothalamic-pituitary-gonadal (HPG) axis is vital as it informs the state of sperm production. Diagnosis of underlying HPG axis abnormalities not only allows an opportunity to explain infertility and improve sperm production but may also identify men with significant medical conditions (hyperprolactinemia, congenital adrenal hyperplasia). Evaluation should include at least a free and total testosterone as well as FSH in men with confirmed oligozoospermia ($<15 \times 10^6$ sperm/ml). Endogenous testosterone is a well-known modulator of spermatogenesis, while FSH provides a reflection on the state of spermatogenesis. With impaired sperm production, FSH should be elevated. Serum LH and prolactin may be obtained if testosterone and FSH are abnormal. Similarly, estradiol may be obtained in men with poor virilization or obesity due to its role as an HPG axis modulator. Additional hormone studies such as thyroid panel and liver function tests should be considered only in setting of known active disease or suspicion of new disease. Common patterns of hormone levels with specific conditions are described in Table 5.5.

In men with infertility and impaired sexual function (low libido or erectile dysfunction), hormonal evaluation is paramount, as it may be a sign of underlying

Table 5.5 Common patterns of hormone levels with specific conditions

Condition	Testosterone	FSH	LH	Prolactin
Normal	NL	NL	NL	NL
Primary testicular failure	Low	High	High/NL	NL
Hypogonadotropic hypogonadism	Low	Low	Low	NL
Hyperprolactinemia	Low	Low/NL	Low	High
Androgen resistance	High	High	High	NL
Exogenous testosterone	High	Low	Low	NL

FSH follicle-stimulating hormone, *LH* luteinizing hormone, *NL* normal endocrinopathy. Nearly 10% of men undergoing hormonal evaluation for infertility are found to have endocrine abnormalities, and nearly 2% are ultimately found to have a significant endocrinopathy.

Genetic Testing

Chromosomal Studies

Between 2% and 15% of men evaluated for azoospermia or severe oligospermia may harbor a sex chromosomal or autosomal abnormality. Cytogenetic testing (karyotype) should be performed on men presenting with suspicion for nonobstructive azoospermia (testis atrophy, elevated FSH). The most frequently identified chromosomal abnormality is Klinefelter syndrome (XXY, sex chromosome) (Fig. 5.4).

Y Chromosome Microdeletion

It is believed that anywhere from 7% to 15% of men with severe oligospermia or azoospermia have underlying microdeletions on the long arm of the Y chromosome in a region termed "azoospermia factor" or *AZF*. There are three primary regions of interest—*AZFa, AZFb, and AZFc*—with deletion of *DAZ* (deleted in azoospermia)

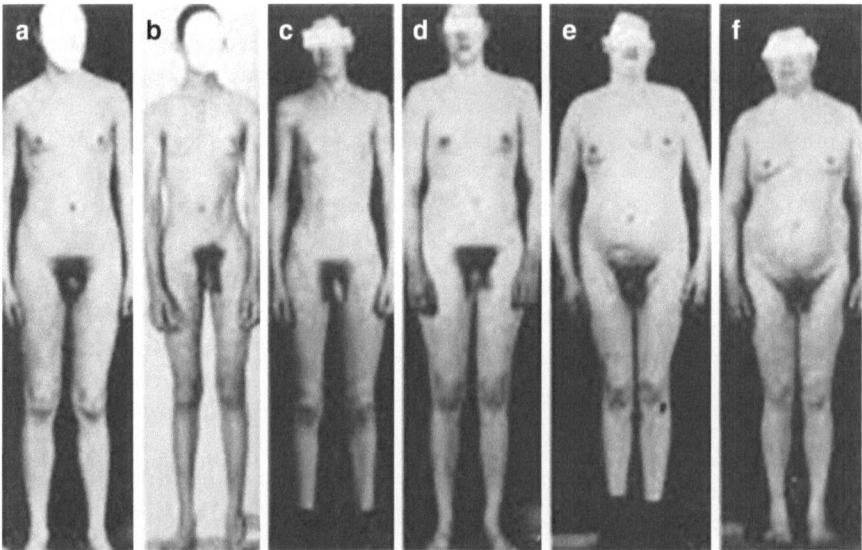

Fig. 5.4 Klinefelter syndrome. Note the eunuchoid habitus, female escutcheon, gynecomastia, and lack of temporal balding. (Reproduced from Bandmann [36])

gene in the *AZFc* region being the most commonly identified microdeletion. Deletions of *AZFc* region may still indicate intact spermatogenesis and possibility of progeny with IVF; however, deletions of *AZFa* and *AZFb* regions have not been found to demonstrate intact spermatogenesis. A polymerase chain reaction (PCR) blood test can evaluate Y chromosomes of peripheral leukocytes for gene deletions. Due to reported high rates, testing is recommended in men with severe oligospermia or azoospermia of nonobstructive etiology.

Cystic Fibrosis Mutation Testing

In men with known cystic fibrosis (CF) or findings of congenital absence of the vas deferens (CAVD), CF testing should be performed. Men with CAVD generally have an atypical form of CF, in which the scrotal vasa are nonpalpable. Nearly 80% of men with nonpalpable vasa will be found to have a CF gene mutation. Recent findings also indicated that men with the triad of chronic sinusitis, bronchiectasis, and obstructive azoospermia (Young syndrome) and men with idiopathic obstructive azoospermia may be at higher risk for CF mutations [37–43].

Additional Testing

Urinalysis

A simple urinalysis can be performed in the office and may inform the presence of infection, hematuria, glucosuria, or renal disease. Any of these findings can be an indication of abnormalities in the urinary tract.

Semen Culture

Semen cultures are obtained in specific conditions when there is concern or evidence of an infection, such as (1) history of genital tract infection, (2) abnormal expressed prostatic secretions, (3) presence of $>1 \times 10^6$ leukocytes/ml in semen (leukocytospermia), and (4) presence of >1000 pathogenic bacteria per ml of semen. Interpretation of results can be inconclusive as the urethra is typically contaminated with bacteria, and approximately 13% of infertile men will have positive semen cultures. The impact of positive semen cultures and infertility is poorly understood and therefore controversial. The most common agents causing genital infections are listed in Table 5.6. Gonorrhea is the most common genital infection, while 10–25% of chlamydial infections may be asymptomatic. *Trichomonas vaginalis*, a protozoan parasite, results in 1–5% of nongonococcal infections that are usually asymptomatic. *Ureaplasma urealyticum* commonly inhabits the urethra in sexually active men (30–50%) and leads to 25% of all cases of nongonococcal infections [21].

Table 5.6 Most common organisms in male genital infection

Neisseria gonorrhoeae	Cytomegalovirus
Chlamydia trachomatis	Herpes simplex II
Trichomonas vaginalis	Human papilloma virus
Ureaplasma urealyticum	Epstein-Barr virus
Escherichia coli (other Gram-negative bacilli)	Hepatitis B virus
Mycoplasma hominis	Human immunodeficiency virus

Radiographic Evaluation

Scrotal Ultrasound

Scrotal imaging has a limited role in the workup for infertility, as the physical exam informs diagnosis and prognostication. However, in some cases, high-frequency ultrasound can aid in the complete evaluation of testicular, paratesticular, and scrotal lesions. Abnormalities such as a hydrocele (when the testis in nonpalpable) or paratesticular masses should prompt an ultrasound evaluation.

Additionally, Doppler ultrasonography has been utilized in the evaluation and confirmation of varicoceles by measuring blood patterns, such as retrograde venous flow as well as vein size and other anatomic considerations. Diagnostic criteria for varicoceles are not clearly established; however, a venous diameter > 3 mm is often used as a threshold for the diagnosis. Retrograde venous flow with Valsalva maneuver is also critical marker of a varicocele (Fig. 5.5).

Transrectal Ultrasound

Transrectal ultrasound (TRUS) is employed to evaluate the prostate, seminal vesicles, and ejaculatory ducts when obstruction is suspected (low-volume ejaculate < 1.5 ml). Dilation of seminal vesicles (>1.5 cm anterior-posterior diameter) or ejaculatory ducts (>2.3 mm) associated with a cyst, calcification, or stones is suggestive of obstruction (Fig. 5.6) [46, 47].

Computed Tomography (CT) or Magnetic Resonance Imaging (MRI) of the Pelvis

Though CT and MRI can be useful in clarifying the reproductive tract anatomy, its use is limited with the ease, availability, and cost efficiency of TRUS.

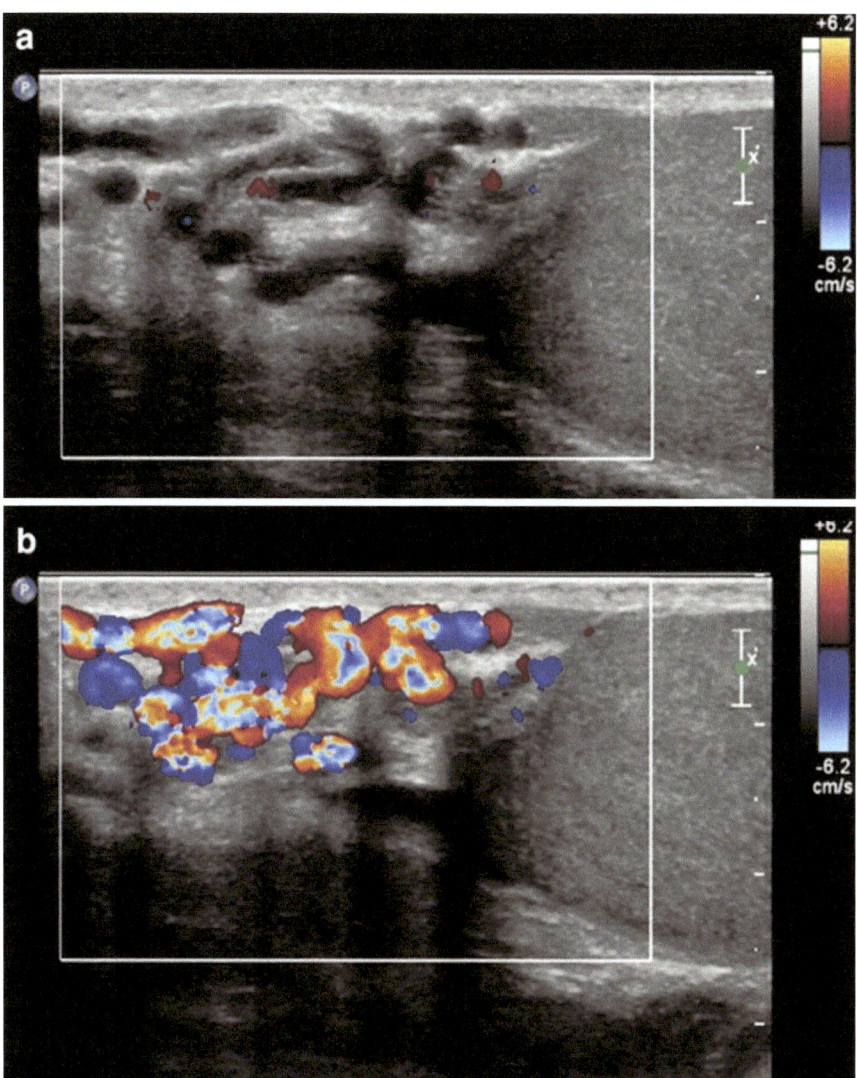

Fig. 5.5 Scrotal ultrasound. Small varicocele lying above the testis (Sarteschi grade II). Color Doppler images obtained at rest (**a**) and during Valsalva (**b**) showing that reflux is detected only during Valsalva. (Reproduced from Freeman et al. [44])

Diagnostic Procedures

Testis Biopsy

A diagnostic testis biopsy provides a direct examination into the state of spermato-genesis, particularly in azoospermic men in whom it is difficult to distinguish

Fig. 5.6 Transrectal ultrasound images transverse on the right and longitudinal on the left, showing a small midline cyst at the distal ejaculatory duct. (Reproduced from Fisch et al. [45])

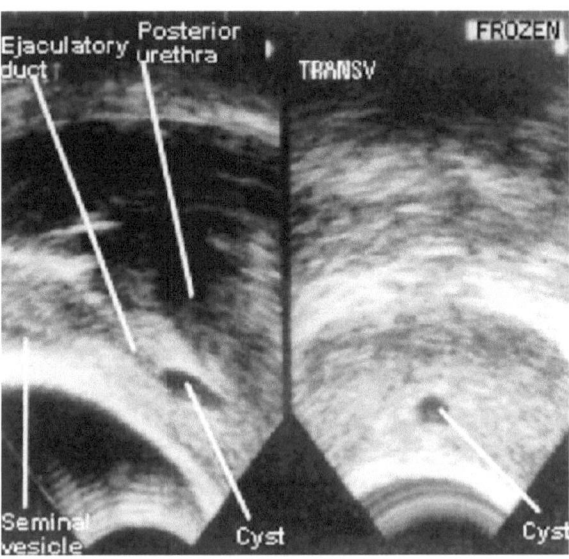

between obstruction and sperm production failure. This procedure is performed under local or general anesthesia and involves a small incision into the scrotal wall and tunica albuginea of the testis. A small tissue sample is obtained and fixed with formalin or Bouin's solution. Histologic examination informs seminiferous tubule architecture and cellular composition and categorizes abnormalities into several patterns. In men with oligospermia, testis biopsy is not indicated, unless it is severe or presents with intermittent azoospermia or cryptozoospermia. Bilateral testis biopsies are warranted when testicular asymmetry is encountered, as asymmetry may indicate obstructed testis on one side and spermatogenesis failure on the other.

Testis biopsy may also function as a sperm retrieval procedure for assisted reproductive technology. Sperm harvested via biopsy are routinely utilized in men with severe male factor infertility in order to perform IVF-ICSI. Sperm retrieval techniques are discussed below. In azoospermic men with normal spermatogenesis by testis biopsy and normal ejaculate volume, investigation of the reproductive tract should be considered in order to identify the site of obstruction [48].

Vasography

If obstruction of vas deferens is suspected, a vasogram is performed by injection of contrast media into the vas deferens toward the bladder followed by plain film radiography or fluoroscopy. Imaging can delineate the reproductive anatomy of the vas deferens to the seminal vesicles and ejaculatory ducts and provide the precise location of obstruction. Similar to a vasogram, chromotubation (injection of dye such as

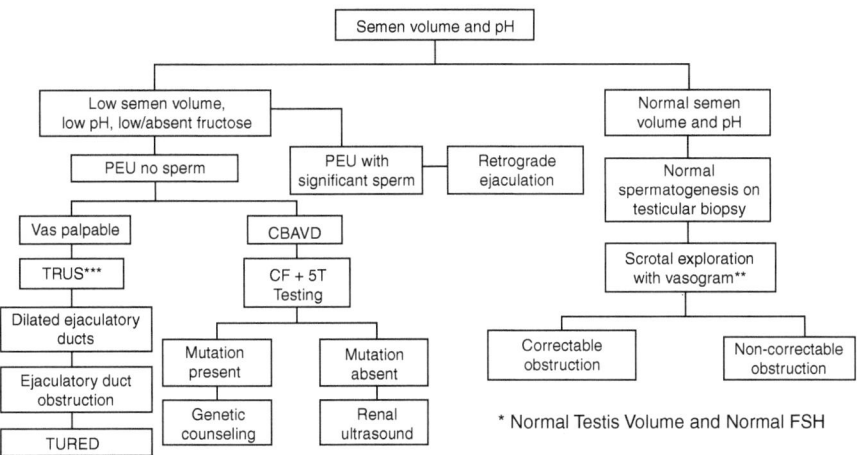

**Vasogram: includes saline, methylene blue, and contrast
***If negative TRUS, Genetic testing is recommended

Fig. 5.7 Algorithm for evaluation of obstructive (**a**) and nonobstructive (**b**) azoospermia. CBAVD congenital bilateral absence of the vas deferens, FSH follicle-stimulating hormone, LH luteinizing hormone, MRI magnetic resonance imaging, CF cystic fibrosis, YCMD Y chromosome microdeletion, micro-TESE microsurgical testicular sperm extraction, IUI intrauterine insemination, IVF/ICSI in vitro fertilization with intracytoplasmic sperm injection. (Adapted from [49])

indigo carmine or methylene blue) may also be performed with simultaneous cysto-urethroscopy to visualize the ejaculatory ducts (Fig. 5.7).

Fine Needle Aspiration (FNA)-Guided Testicular Mapping

In men with spermatogenic failure, testicular sperm retrieval can be highly variable ranging from 25% to 50% success rate. Given the high rate of uncertainty and the associated emotional and financial burdens, percutaneous FNA-guided testicular mapping is being utilized to accurately diagnose the severity of the condition as well as to prognosticate the success of sperm retrieval. Cytologic analysis has been shown to have high concordance with histologic specimen from open testicular biopsies. Furthermore, multisite examination may be more sensitive at detection of focal and heterogeneous pattern of spermatogenesis.

Like testis biopsy, FNA mapping is also performed under local anesthesia. Using a 23G needle, seminiferous tubules are percutaneously aspirated using a standard map from various locations in the testis. Tissue is then smeared on a slide, fixed, and interpreted by an experienced andrologist or cytopathologist for the presence of sperm. The findings of the study are then utilized to inform decisions for patients regarding their chances of sperm retrieval for IVF and ICSI [50] (Fig. 5.8).

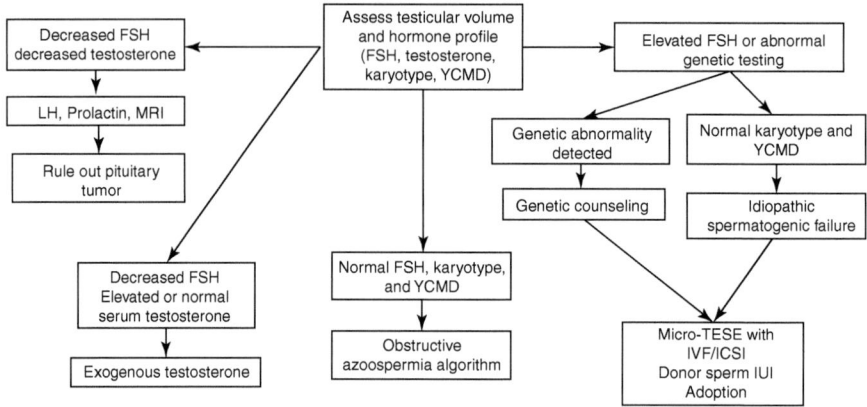

FSH: follicle stimulating hormone; **LH:** luteinizing hormone; **YCMD:** y-chromosome microdeletion; **Micro-TESE:** microsurgical testicular sperm extraction; **CF:** cystic fibrosis; **IVF/ICSI:** in vitro fertilization; Micro-intracytoplasmic sperm injection; **IUI:** intrauterine insemination

Fig. 5.8 Technique of percutaneous fine needle aspiration "mapping" for sperm in the testis. Cytologic samples are taken from various systematically sampled areas of the testis, guided by marks on the scrotum. (Reproduced from Turek et al. [51])

Etiology of Male Infertility

The underlying etiology of male infertility is best explained by site of dysfunction: pretesticular, intratesticular, and posttesticular.

Pretesticular

Pretesticular causes of infertility are secondary to hormonal abnormalities within the HPG axis, outlined in Table 5.7.

Hypothalamic Disease

A. *Gonadotropin Deficiency (Kallmann Syndrome)*

Kallmann syndrome is a condition marked by central hypogonadism, delayed puberty, anosmia, and infertility. Other clinical findings include small testes, occasional renal agenesis, bimanual dyskinesia, cleft lip, and dental agenesis. In the absence of anosmia, the condition is termed idiopathic hypogonadotropic hypogonadism (IHH). The condition is inherited in approximately one third of cases in both X-linked and autosomal fashion. In the X-linked condition, deletions of *KAL1* gene have been identified, which prevents migration of GnRH

Table 5.7 Pretesticular causes of infertility

Hypothalamic disease
Gonadotropin deficiency (Kallmann syndrome)
Isolated FSH deficiency
Isolated LH deficiency ("fertile eunuch")
Congenital hypogonadotropic syndromes
Pituitary disease
Pituitary insufficiency (tumors, surgery, radiation)
Hyperprolactinemia
Growth hormone deficiency
Exogenous hormones (glucocorticoid excess, estrogen/androgen excess, hyper- and hypoparathyroidism)

neurons to the preoptic area of the hypothalamus during embryologic development. Hormonal evaluation is notable for low testosterone, low LH and FSH, and normal prolactin levels. Infertility is reversible in approximately 80% of men with gonadotropin (LH & FSH) replacement over 12–18 months.

B. *Isolated LH and FSH Deficiencies*

Isolated LH deficiency is rare and often partial, such that there is sufficient LH to stimulate intratesticular testosterone production and spermatogenesis, yet insufficient LH to promote adequate circulating testosterone for virilization. As a result, men have a eunuchoid habitus with variable virilization and gynecomastia. Testes are typically normal in size, but sperm concentration is usually low from normal FSH levels but relatively low intratesticular testosterone.

In contrast, patients with isolated FSH deficiency demonstrate a normal body habitus with complete virilization and normal size testes. Both LH and testosterone levels are normal, while FSH levels are uniformly low and unresponsive to GnRH stimulation. Azoospermia or severe oligospermia is a typical finding.

C. *Congenital Hypogonadotropic Syndromes*

Several syndromes are associated with hypogonadotropic hypogonadism. Prader-Willi syndrome (1:20,000) is characterized by mental retardation, obesity, and hypogonadism secondary to GnRH deficiency. The most common causes of the condition are either single-gene deletion or uniparental gene imprinting on chromosome 15. Spermatogenesis can be induced with FSH and LH administration. Bardet-Biedl syndrome (autosomal recessive) results in hypogonadotropic hypogonadism due to GnRH deficiency. It is defined by mental retardation, retinitis pigmentosa, polydactyly, and hypogonadism. Infertility is treatable, like other conditions, with administration of gonadotropins.

Pituitary Disease

A. *Pituitary Insufficiency*

Pituitary insufficiency can be a by-product of many conditions including tumors, surgery, radiation, infarcts, and infiltrative or infectious processes.

Blood dyscrasias such as sickle cell anemia and beta thalassemia can result in pituitary as well as testicular dysfunction. Sickle cell anemia can result in both pituitary and testicular micro-infarcts from sickling of red blood cells, while beta thalassemia can result in micro-infarcts from hemosiderin deposition within the pituitary gland and the testes. Hemochromatosis similarly results in iron deposition within these organs.

B. *Hyperprolactinemia*

Elevated prolactin levels can lead to hypogonadotropic hypogonadism due to suppression of pulsatile GnRH secretion. As a result, both testosterone production and spermatogenesis are suppressed. Prolactin levels should be rechecked when an elevation is encountered, and secondary causes such as anxiety/stress, systemic illnesses, or medications should be excluded. The most notable cause of hyperprolactinemia is a prolactin-secreting pituitary adenoma (prolactinoma). Magnetic resonance imaging (MRI) of the sella turcica is used to distinguish between a microadenoma (<10 mm) and a macroadenoma (>10 mm). Symptoms of hyperprolactinemia may include erectile dysfunction, loss of libido, gynecomastia, and galactorrhea. Referral to endocrinology is advised at this juncture.

C. *Exogenous or Endogenous Hormones*

An imbalance of the testosterone to estrogen ratio (T:E), which is normally 10:1, can result in infertility. Conditions such as liver cirrhosis and obesity can lead to increased endogenous estrogens due to augmented aromatase activity. Less common conditions include adrenocortical tumors, Sertoli cell tumors, and interstitial testis tumors that may produce excess estrogens. Estrogens in turn decrease pituitary gonadotropin secretion, resulting in spermatogenic failure.

Exogenous androgenic steroids (anabolic steroids) are in wide use by athletes from high school all the way up to professional levels and result in sterility due to suppression of the HPG axis. Treatment includes cessation of steroids and semen analysis every 3–6 months until return of spermatogenesis. Excess endogenous androgens most commonly occur in congenital adrenal hyperplasia (CAH) caused by 21-hydroxylase deficiency. Excessive adrenocorticotropic hormone (ACTH) production results in elevated androgenic steroids by the adrenal glands. Androgen excess in prepubertal boys leads to precocious puberty and premature development of secondary sex characteristics, including abnormal enlargement of the phallus [52]. The testes are characteristically small due to central gonadotropin inhibition by androgens. In girls, virilization occurs with enlargement of the clitoris. In classic CAH diagnosed early in childhood, normal fertility has been reported.

Other sources of endogenous androgens include functional adrenal tumors or Leydig cell tumors of the testis. Thyroid abnormalities (hyper- or hypothyroidism) can also impact spermatogenesis both at the pituitary and testicular levels. Thyroid hormone is an important regulatory hormone for normal hypothalamic function [38, 53–59].

Table 5.8 Intratesticular causes of infertility

Klinefelter syndrome (XXY)
XYY syndrome
Y chromosome microdeletions (YCMD)
Noonan syndrome (male Turner syndrome)
Sertoli cell-only syndrome (germ cell aplasia)
Myotonic dystrophy
Gonadotoxins (radiation, chemotherapy)
Systemic disease
Testis injury (orchitis, torsion, trauma)
Cryptorchidism
Varicocele
Idiopathic

Intratesticular

Infertility due to intratesticular conditions is insensitive to hormonal manipulations and is therefore largely irreversible. Table 5.8 highlights common testicular causes.

Klinefelter Syndrome

Chromosomal abnormalities are frequently encountered during workup of male infertility. Studies have shown a nearly 6% overall prevalence of chromosomal abnormalities in men undergoing evaluation for infertility. In men with sperm concentration < 10 million/ml, the prevalence is reportedly 11%, and in men with non-obstructive azoospermia, the prevalence is nearly 21%. Genetic workup (karyotype) is therefore critical and should be considered in men with severe oligospermia and azoospermia.

Klinefelter syndrome has an overall incidence of 1:500 males and remains the most common chromosomal aneuploidy and a significant genetic cause of azoospermia, accounting for up to 14% of cases. Classic findings are small, firm testes, gynecomastia, and azoospermia. Some men may display tall stature, obesity, delayed sexual maturation, and mild cognitive delay. Common medical conditions may include diabetes, leukemia, increased likelihood of extragonadal germ cell tumors, and breast cancer (20-fold higher than in normal males). Although 90% of men with Klinefelter will have an extra X chromosome (47, XXY), nearly 10% will be mosaic (XXY/XY chromosomes).

The testes are usually <2 cm in length and always <3.5 cm. Testis biopsy findings generally show sclerosis and hyalinization with normal numbers of Leydig cells. FSH levels are frankly high with relatively low or normal testosterone and corresponding relatively high LH levels. Serum estradiol levels may also be elevated. There is an expected precipitous decline in testosterone with most men requiring testosterone replacement therapy both for virilization and for normal sexual function. Paternity with this syndrome is low but more likely with mosaicism or milder/earlier course of disease. Some men will have limited spermatogenesis whereby sperm may be retrieved from the testes and used with IVF-ICSI [39, 40].

Y Chromosome Microdeletions (YCMD)

Similar to chromosomal abnormalities, YCMD are also encountered in the workup of male infertility. Nearly 7% of men with oligospermia and 13% with azoospermia have reported alterations in the long arm of the Y chromosome (Yq). Current molecular genetics has allowed us to determine three gene sites in the *AZF* (azoospermia factor) region as the common culprits: *AZFa, AZFb, and AZFc*. The most promising site is *AZFc*, which contains the *DAZ* gene region. Homologs of the *DAZ* gene are found in many other animals, including mouse and *Drosophila*. Currently, blood testing with quantitative polymerase chain reaction assay is performed for diagnosis. Future testing will likely be performed on sperm DNA as part of a semen analysis. Some men with *AZFc* deletions may have sperm in the ejaculate and may also be able to achieve paternity with sperm retrieval and IVF-ICSI. It is important to note and educate patients that these microdeletions can be passed on to the offspring [41, 60–64].

Noonan Syndrome

Noonan syndrome (male Turner syndrome) has a similar presentation to Turner syndrome (45 X) but may also have a mosaic presentation (X/XY). Findings such as webbed neck, short stature, low set ears, wide set eyes, and cardiovascular abnormalities are common. A majority of patients also have cryptorchidism at birth, which limits fertility. FSH and LH levels can be variable based on the degree of testicular dysfunction.

Myotonic Dystrophy

Patients with myotonic dystrophy have various endocrinopathies along with myotonia, cataracts, and muscle atrophy. Apart from endocrinopathies, it is also common to see testis atrophy, which contributes to infertility. The status of fertility is variable, but testis failure is progressive, and hormone levels vary based on testicular function.

Sertoli Cell-Only Syndrome (Germ Cell Aplasia)

Germ cell aplasia implies complete absence of germinal cells on histology based on testicular biopsies, thereby resulting in the presence of Sertoli cells only. Possible causes include genetic defects, abnormal germ cell migration during embryogenesis, autoimmune degeneration, and androgen resistance. Iatrogenic causes such as chemotherapy and irradiation as well as infectious causes such as mumps orchitis should also be considered. Men with this condition appear to have normal virilization with smaller testes of normal consistency. FSH is expected to be typically high in most cases with normal testosterone axis. In some cases, fine needle testicular mapping and microdissection testicular sperm extraction can reverse the misdiagnosis by finding focal spermatogenesis.

Defective DNA Mismatch Repair

Similar to their roles in cancer, defective DNA mismatch repair genes (PMS2, Mlh1) have been linked to infertility in mice. Clinically, both germ cell arrest and Sertoli cell-only syndrome have been noted to have an association with DNA mismatch repair genes.

Gonadotoxins

Medications and radiotherapy are important iatrogenic gonadotoxins leading to infertility. The effects of radiotherapy on spermatogenesis were described in 1983 by Clifton and Bremner, who studied a population of healthy prisoners who were exposed to varying doses of ionizing radiation prior to a vasectomy. They found significant reduction in sperm count with 15 cGy, temporary azoospermia with 50 cGY, and persistent azoospermia at 400 cGy without rebound for at least 40 weeks. Most subjects recovered spermatogenesis to pre-radiation levels with cessation of exposure.

Histologic examination after radiation has shown that spermatogonia are highly sensitive to radiation, while Leydig cells are relatively resistant. During abdominal radiation with gonadal shielding, the estimated mean unintended gonadal exposure is approximately 75 cGy. Importantly, recent data has suggested that environmental or occupational exposure to electromagnetic radiation may also reduce semen quality. There does not appear to be an increase in congenital birth defects in offspring of irradiated men.

Table 5.9 provides a list of gonadotoxic medications. Included medications have different mechanisms by which they cause infertility. Medications that impair testosterone production (steroidogenesis pathway), such as ketoconazole and spironolactone, are commonly implicated in infertility. Spironolactone is widely used for testosterone suppression in transgender females with gender dysphoria. Importantly, many over-the-counter medications may have unknown gonadotoxic potential, and patients that are trying to conceive should be advised to discontinue any unnecessary medications or supplements.

Chemotherapy drugs targeting rapidly dividing cancer cells have an expected, substantial impact on germ cells that are also dividing at a rapid rate. Alkylating agents such as mustard derivatives, cyclophosphamide, and chlorambucil are the

Table 5.9 Medications associated with infertility

Calcium channel blockers	Cimetidine
Sulfasalazine	Valproic acid
Spironolactone	Colchicine
SSRIs	Testosterone
Allopurinol	Alpha blockers
Nitrofurantoin	Lithium
Tricyclic antidepressants	Antipsychotics

most toxic agents. The effects of different agents are widely variable based on type of treatment, dose, duration, and baseline testis health. Despite the toxicity, it is important to mention that there does not appear to be an increase in the incidence of birth defects or genetic disorders in the progeny following exposure to chemotherapy. In general, patients should wait 6 months after chemotherapy to attempt a pregnancy.

Systemic Disease

A. *Renal Failure*

Uremia can cause sexual dysfunction, hypogonadism, and infertility. Testicular hypofunction is noted with decrease in testosterone levels and elevation of LH and FSH levels along with elevation of prolactin levels in some. It is thought that hyperestrogenemia may also be responsible for impaired spermatogenesis. Renal transplantation can improve hypogonadism in patients.

B. *Liver Cirrhosis*

Infertility from liver disease can be secondary to acute liver illness such as hepatitis as well as hypogonadism secondary to chronic liver failure. It is also well understood that testosterone levels are decreased and estrogen levels are increased without expected elevations in LH and FSH levels, suggesting central inhibition of the HPG axis with chronic liver disease.

C. *Diabetes Mellitus*

Peripheral neuropathy secondary to chronic diabetes impacts both erectile and ejaculatory function. Injury to the parasympathetic and sympathetic pelvic plexus leads to hypocontractility of the bladder neck and ejaculatory organs, thereby causing retrograde or anejaculation.

Testis Injury

A. *Orchitis*

Epididymo-orchitis, or inflammation of the testis and epididymis, can occur due to bacterial and viral infections. For example, orchitis occurs in 30% of postpubertal males that acquire mumps parotitis. Testis atrophy can be severe with viral orchitis but less so with bacterial infections.

B. *Torsion*

Testis ischemia secondary to a torsion event is a known surgical emergency and must be corrected within 6 hours of occurrence in order to prevent infarction and testis loss. The by-product of torsion can be inoculation of the immune system with testis antigens and resultant antisperm antibodies, which may cause immunologic infertility in adulthood. It has also been described that the contralateral testis can exhibit histologic abnormalities following a unilateral torsion.

C. *Trauma*

Similar to the immunologic response following torsion, testicular trauma can result in an abnormal systemic immune response that leads to testicular atrophy. When fracture of the testis is suspected, surgical exploration is requisite in order to minimize immunologic exposure of the testis tissue to the body.

Cryptorchidism

Cryptorchidism is observed in about 1% of boys at 1 year of gestational age. Failure of testicular descent increases the risk of testicular cancer as well as germ cell deterioration. Furthermore, the contralateral normal testis is also at risk for germ cell aberration. Thus, boys with unilateral and bilateral cryptorchidism have a higher risk of infertility in their adulthood, and early orchidopexy has been shown to reduce the risk of both testicular cancer and infertility [65–67].

Varicocele

Varicocele is a common condition, found in 15–20% of young, healthy men. The incidence rises to 40% in men with subfertility. Bilateral varicoceles may also be found in nearly 20% of subfertile men. Physiologically, varicoceles are a result of retrograde venous flow due to incompetent valves of the pampiniform venous plexus of the spermatic cord. Varicoceles are a clinical diagnosis based on a highly accurate physical examination, though ultrasound studies are being utilized as adjunct in order to confirm an equivocal examination.

From an anatomic perspective, the predominance of left-sided varicoceles is explained by the fact that the left spermatic vein is not only longer than the right but also joins the left renal vein at a right angle compared to the oblique insertion of the right spermatic vein into the inferior vena cava. This results in high venous pressures within the left spermatic cord veins and retrograde venous flow.

In adolescents, varicoceles can result in testicular atrophy and remains an indication to repair the condition and reverse the damage. There is strong evidence that varicoceles affect semen parameters, including concentration, motility, and morphology, and it is believed that motility is affected the most. Clinical asymmetries of testis size or semen abnormalities are both reasons to repair varicoceles in men seen for infertility.

The mechanism by which varicoceles impact testicular health and spermatogenesis is not well understood. A prevailing theory is that retrograde flow of warmer venous blood leads to disruption of normal countercurrent heat exchange balance and elevation of intratesticular temperature. Other theories include gonadal hormonal dysfunction, metabolic damage via renal-adrenal metabolites, and elevated testicular hydrostatic pressures [68–70].

Idiopathic

At least half of the men with infertility will have no identifiable etiology, and it stands to reason that the causes are multifactorial including genetic, environmental, hormonal, metabolic, and lifestyle factors.

Posttesticular

Posttesticular causes of infertility relate to obstruction of the reproductive anatomy, disorders of sperm function and motility, and disorders of sexual function (Table 5.10) [68, 71–74].

Table 5.10 Posttesticular causes of infertility

Disorders of obstruction
Congenital obstruction
Congenital absence of the vas deferens (CAVD)
Young syndrome
Idiopathic epididymal obstruction
Polycystic kidney disease
Ejaculatory duct obstruction
Acquired obstruction
Vasectomy
Groin surgery
Infection
Functional obstruction
Sympathetic nerve injury
Pharmacologic
Disorders of sperm function and motility
Immotile cilia syndromes
Maturation defects
Immunologic infertility
Infection
Disorders of sexual function
Erectile dysfunction
Hypospadias
Coitus timing and frequency

Congenital Obstruction

A. *Cystic Fibrosis*

Cystic fibrosis (CF) is a common genetic disorder with carrier prevalence of 1:20 among Caucasians in the United States. The condition is characterized by defective chloride ion transport across cell membranes resulting in fluid and electrolyte abnormalities. It is transmitted in an autosomal recessive manner and presents with chronic pulmonary infections, pancreatic insufficiency, and infertility. More than 95% of men with CF will have congenital bilateral absence of the vas deferens (CBAVD). In addition to CBAVD, parts of the epididymis, seminal vesicles, and ejaculatory ducts may also be absent, atrophic, or obstructed. CBAVD accounts for an incidence of 1–2% of infertility cases. Spermatogenesis in CF is quantitatively normal, yet emerging data suggests that the sperm may lack normal capacity to fertilize an egg and carry functional sperm defects. Physical examination confirms absence of one or both sides. Due to global reproductive tract abnormalities, reconstruction is not feasible. While a majority of these men do not have symptoms of CF, up to 80% of men will harbor a CF mutation. Men with unilateral absence of the vas deferens may also have an absent ipsilateral kidney explained by embryologic induction anomalies [37, 42, 43].

B. *Young Syndrome*

Young syndrome is characterized by a triad of chronic sinusitis, bronchiectasis, and obstructive azoospermia. The condition may be explained by abnormal ciliary function or abnormal mucus quality, and obstruction occurs in the epididymis [75].

C. *Adult Polycystic Kidney Disease*

Adult polycystic kidney disease is characterized by innumerable cysts of the kidney, liver, spleen, pancreas, and the reproductive organs—seminal vesicles, epididymides, and testes. Obstructing cysts of the epididymis and seminal vesicles leads to infertility.

D. *Ejaculatory Duct Obstruction*

Ejaculatory ducts are paired, collagenous tubes that attach the vas deferens and seminal vesicles to the urethra. Ejaculatory duct obstruction (EDO) accounts for 5% of azoospermia and can be congenital or acquired. The congenital form is often associated with Mullerian duct cysts, Wolffian duct cysts, or congenital atresia, while the acquired form is secondary to seminal vesicle calculi and postsurgical or inflammatory fibrosis.

Acquired Obstruction

Nearly 500,000 vasectomies are performed each year in the United States, and up to 6% of these men will undergo vasectomy reversal. Other iatrogenic causes of blockage include hernia surgery, which may result in direct injury to vas deferens or indirect blockage secondary to synthetic mesh-related perivasal inflammation.

Bacterial infections (*E. coli* or *Chlamydia trachomatis*) can involve the epididymis, resulting in scarring and obstruction.

Functional Obstruction

Functional obstruction occurs due to impaired contractility of the seminal vesicles. The usual culprits are nerve injury or medication side effects. One of the most well-known examples is ejaculatory dysfunction following retroperitoneal lymph node dissection for testicular cancer. The postganglionic sympathetic fibers overlying the inferior aorta and coalescing as the hypogastric plexus control seminal emission, and damage along this pathway can result in retrograde or anejaculation. Other conditions that may result in ejaculatory dysfunction include multiple sclerosis and diabetes. Medications that cause impaired ejaculation are listed in the section above [46, 75–77].

Disorders of Sperm Function and Motility

A. *Immotile Cilia Syndromes*

Immotile cilia syndromes affect sperm motility due to defects in the motor axoneme in ciliated cells (including sperm). Sperm tails are arranged in a standard "9 + 2" microtubule configuration and connected by dynein arms (ATPase). Defects in the dynein arms cause deficits in ciliary and sperm activity. One of the well-known syndromes, Kartagener syndrome, is characterized by a triad of chronic sinusitis, bronchiectasis, and situs inversus. Men with this condition have a normal sperm concentration and immotile but viable sperm. Diagnosis can be confirmed by electron microscopy of sperm.

B. *Immunologic Infertility*

The blood-testis barrier is composed of Sertoli cell tight junctions, making the testis an immune-privileged site. Following vasectomy, testis biopsy, and testis torsion, exposure to sperm antigens can result in ASAs, which may disturb sperm transport or sperm-egg interaction. Assays that detect sperm-bound ASAs are available and can be clinically relevant.

Disorders of Coitus

Erectile dysfunction and low libido are important conditions to rule out during the evaluation of infertility. A hormonal evaluation should be performed to detect organic causes of these conditions; however, the most common cause is situational due to the anxiety of attempting to conceive. In such instances, sex counseling and the use of oral phosphodiesterase-5 inhibitors are recommended.

A complete evaluation of the couple should assess sexual habits such as coital timing and frequency. Recommended frequency of coitus is every 1–2 days during the periovulatory period. Calculation of ovulatory cycles can be performed by charting of basal body temperature as well as with home kits that measure the LH surge in the urine before ovulation. All synthetic lubricants should be avoided, and unnecessary medications should be stopped. Lifestyle modifications, such as avoidance of hot tubs, saunas, and Jacuzzis as well as tobacco, marijuana, and excessive alcohol, should be suggested.

Management of the Infertile Male

Management of various infertility conditions may be nonsurgical, surgical, or a combination of both. It is important to mention that in many instances, "treatment" of the male may not be possible. Couples are often looking for how to "fix" or "treat" an abnormality, and they should be made aware that such may not be possible and the implications thereof regarding their fertility and general health.

Varicocele

Both surgical and nonsurgical modalities are available for treatment of varicoceles. Surgical varicocelectomy can be performed via three approaches—retroperitoneal, inguinal, or subinguinal. Laparoscopy may also be utilized in the surgical treatment of varicoceles. Microsurgical subinguinal varicocelectomy is the modern surgery of choice due to its minimal comorbidity and complication profile along with high success rates. Radiologic embolization is an accepted alternative to surgical management. The common goal of all treatments is to prevent retrograde venous blood flow through the internal spermatic veins. Table 5.11 provides a comparison of the outcomes. While treatment of varicoceles can yield a higher success rate, patients must also be advised of a 16% pregnancy rate without treatment. Similarly, a pregnancy rate of 35% can be expected with IVF. The overall complication rate of incisional or open approach (1%) is lower than that of laparoscopy (4%) and embolization (10–15%).

Table 5.11 Comparison of the outcomes for modalities available for treatment of varicoceles

	Treatment		
Outcome	Open	Laparoscopic	Radiologic
Improvement of semen parameters	66%	50–70%	60%
Pregnancy rate	35%	12–32%	10–50%
Recurrence	0–15%	5–25%	0–10%
Technical failure	Negligible	Small	10–15%
Pain pills	9.4	11	Minimal
Days to work	5	5.3	1

Vasectomy Reversal

Out of 500,000 men every year that undergo vasectomy in the United States, nearly 6% will undergo vasectomy reversal due to various reasons, including remarriage or loss of a child. Other causes of vasal obstruction, such as trauma, infections, and previous surgery, may also be treated with surgical exploration and vasovasostomy or epididymovasostomy. Obstructive azoospermia is suspected in a man with normal testis size and normal hormones.

Several techniques have been described for vasovasostomy, none superior than the other; however, surgeon experience and use of high-magnification surgical microscope yield higher success rates. Either a modified single-layer or two-layer anastomosis can be performed in patients that fit the criteria for a vasovasostomy. In these patients, a patency rate of 95% or higher can be expected. The absence of sperm below the level of the vasectomy indicates secondary obstruction in the epididymis. It is theorized that a secondary obstruction occurs due to tubular rupture from increased luminal pressure followed by scarring. The most common identifiable factors resulting in epididymal obstruction include prolonged interval of obstruction and low vasectomy site. In the case that epididymal obstruction is suspected, an epididymovasostomy must be performed. Despite being a much more technically challenging operation, the success rate is 60–65% in well-trained and experienced hands.

Pregnancy after a successful vasectomy reversal depends largely on the fertility potential of the couple. Therefore, an understanding of the couple's reproductive health is recommended prior to surgery. Barriers to successful pregnancy after vasectomy reversal include (1) pre-vasectomy semen quality, (2) development of ASAs following vasectomy, (3) delayed obstruction due to anastomotic stenosis, and (4) impaired sperm maturation due to epididymal dysfunction [78–84] (Fig. 5.9).

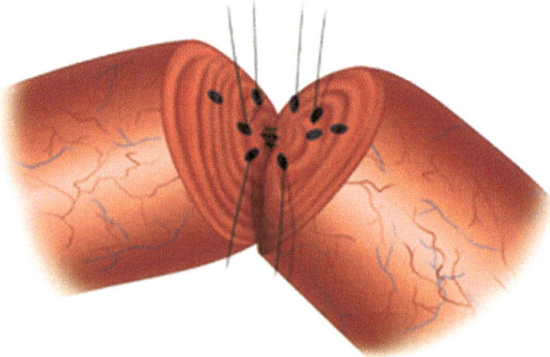

Fig. 5.9 Two-layer microsurgical vasovasostomy. Mucosal stitches of 10-0 nylon are placed in the "back wall" of the vas lumen, incorporating mucosa and a small amount of submucosal tissue. The "front wall" mucosal sutures are then placed. Finally, serosal sutures of 9-0 nylon are placed in the outside wall of the vas deferens to complete the anastomosis. (Reproduced from Marks [85])

Ejaculatory Duct Obstruction

This condition should be suspected when a man presents with normal hormones and low ejaculate volume (<1.5 ml) in the absence of retrograde ejaculation. *Complete EDO* (obstruction of both paired ducts) typically presents with low-volume azoospermia, while *incomplete* or *partial* EDO (obstruction of unilateral duct) is characterized by low-volume ejaculate along with poor sperm count and quality. *Functional* EDO occurs due to hypocontractility of the ejaculatory ducts and is diagnosed when no anatomic obstruction is found on imaging and cystoscopy. Transrectal ultrasound will demonstrate dilated seminal vesicles (diameter > 2.5 cm in anterior-posterior dimension) or dilated ejaculatory ducts with possible midline cystic structure causing obstruction.

Transurethral resection of the ejaculatory ducts (TURED) can be performed, whereby the verumontanum is resected in the midline until the ejaculatory ducts are visualized. Great care must be taken to avoid injury to the external urethral sphincter, similar to transurethral resection of the prostate. A majority of men (70%) will show significant improvement in semen parameters following a TURED with a 30% pregnancy rate. Complication rate is approximately 20%, with most complications being self-limited, which includes hematospermia, hematuria, UTI, and epididymitis. Rare complications include retrograde ejaculation, rectal injury, or urinary incontinence [86, 87] (Fig. 5.10).

Anejaculation

Anejaculation or failure of seminal emission typically occurs due to disruption or dysfunction of pelvic sympathetic nerves, either due to pelvic/retroperitoneal surgery or spinal cord injury. Electroejaculation, performed with a rectal probe, can stimulate these nerves, resulting in the contraction of the vas deferens, seminal

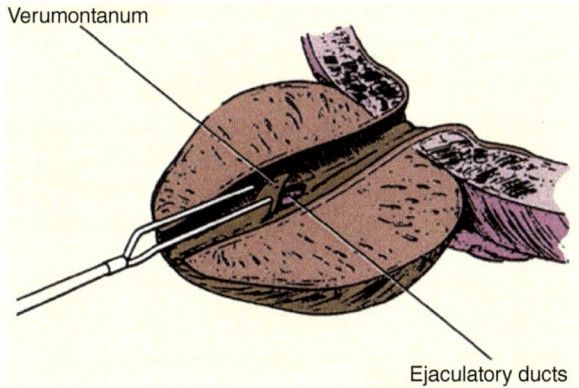

Fig. 5.10 A cystoscope with a resecting loop is used to resect the verumontanum to relieve ejaculatory duct obstruction. (Reproduced from Hendry [88])

Verumontanum

Ejaculatory ducts

vesicle, and prostate. Following induction of ejaculation, semen is collected from
the penis as well as the bladder due to a high rate of retrograde ejaculation. Acquired
sperm may be utilized for both IUI and IVF [89].

Leukocytospermia

The finding of elevated leukocytes (>1 million/ml) in the semen is termed leukocytospermia or pyospermia. This condition is associated with (1) subclinical
genital tract infection, (2) elevated reactive oxygen species, and (3) poor sperm
function. Evaluation for sexually transmitted diseases, penile discharge, prostatitis, or epididymitis should be completed. Expressed prostatic secretion (EPS)
can be obtained for leukocytes, and urine can be assayed for chlamydial, gono-
coccal, and mycoplasma infections. The treatment for nonbacterial leukocytospermia is controversial; however, broad-spectrum antibiotics such as
doxycycline and trimethoprim-sulfamethoxazole are typically used and may
reduce seminal leukocytes. Generally, the female partner is also treated.
Frequent ejaculation (>every 3 days) along with antibiotic therapy may also
provide more durable results. Antioxidant therapy with vitamins (A, C, and E)
as well as glutathione and omega-3 fatty acids (fish oil) may also be utilized. It
is worth noting that the presence of immature (round) germ cells can be confused for leukocytes and should be reviewed with the laboratory. In the setting
of elevated "round" cells, specific testing should be performed to confirm the
presence of leukocytes.

Following retroperitoneal surgery, successful sperm recovery is possible with
electroejaculation in most patients, while in men with spinal cord injuries above the
T5 levels, a reflex ejaculation may be induced with high-frequency penile vibration
(vibratory stimulation). Patients can attempt to conceive at home via vibratory stimulation and cervical insemination using handheld vibrators set to a frequency of
110 cycles/s and amplitude of 3 mm [90, 91].

Antisperm Antibodies

When ASAs are the cause of infertility, treatment poses a significant challenge.
If >50% of sperm are bound with antibodies, treatment should be offered.
Considerations of treatment include steroidal immunosuppression, IUI, and
IVF-ICSI with or without sperm washing. The use of steroidal immunosuppression is rare in clinical practice due to potential side effects. IUI provides pregnancy rate of 10–15% per cycle, while IVF-ICSI can be very effective in this
scenario [31, 90, 91].

Hormonal Abnormalities

A. *Hyperprolactinemia*

   Normal prolactin levels help maintain normal intratesticular testosterone levels and affect growth and secretions of the sex glands. Hyperprolactinemia suppresses normal gonadotropin function by interfering with episodic GnRH release. Microadenomas can be treated with medical therapy (bromocriptine, 5–10 mg daily), while macroadenomas are treated surgically.

B. *Hypothyroidism*

   Thyroid abnormalities can impair spermatogenesis, and reversal of the condition can be effective in treating infertility. Routine screening is not recommended without clinical symptoms.

C. *Testosterone Excess or Deficiency Syndromes*

   The most common form of CAH, 21-hydroxylase deficiency, results in excess androgen production and most commonly presents as precocious puberty. Usual treatment for both the condition and associated infertility is administration of corticosteroids.

Anabolic steroids are a common reason for testicular failure and may be often omitted in patient history. Exogenous testosterone is a potent depressant of the HPG axis, resulting in infertility. Immediate cessation of exogenous testosterone is recommended in order to allow restoration of pituitary gonadal axis and production of endogenous testosterone. Similarly, in men with hypogonadism, testosterone replacement therapy results in infertility via the same mechanism. For both, pituitary stimulation in addition to cessation of exogenous agents may be necessary. Oral clomiphene citrate (discussed below) or injectable hCG is typically used.

Kallmann syndrome presents with HPG inactivity and diminished testosterone due to the lack of GnRH. Infertility due to this condition is effectively treated with hCG (1000–200 U, three times a week) and recombinant FSH (75 IU, twice a week) as replacement for both LH and FSH, respectively. Pulsatile GnRH replacement is also possible (25–50 ng/kg every 2 hours) by portable infusion. Isolated hormonal deficiencies can be treated in a similar manner with therapies described above. Spermatogenesis, and specifically sperm in the ejaculate, can take 9–12 months after initiation of therapy. The injectable treatments are long, cumbersome, and expensive, and therefore sperm cryopreservation is highly recommended.

Idiopathic Infertility

Nearly half the men evaluated for infertility will have no identifiable cause or no specific target for therapy. In these instances, empiric medical therapy may be considered. The goals and timeline of treatment should be established upfront in order to progress the couple toward achieving parenthood via other means.

A. *Clomiphene Citrate*

Clomiphene citrate, a selective estrogen receptor modulator, is a synthetic antiestrogen that blocks the feedback inhibition on the HPG axis, resulting in increased secretions of GnRH, FSH, and LH. The resultant effect is an increase in endogenous testosterone that may improve spermatogenesis. It is only FDA-approved for treatment of female infertility, though it has been in "off-label" use for men for decades. The ideal candidate for clomiphene therapy is a man with low sperm counts in the setting of low-normal LH, FSH, and testosterone levels. Typical dose is 12.5–50 mg/day. Serum gonadotropins and testosterone should be evaluated at 3–4 weeks and dose adjusted to maintain testosterone in the normal range. Higher than normal testosterone levels may lead to hyperestrogenemia and decreased sperm quality. Duration of therapy should be limited to 6 months if no improvement is seen. Results of over 30 studies have been equivocal with regard to effectiveness of clomiphene as an empiric treatment. There is emerging data showing that clomiphene therapy may improve odds of sperm retrieval in men with nonobstructive azoospermia [92].

B. *Antioxidants*

Evidence suggests that nearly 40% of men with infertility have high levels of reactive oxygen species (ROS) within the reproductive tract. ROS (OH, O_2 radicals, hydrogen peroxide) damage sperm membranes via lipid peroxidation resulting in dysmotility and dysfunction. Commonly used agents such as glutathione, vitamins C and E, carnitine, coenzyme Q10, and fish oil may be useful in men with elevated semen ROS; however, high-quality studies demonstrating efficacy are still lacking [90].

Assisted Reproductive Technology

Assisted reproductive technology (ART) can be utilized if no medical or surgical therapy improves chances of natural pregnancy. ART typically refers to IUI and IVF/ICSI.

Intrauterine Insemination (IUI)

IUI is considered a "low-technology" form of ART and involves placement of a washed pellet of ejaculated sperm into female uterus via the cervix. IUI can be used for female factor (cervical conditions) as well as male factor (low sperm quality, immunologic infertility, or inability to deliver sperm through intercourse). At least 5–40 million motile sperm are required in order to have the best odds of success. Pregnancy rates range from 8% to 16% per cycle in couples with male infertility and can be even higher when the female partner is treated to stimulate ovulation [93].

In Vitro Fertilization and Intracytoplasmic Sperm Injection (IVF/ICSI)

IVF is the "high-technology" form of ART, whereby ultrasound-guided egg retrieval is performed with ovarian stimulation followed by fertilization with washed sperm in petri dish. It is important to note that traditional IVF requires 50,000 to 5 million post-wash motile sperm. When faced with severe male infertility, ICSI can be employed. First described in 1992, ICSI involves microscopic injection of a single sperm into the subzonal space of an egg. With the advent of ICSI, the requirement for fertilization has decreased to a single viable sperm. This technology has presented more aggressive options for men with azoospermia and has led to the development of new surgical techniques to retrieve sperm (discussed below). When advanced technology is utilized, barriers to natural selection are limited, such that genetic defects causing infertility may now be passed on to the offspring. Therefore, long-term implications of ICSI on genetic health of the progeny remain to be seen. A higher incidence of hypospadias in babies conceived through ICSI has been documented in some studies. Couples should be made aware that known genetic conditions, such as Y microdeletions, would be passed on to the male offspring when sperm is successfully retrieved from the fathers [94–97].

Sperm Retrieval

Sperm retrieval is indicated when ejaculation of sperm is not feasible or because the couple has elected to use IVF rather than vasectomy reversal. Testicular sperm retrieval may also be possible in men with nonobstructive azoospermia when there is evidence of focal hypospermatogenesis present within the testis. Due to the wide scope of retrieval indications, a variety of techniques have evolved ranging from minimally invasive aspiration to invasive dissection with the use of an operating microscope. Aspiration can be performed from the vas deferens, epididymis, or the testicle. Couple must be advised that IVF is a requisite when sperm retrieval is elected.

A. *Vasal Aspiration*

The vas deferens is delivered through a scrotal incision, and a hemi-vasotomy is made with the use of an operating microscope. Vasal fluid is then aspirated into a culture medium. Once ample sperm is obtained (>10–20 million), the vasotomy is repaired using microscopic sutures. This procedure may be performed as a stand-alone procedure or in conjunction with a vasectomy reversal. It provides the most mature sperm; however, it is fairly invasive and not utilized commonly.

B. *Epididymal Sperm Aspiration*

This technique is performed as a percutaneous or microscopic procedure. A percutaneous epididymal sperm aspiration (PESA) can be performed when the epididymis is palpable and obstruction is suspected. It is less invasive; however,

Fig. 5.11 A variety of sperm retrieval techniques are demonstrated, both percutaneous and microscope-guided based on the specific need of the patient. (Adapted from Turek [98])

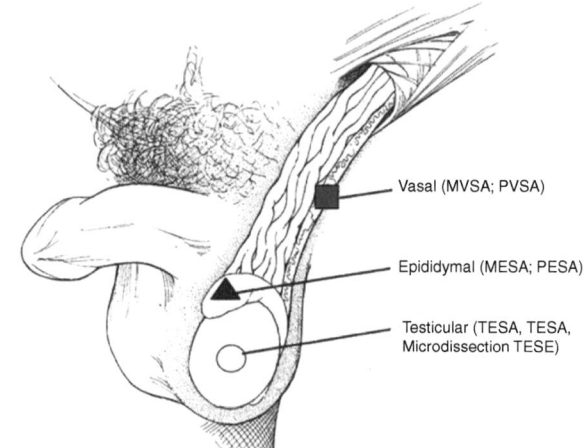

Vasal (MVSA; PVSA)

Epididymal (MESA; PESA)

Testicular (TESA, TESA, Microdissection TESE)

blind insertion of a needle can theoretically result in tubular damage. By contrast, microscopic epididymal sperm aspiration (MESA) involves direct collection of sperm from a single, isolated epididymal tubule with aid of an operating microscope. After enough sperm is obtained, the epididymal tubule is close with microscopic sutures. Of note, both testicular and epididymal sperm are utilized for ICSI as they are not as mature as vasal sperm (Fig. 5.11).

C. *Testicular Sperm Retrieval*

Testicular sperm extraction (TESE) is recommended in the setting of vasal or epididymal obstruction when reconstruction is not desired or technically feasible. It may also be recommended when there is severe testis failure and the low amounts of sperm produced do not reach the ejaculate. Like epididymal procedures, testicular retrievals are also highly variable in technique and invasiveness. A traditional TESE involves a scrotal incision and small opening into the tunica albuginea through which a small section of testis tissue is retrieved and transferred to a buffer solution. When uniform, low-volume spermatogenesis is known or suspected, a testicular sperm aspiration (TESA) can also be performed percutaneously. By contrast, in a man with suspected nonobstructive azoospermia or markedly reduced spermatogenesis, sperm retrieval may be possible with microdissection testicular sperm extraction (microTESE), whereby the testis is bivalved, and tissue is meticulously dissected with the aid of an operating microscope. Finally, testicular fine needle aspiration mapping may also be employed in men with nonobstructive azoospermia in order to guide sperm retrieval.

References

1. World Health Organization (WHO). Infertility: a tabulation of available data on prevalence of primary and secondary infertility. Geneva: WHO; 1991.
2. Tielemans E, Burdorf A, Te Velde E, et al. Sources of bias in studies among infertility clients. Am J Epidemiol. 2002;156:86–92.

3. Turek PJ. Male infertility. In: Tanagho EA, McAninch JC, editors. Smith's urology. 16th ed. Stamford: Appleton & Lange; 2008.
4. Russell L. Sertoli-germ cell interactions: a review. Gamete Res. 1980;3:179.
5. Steinberger E, et al. Molecular mechanisms concerned with hormonal effects on the seminiferous tubule and endocrine relationships at puberty in the male. CH Spilman TJ Lobl KT Kirton et al. Regulatory mechanisms of male reproductive physiology. Excerpta Med Amsterdam. 1976;6:29–34.
6. Eik-Nes KB, et al. Biosynthesis and secretion of testicular steroids. In: Greep RO, Astwood EB, editors. Handbook of physiology. Baltimore: Williams & Wilkins; 1975. p. 95.
7. Hess RA, et al. A role for estrogens in the male reproductive system. Nature. 1997;390:509.
8. Ewing LL, et al. Regulation of testicular function: a spatial and temporal view. In: Greep RO, editor. International review of physiology. Baltimore: University Park Press; 1980. p. 41.
9. Von Eckardstein S, et al. Serum inhibin B in combination with FSH is a more sensitive marker than FSH alone for impaired spermatogenesis in men, but cannot predict the presence of sperm in testicular tissue samples. J Clin Endocrinol Metab. 1999;84:2496.
10. Gui YL, et al. Male hormonal contraception: suppression of spermatogenesis by injectable testosterone undecanoate alone or with levonorgestrel implants in Chinese men. J Androl. 2004;25:720.
11. Setchell BP, Waites GM. The blood-testis barrier. In: Greep RO, Astwood EB, editors. Handbook of physiology. Baltimore: Williams & Wilkins; 1975. p. 143–72.
12. Yanagimachi R, et al. Fertilization. In: Knobil E, Neill JD, Greenwald GS, et al., editors. The physiology of reproduction. New York: Raven; 1994. p. 189–317.
13. Aitken RJ, West K, Buckingham D. Leukocytic infiltration into the human ejaculate and its association with semen quality, oxidative stress, and sperm function. J Androl. 1994;15:343.
14. Carlsen E, et al. Evidence for decreasing quality of semen during the past 50 years. Br Med J. 1992;105:609.
15. Lombardo F, Pallotti F, Cargnelutti F, Lenzi A. Anamnesis and physical examination. In: Simoni M, Huhtaniemi I, editors. Endocrinology of the testis and male reproduction. Cham: Springer; 2017.
16. Jarow JP, et al. Report on optimal evaluation of the infertile male. Fertil Steril. 2006;86:S202–9.
17. Sigman M, Jarow JP. Medical evaluation of infertile men. Urology. 1997;50:659.
18. Honig SC, et al. Significant medical pathology uncovered by a comprehensive male infertility evaluation. Fertil Steril. 1994;62:1028.
19. Carlsen E, et al. History of febrile illness and variation in semen quality. Hum Reprod. 2003;18:2089.
20. Sallmen M, et al. Reduced fertility among overweight and obese men. Epidemiology. 2006;17:520.
21. Turek PJ. Practical approach to the diagnosis and management of male infertility. Nature Clin Pract Urol. 2005;2:1.
22. World Health Organization. WHO laboratory manual for the examination of human semen and sperm-cervical mucus interaction. 4th ed. Cambridge: Cambridge University Press; 1999. p. 60–1.
23. Agarwal A, et al. Clinical relevance of oxidative stress in male factor infertility: an update. Am J Reprod Immunol. 2008;59:2.
24. Chemes HE. Phenotypes of sperm pathology: genetic and acquired forms in infertile men. J Androl. 2000;21:799.
25. Hammoud AO, et al. Impact of male obesity on fertility: a critical review of the current literature. Fertil Steril. 2008;90:897.
26. Guzick DS, et al. Sperm morphology, motility and concentration in fertile and infertile men. N Engl J Med. 2001;345:1388.
27. Kruger TF, et al. Predictive value of abnormal sperm morphology in in vitro fertilization. Fertil Steril. 1988;49:112.
28. Zini A, et al. Prevalence of abnormal sperm DNA denaturation in fertile and infertile men. Urology. 2002;60:1069.

29. Clifton DK, Bremner WJ. The effect of testicular X-irradiation on spermatogenesis in man: a comparison with the mouse. J Androl. 1983;4:387.
30. Gandini L, et al. Effect of chemo- or radiotherapy on sperm parameters of testicular cancer patients. Hum Reprod. 2006;21:2882.
31. Meinertz H, et al. Antisperm antibodies and fertility after vasovasostomy: a follow-up study of 216 men. Fertil Steril. 1990;54:315.
32. Evenson DP, et al. Utility of the sperm chromatin structure assay as a diagnostic and prognostic tool in the human fertility clinic. Hum Reprod. 1999;14:1039.
33. Bungum M, et al. Sperm DNA integrity assessment in prediction of assisted reproduction technology outcome. Hum Reprod. 2007;22:174.
34. Zini A, et al. Sperm DNA damage is associated with an increased risk of pregnancy loss after IVF and ICSI: systematic review and meta-analysis. Hum Reprod. 2008;23:2663.
35. Eisenberg ML, et al. Semen quality and pregnancy loss in a contemporary cohort of couples recruited before conception: data from the Longitudinal Investigation of Fertility and the Environment (LIFE) Study. Fertil Steril. 2017;108(4):613–9.
36. Bandmann H. Klinefelter's syndrome. Berlin, Heidelberg: Springer; 1984.
37. Xu WM, et al. Cystic fibrosis transmembrane conductance regulator is vital to sperm fertilizing capacity and male fertility. Proc Natl Acad Sci U S A. 2007;104(23):9816.
38. Oliveira LMB, et al. The importance of autosomal genes in Kallmann syndrome: genotype-phenotype correlations and neuroendocrine characteristics. J Clin Endocrinol Metab. 2001;86:1532.
39. Bourrouillou G, Bujan L, Calvas P, et al. Role and contribution of karyotyping in male infertility. Prog Urol. 1992;2:189.
40. Oates RD. The natural history of endocrine function and spermatogenesis in Klinefelter syndrome: what the data show. Fertil Steril. 2012;98:266–73.
41. Hopps CV, et al. Detection of sperm in men with Y chromosome microdeletions of the AZFa, AZFb and AZFc regions. Hum Reprod. 2003;18:1660.
42. Chillon M, et al. Mutations in the cystic fibrosis gene in patients with congenital absence of the vas deferens. N Engl J Med. 1995;332:1475.
43. Anguiano A, et al. Congenital bilateral absence of the vas deferens: a primarily genital form of cystic fibrosis. JAMA. 1992;267:1794.
44. Freeman S, Bertolotto M, Richenberg J, et al. Ultrasound evaluation of varicoceles: guidelines and recommendations of the European Society of Urogenital Radiology Scrotal and Penile Imaging Working Group (ESUR-SPIWG) for detection, classification, and grading. Eur Radiol. 2020;30:11–25.
45. Fisch H, Lambert SM, Goluboff ET. Management of ejaculatory duct obstruction: etiology, diagnosis, and treatment. World J Urol. 2006;24(6):604–10.
46. Smith JF, Walsh TJ, Turek PJ. Ejaculatory duct obstruction. Urol Clin North Am. 2008;35(2):221.
47. Jarow JP. Transrectal ultrasonography of infertile men. Fertil Steril. 1993;60:1035.
48. Schoor RA, et al. The role of testicular biopsy in the modern management of male infertility. J Urol. 2002;167:197.
49. Practice Committee of the American Society for Reproductive Medicine in collaboration with the Society for Male Reproduction and Urology. Evaluation of the azoospermic male: a committee opinion. Fertil Steril. 2018;18(5):777–82.
50. Turek PJ, et al. Diagnostic findings from testis fine needle aspiration mapping in obstructed and non-obstructed azoospermic men. J Urol. 2000;163:1709.
51. Turek PJ, Cha I, Ljung BM. Systematic fine needle aspiration of the testis: Correlation to biopsy and the results of organ "mapping" for mature sperm in azoospermic men. Urology. 1997;49:743.
52. Urban MD, Lee PA, Migeon CJ. Adult height and fertility in men with congenital virilizing adrenal hyperplasia. N Engl J Med. 1978;299:1392.
53. Wu SM, Chan WY. Male pseudohermaphroditism due to inactivating luteinizing hormone receptor mutations. Arch Med Res. 1999;30:495.

54. Aiman J, et al. Androgen insensitivity as a cause of infertility in otherwise normal men. N Engl J Med. 1979;300:223.
55. Griffin JE. Androgen resistance: the clinical and molecular spectrum. N Engl J Med. 1992;326:611.
56. Fujisawa M, et al. Growth hormone releasing hormone test for infertile men with spermatogenetic maturation arrest. J Urol. 2002;168:2083.
57. Goffin V, et al. Prolactin: the new biology of an old hormone. Annu Rev Physiol. 2002;64:47.
58. Carter JN, et al. Prolactin-secreting tumors and hypogonadism in 22 men. N Engl J Med. 1978;299:847.
59. Aiman J, Griffin JE. The frequency of androgen receptor deficiency in infertile men. J Clin Endocrinol Metab. 1982;54:725. [PMID: 6801070].
60. Kostiner DR, Turek PJ, Reijo RA. Male infertility: analysis of the markers and genes on the human Y chromosome. Hum Reprod. 1998;13:3032.
61. Pryor JL, et al. Microdeletions in the Y chromosome of infertile men. N Engl J Med. 1997;336:534.
62. Silber SJ, Repping S. Transmission of male infertility to future generations: lessons from the Y chromosome. Hum Reprod Update. 2002;8:217.
63. Kurda-Kawaguchi T, et al. The AZFc region of the Y chromosome features massive palindromes and uniform recurrent deletions in infertile men. Nat Genet. 2001;29:279.
64. Reijo R, et al. Diverse spermatogenic defects in humans caused by Y chromosome deletions encompassing a novel RNA-binding protein gene. Nat Genet. 1995;10:383.
65. Lipshultz LI, et al. Testicular function after orchiopexy for unilaterally undescended testis. N Engl J Med. 1976;295:15. [PMID: 5671].
66. Walsh TJ, et al. Prepubertal orchidopexy for cryptorchidism may be associated with lower risk of testicular cancer. J Urol. 2007;178:1440.
67. Nagler HM, Deitch AD, deVere White R. Testicular torsion: temporal considerations. Fertil Steril. 1984;42:257.
68. Richardson I, et al. Outcomes of varicocele treatment: an updated critical analysis. Urol Clin North Am. 2008;35:191. [PMID: 18423240].
69. Walsh TJ, et al. Differences in the clinical characteristics of primarily and secondarily infertile men with varicocele. Fertil Steril. 2009;91:826.
70. World Health Organization. The influence of varicocele on parameters of fertility in a large group of men presenting to infertility clinics. Fertil Steril. 1992;57:1289.
71. Cayan S, et al. Can varicocelectomy significantly change the way couples use assisted reproductive technologies? J Urol. 2002;167:1749.
72. Cayan S, et al. Response to varicocelectomy in oligospermic men with and without defined genetic infertility. Urology. 2001;57:530.
73. Evers JLH, Collins JA. Assessment of efficacy of varicocele repair for male subfertility: a systematic review. Lancet. 2003;361:1849.
74. Madgar I, et al. Controlled trial of high spermatic vein ligation for varicocele in infertile men. Fertil Steril. 1995;63:120.
75. Handelsman DJ, et al. Young's syndrome: obstructive azoospermia and chronic sinopulmonary infections. N Engl J Med. 1984;310:3.
76. Damani MN, et al. Post-chemotherapy ejaculatory azoospermia: fatherhood with sperm from testis tissue using intracytoplasmic sperm injection. J Clin Oncol. 2002;20:930.
77. Eisenberg ML, et al. Ejaculatory duct manometry in normal men and in patients with ejaculatory duct obstruction. J Urol. 2008;180:255.
78. Belker AM, et al. Results of 1,469 microsurgical vasectomy reversals by the vasovasostomy study group. J Urol. 1991;145:505.
79. Eisenberg ML, et al. Racial differences in vasectomy utilization in the United States: data from the national survey of family growth. Urology. 2009;74:1020.
80. Fuchs EF, Burt RA. Vasectomy reversal performed 15 years or more after vasectomy: correlation of pregnancy outcome with partner age and with pregnancy results of in vitro fertilization with intracytoplasmic sperm injection. Fertil Steril. 2002;77:516.

81. Matthews GJ, Schlegel PN, Goldstein M. Patency following microsurgical vasoepididymostomy and vasovasostomy: temporal considerations. J Urol. 1993;154:2070.
82. Meng M, Green K, Turek PJ. Surgery or assisted reproduction? A decision analysis of treatment costs in male infertility. J Urol. 2005;174:1926.
83. Kapadia AA, Ostrowski KA. Reconsidering vasectomy reversal over assisted reproduction in older couples. Fertil Steril. 2018;109(6):1020–4.
84. Yang G, et al. The kinetics of the return of motile sperm to the ejaculate after vasectomy reversal. J Urol. 2007;177:2272.
85. Marks S. Vasovasostomy: multilayer microsurgical anastomosis. In: Vasectomy reversal. Cham: Springer; 2018.
86. Matsuda T, Horii Y, Yoshida O. Obstructive azoospermia of unknown origin: sites of obstruction and surgical outcomes. J Urol. 1994;151:1543.
87. Kadioglu A, et al. Does response to treatment of ejaculatory duct obstruction in infertile men vary with pathology? Fertil Steril. 2001;76:138.
88. Hendry WF. Disorders of ejaculation: congenital, acquired and functional. Br J Urol. 1998;82(3):331–41.
89. Bennett CJ, et al. Sexual dysfunction and electroejaculation in men with spinal cord injury: review. J Urol. 1988;139:453.
90. Baker WHG, et al. Protective effect of antioxidants on the impairment of semen motility by activated polymorphonuclear leukocytes. Fertil Steril. 1996;65:411.
91. Branigan EF, Muller CH. Efficacy of treatment and recurrence rate of leukocytospermia in infertile men with prostatitis. Fertil Steril. 1994;62:580.
92. Patel DP, et al. The safety and efficacy of clomiphene citrate in hypoandrogenic and subfertile men. Int J Impot Res. 2015;27(6):221–4. https://doi.org/10.1038/ijir.2015.21. Epub 2015 Aug 20.
93. Guzick DS, et al. Efficacy of superovulation and intrauterine insemination in the treatment of infertility. National Cooperative Reproductive Medicine Network. N Engl J Med. 1999;340:177.
94. Kenti-First MG, et al. Infertility in intracytoplasmic-sperm-injection-derived sons. Lancet. 1996;348:332.
95. Walsh TJ, et al. The genetics of male infertility. Semin Reprod Med. 2009;27(2):124.
96. Xu EY, Moore FL, Reijo Pera RA. A gene family required for human germ cell development evolved from an ancient meiotic gene conserved in metazoans. Proc Natl Acad Sci U S A. 2001;98:7414.
97. Cox G, et al. Intracytoplasmic sperm injection may increase the risk of imprinting defects. Am J Hum Genet. 2002;71:162.
98. Turek PJ. Sperm retrieval techniques. In: Carrell DT, Peterson CM, editors. Reproductive endocrinology and infertility. New York: Springer; 2010.

Chapter 6
Evaluation and Management of Erectile Dysfunction

Christopher I. Sayegh, Joseph M. Caputo, Vinson Wang, and Denise Asafu-Adjei

Epidemiology and History of Erectile Dysfunction

Erectile dysfunction (ED) is the most studied sexual dysfunction and one of the most common medical conditions, affecting about 52% of men between ages 40 and 70 [1]. The societal burden of ED is significant, and it is estimated that 322 million men will be affected worldwide by 2025 [2]. In the United States, ED affects approximately 18 million men [3]. The prevalence among adult men is estimated at about 20% worldwide, with higher prevalence rates among older age cohorts [4]. In one study, the crude ED incidence rate was 25.9 cases/1000 man-years among men aged 40–69 [5]. If all affected men in the United States sought some type of ED therapy, treatment costs would theoretically approach a staggering $15 billion [6].

ED management has evolved in the last several decades. In the pre-1970s era, the sole diagnostic tool available to the physician was taking a psychosexual history. More of these diagnostic tools have become available over the past half century. Providers can now perform a complete medical and psychosexual history, physical examination, endocrine evaluation, and penile duplex ultrasound, as well as perform in-office intracavernosal injections, just to name a few. Similarly, an increasing number of therapies have become available over the years, which will be the focus of this chapter. With all of these available diagnostic tools and therapeutic options, multiple professional governing medical bodies now contribute to ED management guidelines and recommendations, including the American Urological Association (AUA), Sexual Medicine Society of North America, American Academy of Family Physicians, European Association of Urology, and the Canadian Urological Association.

C. I. Sayegh (✉) · J. M. Caputo · V. Wang · D. Asafu-Adjei
Columbia University Irving Medical Center, Department of Urology, New York, NY, USA
e-mail: Cs2948@cumc.columbia.edu

© Springer Nature Switzerland AG 2021   93
J. P. Alukal et al. (eds.), *Design and Implementation of the Modern Men's Health Center*, https://doi.org/10.1007/978-3-030-54482-9_6

Principles of Management

Erectile dysfunction is a unique medical entity in that its diagnosis is largely based on the merit of subjective complaints. Often times, ancillary diagnostic tools that are otherwise commonly used have limited utility in its diagnosis. These notions have implications for how to approach and appropriately manage patients who come to the clinic with complaints of ED. Although treating ED with oral pharmacotherapy is often successful, adequate time should be taken to systematically review a patient's history in order to arrive at the most optimal therapeutic outcome and to ensure treatment of the problem and not just the symptom.

Early Detection of ED

Several investigations have uncovered the notion that many patients who suffer from ED also have other common medical cómorbidities. These risk factors for erectile dysfunction include diabetes, hypertension, cardiovascular disease, hypercholesterolemia, benign prostatic hyperplasia (BPH) with urinary symptoms, current cigarette smoking, being overweight, leading a sedentary lifestyle, and antidepressant use [3, 7]. Providers are thus afforded the opportunity to screen patients for these comorbidities who come to the clinic complaining of ED. In identifying the presence of these risk factors, providers can further tailor the management of their patients.

Goal-Directed Management with Shared Decision-Making and the Role of the Partner Interview

A goal-directed method of managing patients with ED has been a largely accepted tactic for decades [8]. The aim of this approach is to develop a therapeutic plan that is catered specifically to the patient, allowing for the best outcome in terms of sexual function. The provider is charged with the responsibility to provide all appropriate treatment options, recognizing that the goals and expectations of patients will vary on a case-by-case basis. All risks, benefits, advantages, and disadvantages for each option should be discussed in order to allow the patient and provider to make the most appropriate informed and shared decision.

The partner can also be a significant source of relevant information regarding the patient's ED and can help with guiding treatment. Information shared by the partner can help provide insight into the couple's relationship, the patient's sexual dysfunction, and the ultimate goal for both the patient and partner in treating ED. In fact, the role of the partner interview has been shown to influence both the diagnosis and management of ED in nearly 60% of cases [9]. The partner can also be helpful in maintaining the patient's treatment adherence.

Referring to a Specialist and Follow-Up Care

Due to the ease of use and efficacy of oral pharmacotherapy for ED, many primary providers have found comfort in managing most straightforward cases without specialty referral. Despite this, there still exist many presentations that are more complex and likely require the assistance of a specialist. These multidisciplinary teams for less straightforward cases of ED can be comprised of cardiologists, endocrinologists, psychiatrists, psychologists, other surgeons, and urologists. Some potential indications for referral include failure of initial treatment, younger patients, those with a history of pelvic trauma, anatomic deformities (e.g., Peyronie's disease), endocrinopathies (e.g., pituitary adenomas and secondary hypogonadism), psychosexual disorders, and severe cardiovascular disease.

Follow-up care is an essential aspect of the treatment strategy for patients with ED. Without adequate systematic follow-up, studies have demonstrated that patients tend to be less adherent, with high treatment discontinuation rates [10]. Follow-up also allows for the provider to titrate medication doses and address any potential ongoing psychosexual issues that may be contributing to the patient's sexual dysfunction.

Diagnostic Evaluation

A comprehensive medical, psychosocial, and surgical history, focused physical examination, and appropriate laboratory testing are crucial in the evaluation of patients presenting with ED. Due to the sensitive nature associated with ED and sexual dysfunction, it is essential to approach the patient encounter with the utmost professionalism to foster trust and encourage a strong doctor-patient relationship. Therefore, it is necessary to ensure that all history is obtained privately with the patient, assuring confidentiality.

It is believed that sexual dysfunction is underdiagnosed because physicians often do not include sexual histories in the patient encounter [11]. Some have proposed a standardized template for obtaining a sexual history for all providers to ensure sexual dysfunctions are being adequately captured and appropriately treated. Furthermore, the use of questionnaires for evaluating and managing sexual issues has been validated with reportedly high patient satisfaction rates [12].

Medical History and Cardiac Risk Assessment

A thorough medical and surgical history needs to be obtained in patients presenting with ED. As mentioned in the "Principles of Management" section of this chapter, the diagnosis of ED carries with it the inherent risk of other comorbidities that are yet to be diagnosed. The association of ED with cardiovascular disease is of particular importance. A multidisciplinary forum, known as the Princeton Consensus, was developed and convened for several discussions regarding this link between sexual activity and cardiac risk. One of the fundamental notions to come out of these conferences was that all men with ED, even in the absence of active cardiac symptoms, should be considered at risk for cardiovascular disease [13]. Therefore, it is the role of the provider to ensure that a complete medical history is obtained and the patient has been seen by the appropriate practitioner.

The most updated Princeton Consensus guidelines from 2012 state that all ED patients should undergo a thorough evaluation in order to stratify their cardiovascular risk as either high, intermediate, or low. High-risk individuals include those patients who have unstable or refractory angina, recent myocardial infarction (MI), uncontrolled hypertension (HTN), New York Heart Association (NYHA) class IV congestive heart failure (CHF), or certain high-risk arrhythmias. For all high-risk patients, sexual activity with any ED therapy should be delayed until the respective cardiac condition is stabilized via cardiology referral. Intermediate-risk patients include those with mild to moderate stable angina, MI within the past 2–8 weeks without intervention, NYHA class III CHF, and noncardiac vascular disease. Intermediate-risk patients should receive the minimum standard of care in terms of their cardiovascular management prior to initiating therapy for ED. Low-risk individuals include successfully revascularized patients, those with asymptomatic controlled HTN or mild valvular disease, and patients with NYHA class I and II CHF. Generally, low-risk patients can usually be sexually active and begin an ED treatment without further evaluation. Regardless of the patient's cardiovascular risk category, the Princeton Consensus suggests that behavioral modifications, such as improved physical activity and weight control, are fundamental interventions for all patients with ED [14].

Taking a thorough surgical history is another crucial aspect to the patient's evaluation. It primarily assists in determining the etiology for the ED. Specifically, it is important to ask about prior pelvic surgery (i.e., cystectomy, prostatectomy) and prior penile surgery. Furthermore, patients should be asked about a prior history of pelvic radiation, as radiation exposure can result in nerve damage and subsequent ED. A history of any prior trauma resulting in either spinal cord injury or pelvic/genital injury should also be obtained as these are risk factors for ED. Lastly, a medication history should be obtained in order to elicit medications that are known to be associated with ED. See Table 6.1 for different agents that can impact erectile function.

Table 6.1 Abbreviated list of drugs found to be associated with erectile dysfunction

Drug class	Specific drugs
Antihypertensives	Thiazide diuretics, loop diuretics, non-selective beta-blockers
Antidepressants	Tricyclics; selective serotonin reuptake inhibitors; serotonin and norepinephrine reuptake inhibitors
Antipsychotics	Phenothiazines
Antiulcer drugs	H_2 receptor antagonists (cimetidine)
Cytotoxic agents	Cyclophosphamide, methotrexate
Opiates	Morphine, oxycodone, hydrocodone

This is an adapted figure originally published in Campbell-Walsh Urology, 11th Edition, Wein et al., Chapter 27: Evaluation and Management of Erectile Dysfunction, Page 645, Copyright Elsevier 2016 [15]

Psychosocial History

Obtaining an accurate psychosocial history for all patients presenting with ED cannot be stressed enough. It is important to note that there is a definite link between sexual function and mental well-being and that particular psychosocial situations can adversely affect sexual function. Specific questions regarding emotional stressors, relationship difficulties, and body image concerns should be addressed in their relation to the timing of ED onset. Please see the "Mental Health" section of this chapter for more details.

Sexual History

The sexual history serves to completely characterize the patient's ED including symptom onset, duration, severity, progression, and situational differences (partner vs alone, nocturnal erections, etc.). It is important to also understand if the patient's ED is interfering with sexual intercourse, as often patients with mild ED symptoms are still able to achieve erections satisfactory for intercourse. Some patients may not be comfortable talking in depth about their sexual history. Ensuring them that this is an essential part of the history and physical exam is important. Starting with open-ended questions before asking more detailed questions may also help to put the patient at ease.

Patients should be asked about prior treatments for ED including any pharmacologic therapy (oral, intracavernosal, intraurethral), vacuum erection devices, and surgery. For those who report treatment failure with phosphodiesterase type 5 (PDE5) inhibitors, it is important to ensure that they are taking these medications properly. In fact, studies report that incorrect use of PDE5 inhibitors accounts for 56–81% of treatment failures [16–19]. Dosage, time relation to food consumption, time relation to desired sexual activity, and the use of sexual stimulation should all be verified.

All patients should be asked about sexual preference, sexual partners, and concern for sexually transmitted diseases. Finally, it is important to inquire about pain with intercourse and penile curvature, as this may be a sign of Peyronie's disease, a known cause of ED.

Questionnaires

Questionnaires have been used for many years to assist in obtaining the sexual history for patients with ED. In the 1970s, the Derogatis Sexual Functioning Inventory was used [20]. This questionnaire consisted of 245 questions and was largely impractical for patients to complete. In the 1980s, the Golombok Rust Inventory of Sexual Satisfaction (GRISS) was introduced [21]. This was made up of 28 questions. Similar to the Derogatis Sexual Functioning Inventory, this aimed to differentiate psychogenic ED from non-psychogenic ED. Since the introduction of these early instruments, an array of other tools have been developed.

The more commonly used instruments are the International Index of Erectile Function (IIEF), the Brief Male Sexual Function Inventory (BMSFI), the Erection Hardness Score (EHS), and the Male Sexual Health Questionnaire (MSHQ) [22–25]. The IIEF contains 15 questions, shown in Table 6.2, that are divided into five domains: erectile function (Q1–5, Q15), sexual desire (Q6, Q11–12), satisfaction with intercourse (Q7–8), overall satisfaction (Q13–14), and orgasmic function (Q9-10). ED is classified into five categories based on overall responses: no ED (22–25), mild (17–21), mild to moderate (12–16), moderate (8–11), and severe (5–7). An abridged 5-question version called the IIEF-5 or the Sexual Health Inventory for Men (SHIM) includes questions specifically pertaining to the domain of erectile function. This was developed to diagnose the presence and severity of ED and is a quicker questionnaire to complete, making its use widely practical in many clinics [26]. The SHIM and IIEF are very commonly used as outcome measures in ED studies.

Table 6.2 Individual items of International Index of Erectile Function Questionnaire and response options

Questions	Response options	Questions	Response options
Q1. How often were you able to get an erection during sexual activity? **Q2.** When you had erections with sexual stimulation, how often were your erections hard enough for penetration?	0 = No sexual activity 1 = Almost never/never 2 = A few times (much less than half the time) 3 = Sometimes (about half the time) 4 = Most times (much more than half the time) 5 = Almost always/always	**Q8.** How much have you enjoyed sexual intercourse?	0 = No intercourse 1 = No enjoyment 2 = Not very enjoyable 3 = Fairly enjoyable 4 = Highly enjoyable 5 = Very highly enjoyable
Q3. When you attempted sexual intercourse, how often were you able to penetrate (enter) your partner? **Q4.** During sexual intercourse, *how often* were you able to maintain your erection after you had penetrated (entered) your partner?	0 = Did not attempt intercourse 1 = Almost never/never 2 = A few times (much less than half the time) 3 = Sometimes (about half the time) 4 = Most times (much more than half the time) 5 = Almost always/always	**Q9.** When you had sexual stimulation *or* intercourse, how often did you ejaculate? **Q10.** When you had sexual stimulation *or* intercourse, how often did you have the feeling of orgasm or climax?	0 = No sexual stimulation/intercourse 1 = Almost never/never 2 = A few times (much less than half the time) 3 = Sometimes (about half the time) 4 = Most times (much more than half the time) 5 = Almost always/always

Table 6.2 (continued)

Questions	Response options	Questions	Response options
Q5. During sexual intercourse, *how difficult* was it to maintain your erection to completion of intercourse?	0 = Did not attempt intercourse 1 = Extremely difficult 2 = Very difficult 3 = Difficult 4 = Slightly difficult 5 = Not difficult	**Q11.** How often have you felt sexual desire?	1 = Almost never/never 2 = A few times (much less than half the time) 3 = Sometimes (about half the time) 4 = Most times (much more than half the time) 5 = Almost always/always
Q6. How many times have you attempted sexual intercourse?	0 = No attempts 1 = One to two attempts 2 = Three to four attempts 3 = Five to six attempts 4 = Seven to ten attempts 5 = 11 + attempts	**Q12.** How would you rate your level of sexual desire?	1 = Very low/none at all 2 = Low 3 = Moderate 4 = High 5 = Very high
Q7. When you attempted sexual intercourse, how often was it satisfactory for you?	0 = Did not attempt intercourse 1 = Almost never/never 2 = A few times (much less than half the time) 3 = Sometimes (about half the time) 4 = Most times (much more than half the time) 5 = Almost always/always	**Q13.** How satisfied have you been with your overall *sex life*? **Q14.** How satisfied have you been with your *sexual relationship* with your partner?	1 = Very dissatisfied 2 = Moderately dissatisfied 3 = About equally satisfied and dissatisfied 4 = Moderately satisfied 5 = Very satisfied
		Q15. How do you rate your *confidence* that you could get and keep an erection?	1 = Very low 2 = Low 3 = Moderate 4 = High 5 = Very high

Precede all questions listed below with the phrase, "Over the past 4 weeks…." Use the scale to the right of each question in determining response

Reprinted from Rosen et al. [22], Copyright 1997, with permission from Elsevier

Physical Exam

The physical exam provides information for possible etiologies of ED. Considering that the potential causes of organic ED may be broken down into a few general categories including vascular, neurologic, endocrine, and anatomic, the physical exam will provide insight into which category the patient falls into. Of course, patients may fit into more than one of these categories.

Obesity, hypertension, or diminished extremity pulses are all representative of a likely vascular cause of ED. As discussed earlier, it is essential to ensure that these patients are provided with appropriate medical follow-up/evaluation. Much in the way that diabetic retinopathy is a sequela of poorly controlled diabetes, ED can be a sequela of undiagnosed cardiovascular disease. Poor sensation in the perineum or lower extremities may be consistent with peripheral neuropathy, as is seen with patients with diabetes. Signs of hypogonadism (gynecomastia, small testes, poor masculinization) may be signs of an endocrine cause of ED. Penile abnormalities (penile plaque, micropenis, chordee) are all possible signs that ED is anatomic in origin. The penis should be held taut and palpated along the corpora to assess for any plaques. In uncircumcised men, the foreskin should be examined for phimosis. Patients with severe phimosis may have difficulty and pain with erections and intercourse.

Laboratory Testing

There is not much of a consensus among various societal guidelines regarding laboratory testing in patients with ED. We believe that total testosterone should at least be obtained in all men with ED. This is supported by the AUA guideline on the evaluation of ED because sexual symptoms tend to be worse with lower testosterone levels [27, 28]. Testosterone should be checked in the early morning since diurnal variations can be up marked, with up to 25% lower values obtained in the late afternoon [29].

Other laboratory testing can be considered and is based on the physician's discretion and the particular clinical scenario. These include fasting glucose, hemoglobin A1c, thyroid function tests, prolactin, and luteinizing hormone.

Vascular Evaluation

One of the most common tests performed to evaluate for vasculogenic ED is an in-office intracavernosal injection of an erectogenic agent with simultaneous duplex ultrasonography (DUS). The aim of this evaluation is to assess the vascular requirements involved in erectile function: arterial inflow and veno-occlusion within the corpora. Penile DUS therefore provides information regarding possible arterial insufficiency or veno-occlusive dysfunction. During the DUS, the two key parameters measured are the peak systolic velocity (PSV) and the end diastolic velocity (EDV) in assessing penile vascular dynamics. PSV is the cavernosal artery blood flow rate at the start of systole and EDV is the cavernosal artery blood flow rate at the end of diastole. Normative values have neem described with a PSV < 25–30 cm/s consistent with arterial insufficiency and EDV > 5 cm/s consistent with veno-occlusive dysfunction.

Lifestyle Management

Lifestyle modifications can have a major impact on sexual function and are first-line recommendations for ED. Many risk factors for ED are preventable, implying that modifying these risk factors can prevent ED or at least improve erectile function.

Physical Activity

Several studies have shown improvement in sexual dysfunction with exercise and associated weight loss [30]. Physical activity is the most effective way to increase nitric oxide and strengthen endothelial function, with direct implications on erectile function. Exercise can also increase testosterone and positive body image, which can also impact erectile function. Physical activity interventions have demonstrated significant efficacy in the treatment of ED, with varying effects dependent on exercise modalities.

Diet

Certain diets have shown promising potential and results in regard to ED treatment [31]. The Mediterranean diet, which consists of fish, fruits, vegetables, and whole grains, were shown in the PREDIMED randomized controlled trial to lower the incidence of type 2 diabetes, metabolic syndrome, and cardiovascular events [32, 33]. Plant-based or vegetarian diets also have well-established benefits on cardiovascular disease, which in turn affect erectile function [31]. Additionally, polyphenols in plant-based diets suggest reduction in reactive oxygen species and activation of endothelial nitric oxide synthase [34]. There is continued need for research on the direct implications of these diets on ED.

Mental Health

Given the inherent overlap of sexual dysfunction with associated psychological and emotional concerns, it should come as no surprise that mental health maintenance is a pillar in the treatment of erectile dysfunction. If psychological factors seem to be the sole contributor to the patient's ED after performing a thorough psychosocial history, then they are deemed to have psychogenic ED. Although the data is lacking in this area, it is generally accepted that psychosexual therapy with trained professionals is very effective at managing these patients. Examples of psychosexual therapies include systematic desensitization, anxiety reduction, sensate focus, interpersonal therapy, behavioral assignments, sex education, couples' communications and sexual skills training, and masturbation exercises [35]. Although it has been difficult to quantify the significance of any of these interventions on the treatment of psychogenic ED, some studies do exist that demonstrate a qualitative improvement in sexual function based on validated questionnaires [36].

It is indeed possible that psychogenic ED can occur in combination with organic causes as well. In these cases, medical treatments alone may be insufficient, and an integrated approach should be taken. This notion is supported by the fact that despite medical treatments being efficacious up to 90% of the time, nearly half of patients will still discontinue their medical therapy for ED [37]. It is clear from this that clinicians should be doing a better job at addressing the patient's entire sexual history, taking time to incorporate any relevant psychological or interpersonal issues that the patient may be experiencing. More specifically, performance anxiety, depression, unrealistic expectations, feelings of inadequacy, the patient's overall relationship with his partner, and life stressors are just some of the issues that the provider needs to address. Integrated treatments, combining behavioral therapies with medical therapy, have shown promise in managing patients with ED in the setting of potential psychosexual concerns [35, 38]. Although these social and emotional matters may be difficult to discuss, providers should be able counsel patients with mild psychosexual symptoms. Those with a more significant psychogenic component to their ED should be referred to mental health providers who are more familiar with psychosexual therapy.

Oral Therapy

Oral pharmacologic therapy is often the first type of medical therapy recommended for patients suffering from ED due to its high efficacy, convenience, noninvasiveness, and favorable adverse-effect profile. Patients with ED will frequently request these oral medications, as their popularity has grown over the years. Thus, it goes without saying that both providers and patients should be fully aware of the risks, benefits, and contraindications to this commonly utilized class of medications.

Phosphodiesterase Type 5 Inhibitors

The mechanism in which phosphodiesterase type 5 (PDE5) inhibitors are able to influence erectile physiology is by taking advantage of the nitric oxide-induced vasodilatory pathway. Normally, nitric oxide acts as a substrate for the cavernosal smooth muscle plasma membrane enzyme guanylate cyclase. Upon binding, cyclic guanosine monophosphate (cGMP) is synthesized, which leads to decreased intracellular calcium. This then yields a relaxation of the cavernosal smooth muscle cells, resulting in an erection. Detumescence is associated with the enzyme PDE5, which triggers the catabolism and breakdown of cGMP. PDE5 inhibitors act on this pathway and competitively inhibit the PDE5 enzyme, thereby increasing both the number and duration of erections [39, 40]. An important point to note is that PDE5 inhibitors function by enhancing, but not inducing, the erectile physiologic pathway. Therefore, patients must be aware of the fact that the nitric oxide pathway must still be initiated by a patient's intact penile nerve endings in the setting of sexual stimuli [41].

After the initial FDA approval of sildenafil citrate for ED in 1998, three other PDE5 inhibitors have also emerged as viable options over the years: vardenafil hydrochloride, tadalafil, and avanafil. All four of these medications have proven to demonstrate equivalent efficacy with similar adverse-effect profiles, and they have generally resulted in success rates of around 70% [42–44]. In patients with medical comorbidities, improvements in their conditions (such as optimal glycemic control, hyperlipidemic control, and androgen replacement) have resulted in improved responses to PDE5 inhibition [45].

Despite their common ability to inhibit the PDE5 enzyme in assisting with the erectile pathway, these four drugs do indeed differ in their biochemical properties (Table 6.3). One notable distinction is that sildenafil and vardenafil cross-react and inhibit PDE type 6, which is expressed in the retina, and likely accounts for the complaint of visual disturbances with these two medications versus tadalafil and avanafil. Additionally, the longer half-life of tadalafil suggests a longer therapeutic window, which offers an increased benefit for patients. Another notable difference

Table 6.3 Comparison of the four phosphodiesterase type 5 inhibitors

Drug	Sildenafil	Vardenafil	Tadalafil	Avanafil
Trade name(s)	Viagra®	Levitra® Staxyn®	Cialis®	Stendra®
Tmax (h)	0.8	0.7–0.9	2	0.3–0.5
Onset of action (min)	15–60	15–60	15–120	15–60
Half-life (h)	3–5	4–5	17.5	3–5
Fatty food	Reduced absorption	Reduced absorption	No effect	Reduced absorption
Doses	25, 50, 100 mg	5, 10, 20 mg	5, 10, 20 mg	50, 100, 200 mg
Contraindicated with nitrates	Yes	Yes	Yes	Yes
Side effects:				
Headaches, dyspepsia, flushing	Yes	Yes	Yes	Yes
Backaches, myalgias	Rarely	Rarely	Yes	Rarely
Blurred/blue vision	Yes	Rarely	Rarely	No
Precaution with antiarrhythmics	No	Yes	No	No

This is an adapted figure originally published in Campbell-Walsh Urology, 11th Edition, Wein et al., Chapter 27: Evaluation and Management of Erectile Dysfunction, Page 662, Copyright Elsevier 2016 [15]

is that tadalafil is the only medication whose absorption is not impacted by the presence of fatty food in the gastrointestinal tract. Therefore, providers must remember to instruct patients to have a relatively empty stomach when taking sildenafil, vardenafil, or avanafil. As a general rule, providers are encouraged to recommend starting a patient on the lowest available dose for any of these medications and titrating up as necessary in order to achieve a satisfactory erection that does not last more than 4 hours with limited side effects. All four options are often suggested to be taken between 30 minutes and 1 hour prior to anticipated sexual activity in order to achieve peak (or near peak) serum concentrations. Avanafil tends to have a slight advantage in terms of time to peak concentration, with some reports of just 10–20 minutes [46].

Risks and Adverse Effects of Phosphodiesterase Type 5 Inhibitors

When considering prescribing PDE5 inhibitors, the patient should be made aware of the risks involved with this class of medications. Given the inherent cardiovascular risk of sexual activity alone, a cardiovascular risk evaluation should be considered in all men before starting therapy. When specifically weighing the risks of myocardial infarction or death, PDE5 inhibition has not been found to be associated with these catastrophic events as compared to controls [43, 47]. Caution should still be taken with any of the PDE5 inhibitors in patients with severe cardiovascular disease (e.g., aortic stenosis, left ventricular outflow obstruction, hypotension, and hypovolemia). Vardenafil specifically is not recommended to be prescribed in patients taking type 1A or type 3 antiarrhythmics.

Perhaps the most important cardiovascular implication in prescribing PDE5 inhibitors is the absolute contraindication for their use in patients taking nitrates. This includes nitrates in any form (e.g., sublingual nitroglycerin, isosorbide dinitrate, etc.) that are used in patients who are high risk for myocardial infarction, angina, and other acute cardiac events. It is important that both the provider and patient understand that an antidote does not exist for the interaction between a nitrate and PDE5 inhibition. If a patient begins to experience angina during sexual activity while having taken a PDE5 inhibitor, they should stop and seek emergency care immediately. In these cases, any nitrate treatment should be delayed. This delay should be about 24 hours if sildenafil or vardenafil was taken, and 48 hours if tadalafil was taken due to its longer half-life [48].

Other common side effects of PDE5 inhibitors include flushing, headaches, dyspepsia, myalgias, back pain, nasal congestion, and visual disturbances. Sudden hearing loss has also been reported in those who have taken sildenafil, vardenafil, and tadalafil, albeit very rarely and without proof of a causal relationship [49]. Despite an initial concern for an association between PDE5 inhibitors and the development of nonarteritic anterior optic neuropathy, many reviews have actually not shown this suspected relationship to be true [50].

Other Considerations for Phosphodiesterase Type 5 Inhibitors in Urologic Patients

It is fairly common for a patient being evaluated for ED to have other urologic complaints as well. Men with BPH will often be taking an alpha-adrenergic antagonist (e.g., tamsulosin, alfuzosin, silodosin, terazosin, and doxazosin) to help with their lower urinary tract symptoms. Caution should be taken when considering prescribing a PDE5 inhibitor to these patients, as the combination of these two medications carries the risk of symptomatic hypotension. The lowest dose for any particular PDE5 inhibitor should be utilized in these patients, and studies have shown that tamsulosin and silodosin tend to be associated with less or no hypotension compared to the other alpha-adrenergic blockers [51, 52]. Another urologic complaint that men will have is that of low testosterone levels, which often coexists with ED in older men. As mentioned in the "Diagnostic Evaluation" section, the AUA guideline recommends that all men with ED should have a morning serum total testosterone measured [27]. This is largely due to the fact that testosterone replacement has been shown to improve libido and erectile function in hypogonadal men [53]. Despite conflicting data, there is emerging evidence suggesting that combination therapy of testosterone replacement with PDE5 inhibition may be beneficial in hypogonadal men who do not initially respond to PDE5 monotherapy [54].

The Role of Yohimbine

Yohimbine, an alpha-2 adrenergic antagonist, has been heavily studied in the treatment of ED and has classically been purported to be an aphrodisiac agent. Although it has been suggested that yohimbine has a significant effect on erectile function compared to placebo, the data has been conflicting, and it actually does not seem to demonstrate an improvement in the ability to enable sexual intercourse [55, 56]. Yohimbine is generally well tolerated with side effects often limited to hypertension, tachycardia, anxiety, and headache. In spite of the conflicting data, there does appear to be a role for yohimbine strictly in the treatment of psychogenic ED [50, 57].

Intracavernosal Injections

Intracavernosal injections (ICI) are an alternative to oral medications in the armamentarium available to treat ED. ICIs are administered by self-injecting a medication directly into the cavernosa of the penis in order to develop an erection. Typically, the medication is injected at the lateral base of the penis, often referred to as the "3 o'clock" or "9 o'clock" positions. Care must be taken to avoid the urethra ventrally and the neurovascular bundles dorsally. The AUA guideline for ED states that an in-office injection test should be administered in men who are considering ICI as a treatment modality [27]. This allows for dose optimization with the goal of attaining an erection for no more than 1 hour, as well as ensuring the patient does not develop priapism or other systemic effects [58].

Alprostadil (prostaglandin E_1) is currently the only medication that is FDA-approved for ICI, and it is the only medication utilized as a single agent for administration. Alprostadil works to increase cAMP in the cavernosal smooth muscle cells, which decreases intracellular calcium and therefore relaxes smooth muscle, resulting in an erection. Other medications utilized as combination ICI therapy in common practice include papaverine (a phosphodiesterase inhibitor) and phentolamine (an alpha-adrenergic antagonist). Combination therapy carries with it the benefit that multiple vasoactive agents can synergistically influence different aspects of the erectile physiologic pathway, thereby eliciting a maximal erectile response (Fig. 6.1). Patients are often started on alprostadil alone, and if they fail the monotherapy, they are transitioned to some form of combination therapy. See Table 6.4 as a reference for the different ICI therapies currently available in the United States. In general, there is usually an improved erectile response as more medications are used in combination for ICI, although the data are conflicting. One study found that trimix resulted in a superior erectile response compared to either bimix or alprostadil monotherapy; however, no difference was found between alprostadil monotherapy and bimix [59].

ICI is a useful alternative approach for ED treatment, particularly in those patients where oral therapy is either contraindicated or ineffective. Other indications for ICI include mild-to-moderate vasculogenic ED, psychogenic ED refractory to psychotherapy, drug-induced ED, and mixed forms of ED. Since the medication is being administered directly into the cavernosa, it is able to act directly on the substrates involved in the physiology of an erection. This theoretically may make ICI a better option in patients who suffer from damage to the nerves involved with penile sensation and erectile stimulation [58].

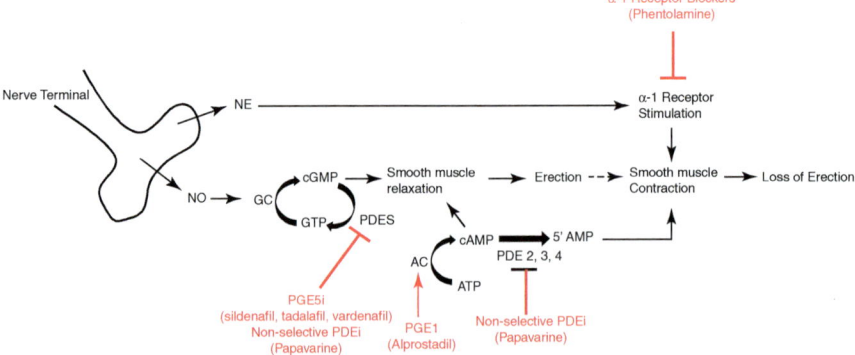

Fig. 6.1 Normal physiology of erections and the mechanism of action of medications that treat erectile dysfunction. (Reprinted from: Krzastek et al. [58])

Table 6.4 Available ICI therapies and associated doses

Trade name(s)	Generic name	Available doses
Caverject Edex	Alprostadil	5–40 µg/mL
Bimix	Papaverine + phentolamine	30 mg/mL + 0.5 mg/mL
Trimix	Alprostadil + papaverine + phentolamine	10 µg/mL + 30 mg/mL + 1 mg/mL

This is an adapted figure originally published in Campbell-Walsh Urology, 11th Edition, Wein et al., Chapter 27: Evaluation and Management of Erectile Dysfunction, Page 664, Copyright Elsevier 2016 [15]

Risks and Adverse Effects of Intracavernosal Injections

The largest burden a patient has to face is the anxiety associated with self-injecting into the corpora. Perhaps the most serious adverse effect associated with ICI is the development of priapism. Other adverse effects include pain at the injection site and the development of penile fibrosis or plaques from chronic injections. For this reason, it is often recommended that patients inject in different sites when anticipating sexual activity. Contraindications for ICI include men with psychological instability, severe coagulopathies, unstable cardiovascular disease, a history or risk for priapism, poor manual dexterity, and the use of monoamine oxidase inhibitors. The last contraindication is due to the risk of a hypertensive crisis in the event that a patient requires alpha-adrenergic injections to reverse an episode of priapism [60].

Intraurethral Alprostadil

Intraurethral (IU) delivery of vasoactive agents is another pharmacologic technique to treat ED. It was introduced with the intention to avoid intracavernosal injections and relies on the absorption of medication into the corpus spongiosum and eventually into the corpora cavernosa. Prostaglandin E_2 was first demonstrated in the early 1990s in a series of 20 men with ED and showed a 70% partial response and 30% complete response [61]. Subsequently, a synthetic formulation of prostaglandin E_1, known as medicated urethral system for erections (MUSE), was FDA-approved in 1996. Compared to placebo, IU alprostadil does indeed result in higher rates (65–69% vs 11–19%) of sufficient erections for intercourse, confirming its efficacy [62, 63].

The current data on IU alprostadil provides a few noteworthy points to discuss. First, the randomized studies examining this modality have only included patients that had an initial in-office response to therapy, and therefore comparisons of treatment modalities are based on those individuals with a positive in-office response. The at-home response rates, however, range from 20% to 65%, and therefore patients should be aware that a positive in-office response does not mean that they will be successful at home. Another point to consider is that randomized trials have demonstrated lower success rates ranging between 53% and 60% with IU alprostadil in comparison to success rates reported as high as 82.5–90% with intra-cavernosal alprostadil [64, 65]. The advantage of IU alprostadil seems to stem from the adverse event profile, with less severe side effects reported with IU alprostadil. Most commonly, patients complain of penile and urethral pain. No episodes of priapism have been reported in these trials.

Administration of IU Alprostadil

In the office, patients should be counseled on proper administration. They should void before administration because urine aids in the dissolution of the medicine. The penis should be held straight pointing up. The applicator should then be advanced 3 cm into the urethra and the medication delivered. The penis is then rolled between the hands still being held upright to prevent leakage of medication from the urethra. In order to increase blood flow, the patient is instructed to walk or stand for about 10 minutes.

Vacuum Erection Devices

For men that are not interested in pharmacologic therapy or for which contraindications exist, a vacuum erection device (VED) is another possible option. VEDs are arguably one of the safest and most cost-effective therapies for ED.

Device Design and Mechanism

There are many available VEDs, all of which result in an erection by entrapping blood within the penis. The device usually consists of a suction cylinder, a constriction band, and a handheld or motorized pump (Fig. 6.2). The cylinder is placed over the flaccid penis, and blood engorgement is achieved by creating negative pressure via the manual or motorized pump. All FDA-approved devices have a pressure limiter in order to regulate the degree of vacuum pressure. It is important that only FDA-approved VEDs are utilized. A clamp or ring is left in place at the base of the penis in order to prevent the pooled blood from draining.

VEDs for Management of ED

Most of the data on VEDs are driven by observational studies with few randomized trials. Studies report success rates as high as 90% [67, 68].

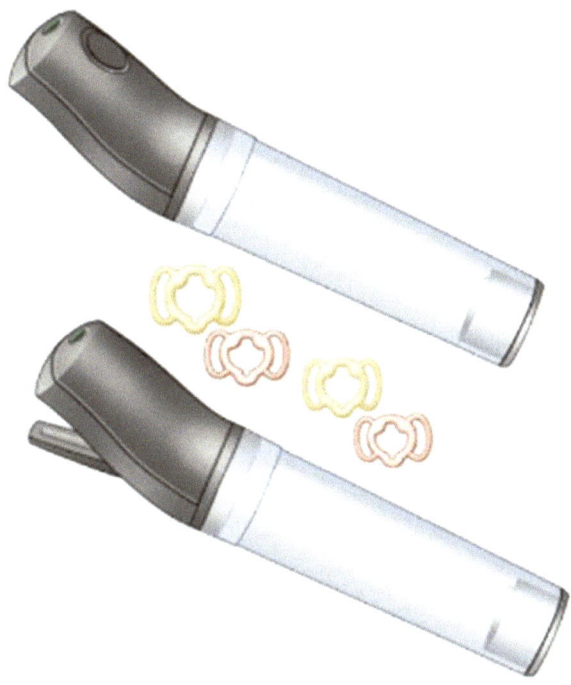

Fig. 6.2 Vacuum erection device: components include a cylinder, motorized pump, and elastic constriction bands. (Reprinted/adapted with permission from Springer Nature: Springer, *Contemporary Treatment of Erectile Dysfunction: A Clinical Guide*. 2nd Edition, Vacuum Therapy for Erectile Dysfunction, Hecht et al., Copyright 2016 [66])

VEDs have also been studied in combination with oral PDE5 inhibitors, intra-cavernosal therapy, and intraurethral therapy. One study reported that the addition of a VED for those that failed maximal doses of PDE5 inhibition resulted in a significant improvement in reported sexual symptoms [69]. Another study reported that patients on combination therapy with sildenafil and VED were more satisfied than being on either treatment alone [70]. When specifically considering diabetic patients who suffer from ED, combination therapy with PDE5 inhibition and VED has shown improved outcomes compared to PDE5 inhibitors alone [71]. Other studies examining VED combination therapy with concomitant intracavernosal therapy or intraurethral prostaglandin therapy have reported similar outcomes [72–74].

VED Complications and Contraindications

Patients should be informed that complications from VEDs are relatively minor. These include penile bruising, difficult ejaculation secondary to the constriction band, and penile pain. All patients must be counseled on removing the constriction band within 30 minutes to avoid penile ischemia. There are no absolute contraindications to VED usage; however, patients on blood thinners should be warned about the risk of bruising and bleeding [75]. Furthermore, patients with poor sensation (e.g., spinal cord injury and diabetic patients) are at increased risk of complication due to the constriction band being too tight.

Transdermal Therapy

While topical therapies have been shown to be useful elsewhere in the body, the same principles apply when considering their utility in erectile dysfunction. Transdermal treatment, either with creams or gels, are easy to use, safe from a systemic standpoint, and generally effective. However, one must consider specifically for ED the fact that vasoactive drugs are being used in a sensitive location. Many transdermal options have been explored for the treatment of ED, although there have been difficulties in limiting the adverse reactions, which has curbed their popularity.

Nitroglycerin, in a 2% paste formulation, has been shown to increase blood flow and improve tumescence; however, there have been conflicting data on whether the resultant rigidity is sufficient enough for intercourse [76]. Headaches have often been reported for both the patient and partner, and the potential for systemic absorption of a potent vasodilator has largely led to topical nitroglycerin falling out of favor for managing ED [77]. Papaverine, used as a topical gel, was also investigated and showed initial promise with improved blood flow. However, its use was also halted when it was demonstrated that its relatively large molecular weight (376 Da) precluded adequate transdermal absorption [78].

Alprostadil applied to the glans penis or intrameatally has been shown to be more successful than any of the other topical formulations for the treatment of ED. It is used in combination with a proprietary transdermal permeation enhancer: either Vitaros (Apricus Biosciences Inc., San Diego, CA) or alprostadil combined with NexACT, also known as Alprox-TD (NexMed Inc., Robbinsville, NJ, USA). This transdermal delivery enhancer is able to improve penetration of alprostadil by altering the lipid fluidity in the epidermis. Several studies have shown that different topical alprostadil formulations have resulted in improved erections with rigidity sufficient enough for penetration as compared to placebo. The adverse effects have been mild and are limited to penile warmth or burning at comparable rates to that of placebo, as well as vaginal burning or itching in the partners [79–81].

A prodrug of prostaglandin E_1 was subsequently developed through esterification in an effort to maximize transdermal permeation. One randomized study demonstrated that prostaglandin E_1 ethyl ester applied to the shaft of the penis was able to achieve significantly higher rigidity scores compared to placebo. Despite these higher rigidity scores, penetration could not be performed significantly more frequently. However, about half of patients considered the treatment successful [82]. It is for these reasons that transdermal alprostadil shows the most promise among topical therapies for ED, and with more future data, it may be increasingly recommended within the ED treatment algorithm.

Introduction to Surgical Options for Erectile Dysfunction

There is a vast array of surgical options available to the patient suffering from ED. Surgery is often reserved for patients with penile trauma or those who have structural penile deformities due to Peyronie's disease, as well as those patients with peripheral vascular disease or a history of ischemic priapism all resulting in cavernosal fibrosis. Surgery can also be considered in patients who fail, are unfit for, or do not desire to pursue medical therapy.

Penile Prosthesis Surgery

Penile implants have been utilized for the surgical treatment of ED since the 1950s. Originally placed in a subcutaneous fashion before transitioning to an intracorporal approach, acrylic splints, silicone implants, and polyethylene rods were the materials of choice [83]. Marked improvements have been made to the implants over the years, particularly with the advent of the inflatable penile prosthesis. Today, approximately 20,000 penile implants are inserted in the United States annually [84]. Although at times penile prostheses have been associated with a negative connotation leading to patient apprehension, they have actually been found to have the highest patient satisfaction rates [85].

The goal of penile implant placement is to achieve artificial erections that are similar to natural erections in terms of appearance, rigidity, and functionality. Insertion of a penile prosthesis indeed results in an erection that is fundamentally different from a physiologic or pharmacologically induced erection. Despite this, the patient is still left with a natural appearance and normal sensation. Indications for prosthetic placement include failure of or unwillingness to utilize more conservative measures, those with Peyronie's disease with concomitant ED or penile deformity significant enough to prevent adequate penetration, severe and irreversible organic ED, cavernosal fibrosis, and those undergoing phalloplasty either for gender reassignment surgery or post-radical penectomy [27, 86].

Outside of undergoing the surgery itself, the patient will not experience any pain or discomfort immediately prior to intercourse (as is the case with intracavernosal injections, intraurethral suppositories, or the application of external devices). Two types of penile prostheses are available for placement: semirigid and inflatable. The selection of either type is determined by a patient's history, preference, anatomical considerations, insurance coverage, and, perhaps most importantly, the surgeon's experience.

Semirigid Penile Prostheses

Semirigid rods are paired, solid cylinders implanted in the corpora cavernosa that do not permit flaccidity. Two subtypes include silicone malleable rods and positional rods, the latter consisting of a series of articulating polyethylene disks with a central

Spectra™ Positional Prosthesis*	Tactra™ Malleable Prosthesis*	Genesis** Malleable Prosthesis*
AMS, Minnetonka, MN	AMS, Minnetonka, MN	Coloplast Corp., Minneapolis, MN

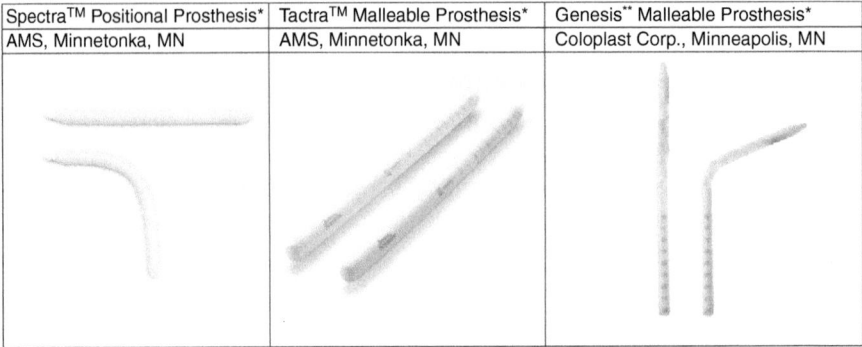

Fig. 6.3 Examples of available semirigid prostheses. (*Reprinted with permission from Boston Scientific Corporation. Boston Scientific Corporation is the owner of all Trademarks, whether or not registered. All product images and accompanying text are copyrighted by Boston Scientific Corporation. **Reprinted with permission from Coloplast Corporation. Coloplast A/S is the owner of all Trademarks, whether or not registered. All product images and accompanying text are copyrighted by Coloplast Corporation)

metal cable support. These articulating disks make the prosthesis better able to maintain upward and downward positions. They are often available in several different diameters and lengths. Advantages of semirigid implants include their low cost and relative ease of implantation with a low chance of mechanical failure. The disadvantages include that they do not allow for flaccidity, resulting in a constant simulated erection that is difficult to conceal, and that the cosmetic results are often less than ideal [87]. Another major concern is the potential for distal migration into the glans or even erosion of the device through the urethral meatus due to the tunica albuginea's tendency to want to retract when stretched to erectile length, resulting in potential migration of the device distally.

Examples of semirigid penile prostheses are shown in Fig. 6.3 and include the American Medical Systems (AMS, Minnetonka, MN) Spectra™ positional implant and the Tactra™ malleable implant. Coloplast (Coloplast Corp., Minneapolis, MN) manufactures the Genesis® malleable implant.

Inflatable Penile Prostheses

Inflatable penile prostheses (IPPs) aim to replicate normal erectile function more closely by allowing girth and length expansion during an erection and by also permitting penile flaccidity when not in use. Two cylinders are placed intracorporally and have the ability to be filled with saline solution via a pump mechanism, resulting in penile rigidity when desirous of sexual activity. IPPs can be further subdivided into three-piece and two-piece implants.

Three-piece implants are more commonly used and tend to dominate the market. They are comprised of the penile cylinders, scrotal pump, and a fluid reservoir often placed in the lower abdomen, all of which are connected via silicone tubing. Two-piece implants combine the function of the scrotal pump and fluid reservoir, obviating the need to violate the lower abdomen. Two-piece devices are thus more desirable when patients have a history of extensive abdominopelvic surgery or have undergone a kidney transplant. Two-piece devices are also often easier to inflate with fewer squeezes of the pump mechanism. However, the pump in a two-piece is often very small and difficult to manipulate, and two-piece devices tend to require larger incisions of the tunica albuginea. Overall, three-piece implants do a better job at simulating a natural appearing erection, are more rigid when inflated, and are more flaccid when deflated.

In both three-piece and two-piece implants, the scrotal pump is pressed repeatedly, which then activates a valve mechanism allowing saline to enter the cylinders from the pump or reservoir. A release valve, which varies depending on the model being utilized, then allows for the device to be deflated. Cylinders are usually available in different widths and lengths, and reservoirs are also available with different volumes, all to tailor to each patient individually.

Examples of inflatable penile prostheses are shown in Fig. 6.4 and include the three-piece AMS 700™ Inflatable Penile Prosthesis and the two-piece AMS Ambicor™ Inflatable Penile Prosthesis. Coloplast also manufactures two different three-piece IPPs: the Titan® and the Titan® Touch, the latter of which has an improved one-touch release to help deflate the implant.

Approximately 75% of all penile implants are sold in the United States, with the three-piece IPP comprising about 70% of all implants placed. Roughly 20% of implants placed are two-piece IPPs, and the rest are semirigid rods. Outside of the United States, inflatable devices and semirigid rods are placed with equal frequency, often due to cost [88].

Preoperative Evaluation and Counseling

Prior to moving forward with placement of a penile prosthesis, careful evaluation and counseling must occur due to the fact that it is an irreversible process and carries many associated risks. Thorough evaluation via a multi-visit process allows for appropriate patient selection, as well as maximization of patient confidence in the decision to move forward. A patient's first visit regarding penile implant surgery should be largely informational in nature. Allowing the patient to handle a prosthetic sample in the office is critical to the patient's understanding of its functionality and postoperative satisfaction rates [89]. Keep in mind that doing this on the first visit may be extremely intimidating for the patient and that they may be better served by referring to educational handouts or videos prior to physically handling a sample. It is also important to stress to the patient that after an implant is placed, they will indeed retain the ability to have normal sensation, orgasm, and ejaculatory function.

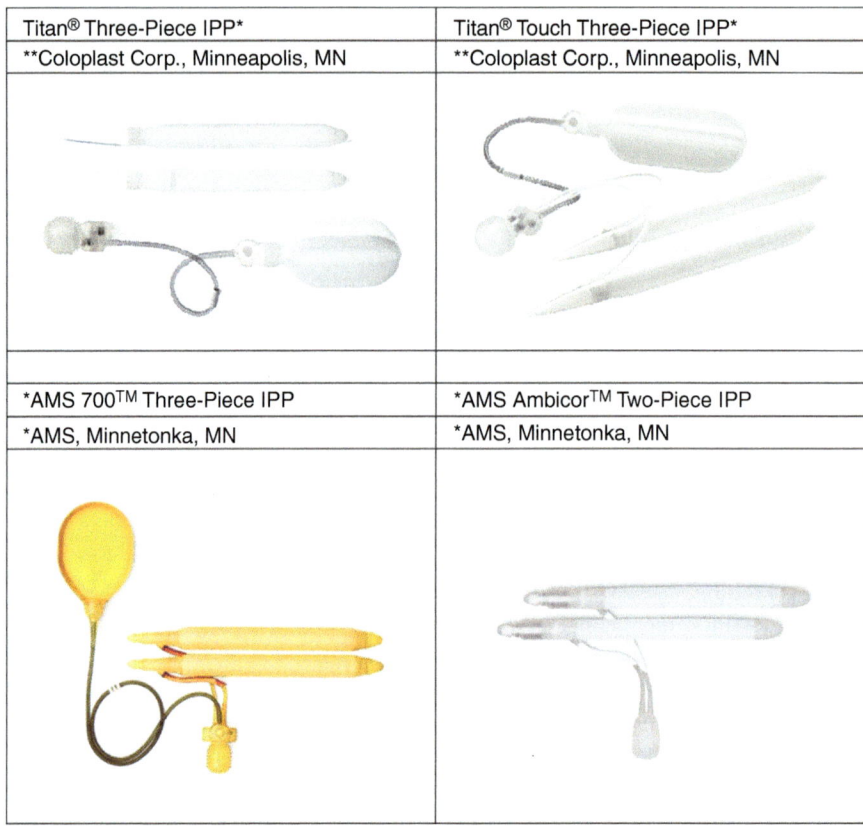

Titan® Three-Piece IPP*	Titan® Touch Three-Piece IPP*
**Coloplast Corp., Minneapolis, MN	**Coloplast Corp., Minneapolis, MN
*AMS 700™ Three-Piece IPP	*AMS Ambicor™ Two-Piece IPP
*AMS, Minnetonka, MN	*AMS, Minnetonka, MN

Fig. 6.4 Examples of available inflatable penile prostheses. (*Reprinted with permission from Boston Scientific Corporation. Boston Scientific Corporation is the owner of all Trademarks, whether or not registered. All product images and accompanying text are copyrighted by Boston Scientific Corporation. **Reprinted with permission from Coloplast Corporation. Coloplast A/S is the owner of all Trademarks, whether or not registered. All product images and accompanying text are copyrighted by Coloplast Corporation)

Before proceeding with surgery, a thorough review of the patient's medical, sexual, and surgical history should take place. In doing so, this allows for the practitioner to select the best and most appropriate type of prosthesis while highlighting any possible contraindications for surgery. Contraindications to penile implant surgery include, but are not limited to, potentially reversible ED, ED due to relationship conflicts, inability to follow instructions, limited dexterity, spinal cord injury, poor hygiene maintenance, noncompliance with medications, and uncontrolled diabetes. Implantation of a penile implant is also contraindicated in the presence of any infection: be it systemic, urinary, cutaneous, or pulmonary. The genitalia must be free of any skin abrasions, wounds, dermatitis, or other lesions.

The preoperative visit should also include a thorough penile exam. One can use vasodilating agents intracorporally to assess penile vascular status with the aid of a penile Doppler ultrasound. At this time, preoperative measurements of the penis on full stretch can be made in anticipation of what size implant may be necessary intraoperatively. Furthermore, it is during this office visit where any other anatomic deformities can be noted for proper surgical planning.

Informed consent should address the surgical technique and the expectations in the immediate- and long-term postoperative setting. Establishing appropriate and realistic expectations in advance of the surgery helps with patient outcomes and satisfaction postoperatively [90]. A discussion of potential complications should occur, particularly calling attention to those that may require subsequent surgical intervention. Reiterating the notion that prosthesis implantation causes irreversible changes to the cavernosa resulting in a loss of any preexisting organic erectile function is of the utmost importance. Lastly, patients must be made aware of the potential for slight penile shortening and glans softening after prosthesis placement [91].

Postoperative Expectations

Outcomes after penile prosthesis placement may have small variations based on the surgical technique and approach. Often times, the patient will be discharged home on the same day of surgery or may be admitted for one night. Despite the controversy surrounding prophylactic antibiotics in the immediate postoperative period, many urologists will still prescribe a short course after surgery to minimize the theoretical risk of infection [92]. The first postoperative visit usually occurs somewhere between 7 and 14 days after surgery in order to assess wound healing and any signs of device malfunction and to rule out signs or symptoms of early infection. Then after around 4–6 weeks from the date of surgery, the patient will return to the office to learn how to control the device.

Complications of Penile Prosthesis Surgery

Infection

Infection can be an extremely devastating complication after penile prosthesis placement. Often an infection will arise from the space between the pseudocapsule that normally forms around the implant and the implant itself. Implant infections can occur in approximately 2–4% of new implants as well as up to 10–13% of revision implants [93, 94]. While most infections are the result of the implant procedure itself, they can still occur many years following surgery likely via secondary bloodborne pathogens. When an implant is felt to be infected, the management is to remove the implant in its entirety. Traditionally, urologists would delay replacement of an implant for at least 6–12 months following device removal. However, more recent practices have been in favor of replacing implants sooner due to the significant fibrotic changes that would occur in the cavernosa following initial device removal, making delayed implant placement extremely difficult [95].

Device Malfunction

Device malfunction is another complication that can occur following implant placement. While the types of malfunction vary based on the model implanted, the most common types of malfunction include cracks in the silicone tubing, leaks at the tube connection sites, cylinder leaks or aneurysms, and pump disruption [84]. Autoinflation, where the saline fluid inadvertently enters the cylinders often due to higher intra-abdominal pressures surrounding the reservoir, has also been reported. However, autoinflation rates have drastically improved with the advent of lockout valves. Overall, surgical revision has been required specifically for device malfunction in about 15% of cases in the first 5–6 years after initial placement [96].

Other Complications

Other complications of IPP placement occur much less frequently. These include erosion, the development of an S-shaped penile deformity, poor glans support, and scrotal hematoma. If any part of the implant is found to be eroding into neighboring structures, treatment is complete removal of all components of the prosthesis.

Penile Vascular Surgery

Penile Arterial Reconstruction

In cases of arteriogenic insufficiency, arterial blood flow to the corpora cavernosa may be improved through penile arterial reconstruction. Penile arterial reconstruction was first described in 1973 where blood was diverted from the inferior epigastric artery to the corpora cavernosa [97]. Subsequent modifications were incorporated to improve outcomes by anastomosing the inferior epigastric artery to the deep dorsal vein, with or without extensive venous ligation [98]. Over 30 studies have reported outcomes for arterial reconstruction procedures, but these outcomes have varied significantly due to patient factors, surgical technique, follow-up duration, and different definitions of success [27, 99, 100]. Some studies include men with veno-occlusive dysfunction and vascular comorbidities. Overall surgical success was generally defined as being able to have sexual intercourse without the use of PDE5 inhibitors or vacuum devices [27]. Surgical success rates have varied widely, ranging from 10% to 90% [27, 98]. In a more recent study, surgical success was defined as an International Index of Erectile Function (IIEF-5) score of >26. Success rates were 77.2% at 1 year, 70% at 2 years, and 64% at 5 years [101]. In general, surgical response rates tend to decline at longer intervals of follow-up.

Short-term complications include postoperative edema and bleeding (9%), dysuria (7%), and wound infection (3%) [27, 100]. Long-term complications include loss of penile length (9%), decreased penile sensation (7%), glans hypervascularization (13%), and anastomotic occlusion (18%) [27, 100, 101]. The AUA guideline states that penile arterial reconstruction may be considered in young men with erectile dysfunction and focal pelvic or penile arterial occlusion without generalized vascular disease or veno-occlusive dysfunction [27].

Penile Venous Surgery

For men with ED secondary to veno-occlusive disease, ligation of the dorsal penile vein became more popular in 1985 [102]. Venous leak surgery expanded to include more elaborate techniques that involved ligation of the deep dorsal vein, cavernous veins, and large accessory veins [103]. Many studies have reported various techniques for penile venous ligation [27, 104–108]. Similar to penile arterial reconstruction, surgical outcome definitions were widely variable from study to study but primarily focused on the ability for unassisted sexual intercourse. Surgical success rates again varied significantly from 10% to 80% [27]. Furthermore, success rates were generally highest in the short term and decreased with length of follow-up, with poor evidence of sustained long-term success [104].

Complications of penile venous surgery include decreased penile sensation, irreversible deformity, and lymphedema secondary to damage to the penile lymphatic system [108]. Given the lack of sustained long-term success and risk for significant complications, the general consensus is that penile venous surgery is not recommended, which is reflected in the 2018 AUA guidelines [27].

Investigational Therapies for Erectile Dysfunction

Extracorporeal Shock Wave Therapy

Extracorporeal shock wave therapy has long been used in medicine for the treatment of kidney, gallbladder, and pancreatic stones. Research in animal models at lower energy levels led to the observation that shock waves at lower intensity can lead to neovascularization and tissue healing and were associated with anti-inflammatory properties [109, 110]. Low-intensity extracorporeal shock wave therapy is now commonly used to treat a number of orthopedic disorders including plantar fasciitis [111, 112].

Several randomized controlled trials have been conducted to evaluate the efficacy of shock wave therapy for ED [113–116]. Shock wave therapy varied by study but generally utilized a 5–6-week regimen with one to two treatment sessions per week. Anywhere between 600 and 3000 shock pulses were applied at low intensity (<0.2 mJ/mm^2). A variety of outcome measures were utilized to assess success rates, including IIEF-EF validated questionnaires, erectile hardness score, and changes to peak systolic flow. Statistically significant improvements were observed in response to shock wave therapy, but no trial reported a return of unassisted erectile function (IIEF-EF score of ≥26). However, follow-up at 1 year following shock wave therapy showed a decline in IIEF-EF scores [115]. There were no significant adverse events reported in these studies, and extracorporeal shock wave therapy is generally regarded as safe. Further research is required to evaluate the efficacy of shock wave therapy compared to other established treatment modalities and long-term outcomes. Given the limited research on extracorporeal shock wave therapy and the fact that its use is not FDA-approved in this setting, the AUA guideline on ED concludes that therapy should be conducted in an investigational manner only [27].

Intracavernosal Stem Cell Therapy

Stem cell-based therapies have received much attention in medicine given their multipotent potential and ability for self-renewal. Stem cell therapies have been reported to improve vasculopathies through promoting angiogenesis and neuropathies through promoting neural regeneration [117, 118]. There are a variety of adult stem cell types, such as bone marrow, adipose, and umbilical cord-derived stem cells. Following stem cell extraction, stem cells are injected into both corpora cavernosa of each patient.

There are several studies utilizing stem cell injections in men with refractory erectile dysfunction. One study reported the use of umbilical cord stem cells in seven men with erectile dysfunction who were scheduled to undergo penile prosthesis surgery, and a control group of three men were administered intracavernosal saline injections [119]. Morning erections were regained in six of the seven men by the third month following stem cell therapy. Rigidity increased following stem cell therapy but was insufficient for penetration. Two of the seven men were able to achieve erections rigid enough for penetration with the addition of 100 mg sildenafil. However, one of the two men lost that ability by 9 months. Of the original seven men, only one was able to maintain erections sufficient for intercourse at 9-month follow-up. In a dose escalation study, the safety profile of intracavernosal bone marrow stem cell injection was investigated [120]. Twelve men with ED following radical prostatectomy were injected with one of four doses of intracavernosal bone marrow stem cell injections. No significant side effects were observed following therapy with 12 months of follow-up. Secondary endpoints included

IIEF-EF scores, erectile hardness score, and peak systolic flow rates. At 6-month follow-up following stem cell therapy, IIEF-EF scores with PDE5 inhibitors increased from 7.3 to 17.4 ($p = 0.006$), erectile hardness score with PDE5 inhibitors increased from 1.3 to 2.6 ($p = 0.008$), and peak systolic velocity increased from 21.6 cm/s to 32.1 cm/s ($p = 0.03$). Several other studies have reported mixed outcomes following intracavernosal stem cell therapy [121, 122]. Given the limited long-term safety and efficacy data, intracavernosal stem cell therapy should still be considered only in the investigational setting but may become a more widespread treatment for erectile dysfunction as the body of literature matures.

Experimental Therapies for Erectile Dysfunction

Platelet-Rich Plasma Therapy

Platelets have various growth factors that are involved in angiogenesis, wound healing, and recruitment of stem cells [123]. Therefore, it is theoretically possible that platelet-rich concentrates injected into the corpora cavernosa can promote vascular and neurogenic regeneration, thereby improving erectile function. Platelet-rich plasma concentrates can be produced by centrifugation of a patient's own whole blood. Once platelets are separated from red blood cells and plasma, the platelets can then be activated prior to intracavernosal injection.

The effects of platelet-rich plasma on erectile function are poorly understood as there are currently no clinical trials evaluating the efficacy and safety of platelet-rich plasma. Animal model studies have examined the effects of platelet-rich plasma in rats with a cavernous nerve injury model. One study reported that rats that received platelet-rich plasma treatments had higher intracavernosal pressure and more myelinated axons of the cavernous nerves [124]. Similarly, another study reported significantly improved erectile function in rats that received platelet-rich plasma treatments [125].

Given the paucity of literature supporting platelet-rich plasma use in treating ED in humans, the AUA guideline recommends against utilizing this therapy for the treatment of ED outside of an experimental research context [27]. Despite this, there is an increasing number of patients demanding novel treatment options and overly optimistic marketing of regenerative alternatives. In the United States, platelet-rich plasma is exempt from regulation and thus is not required to conform to the FDA's regulatory pathway [126]. Clinicians can offer platelet-rich plasma off-label without the standard clinical trials demonstrating a therapy's efficacy. Furthermore, costs for platelet-rich plasma therapy range from $1500 to 2200 per procedure, and these costs are not covered by insurance [126]. Considering the high cost to patients and the unproven effectiveness, platelet-rich plasma therapy should not be offered to patients for the treatment of ED outside of a clinical trial.

Chapter Summary Points
1. Erectile dysfunction is an extremely prevalent medical condition among adult men.
2. The cause of erectile dysfunction can be multifactorial in nature. Thus, a systematic approach considering a patient's medical, psychosocial, and surgical history in making the diagnosis and developing treatment strategies is warranted.
3. All men with erectile dysfunction should be considered at risk for cardiovascular disease, even in the absence of active cardiac symptoms.
4. Several drugs and agents have been shown to be associated with erectile dysfunction.
5. Improvements in physical activity and diet are associated with improvements in erectile function.
6. Psychosexual therapies may help patients who suffer from erectile dysfunction with an underlying psychogenic component. Referral to mental health providers may help those patients with severe psychosexual symptoms.
7. Oral pharmacologic therapy is the most frequently utilized medical therapy in a provider's armamentarium to treat erectile dysfunction and has substantial efficacy. However, all providers must be aware of the cardiovascular adverse effects with PDE5 inhibitors, namely, the absolute contraindication for use in those taking concomitant nitrates.
8. Other pharmacological therapies and vacuum erection devices are available for those patients in whom oral therapy is not indicated or well tolerated. Vacuum erection devices can also be used in combination with pharmacological therapies.
9. Inflatable penile prostheses have been found to have the highest patient satisfaction rates, although the risks of infection and device malfunction must be considered.
10. Experimental therapies, such as platelet-rich plasma therapy, should not be offered to patients with erectile dysfunction outside of a clinical trial.

References

1. Feldman HA, Goldstein I, Hatzichristou DG, et al. Impotence and its medical and psychosocial correlates: results of the Massachusetts Male Aging Study. J Urol. 1994;151:54.
2. Ayta IA, McKinlay JB, Krane RJ. The likely worldwide increase in erectile dysfunction between 1995 and 2025 and some possible policy consequences. BJU Int. 1999;84:50.
3. Selvin E, Burnett AL, Platz EA. Prevalence and risk factors for erectile dysfunction in the US. Am J Med. 2007;120:151.
4. Lewis RW, Fugl-Meyer KS, Corona G, et al. Definitions/epidemiology/risk factors for sexual dysfunction. J Sex Med. 2010;7:1598.

5. Johannes CB, Araujo AB, Feldman HA, et al. Incidence of erectile dysfunction in men 40 to 69 years old: longitudinal results from the Massachusetts male aging study. J Urol. 2000;163:460.
6. Wessells H, Joyce GF, Wise M, et al. Erectile dysfunction. J Urol. 2007;177:1675.
7. Francis ME, Kusek JW, Nyberg LM, et al. The contribution of common medical conditions and drug exposures to erectile dysfunction in adult males. J Urol. 2007;178:591.
8. Lue TF. A patient's goal-directed approach to erectile dysfunction and Peyronie's disease. Can J Urol. 1995;2:13.
9. Tiefer L, Schuetz-Mueller D. Psychological issues in diagnosis and treatment of erectile disorders. Urol Clin North Am. 1995;22:767.
10. Albaugh J, Amargo I, Capelson R, et al. Health care clinicians in sexual health medicine: focus on erectile dysfunction. Urol Nurs. 2002;22:217.
11. Althof SE, Rosen RC, Perelman MA, et al. Standard operating procedures for taking a sexual history. J Sex Med. 2013;10:26.
12. Hartmann U, Burkart M. Erectile dysfunctions in patient-physician communication: optimized strategies for addressing sexual issues and the benefit of using a patient questionnaire. J Sex Med. 2007;4:38.
13. DeBusk R, Drory Y, Goldstein I, et al. Management of sexual dysfunction in patients with cardiovascular disease: recommendations of the Princeton Consensus Panel. Am J Cardiol. 2000;86:62F.
14. Nehra A, Jackson G, Miner M, et al. The Princeton III Consensus recommendations for the management of erectile dysfunction and cardiovascular disease. Mayo Clin Proc. 2012;87:766.
15. Partin AW, Wein AJ, Kavoussi LR, et al. Campbell-Walsh urology E-book. Philadelphia: Elsevier Health Sciences; 2015.
16. Atiemo HO, Szostak MJ, Sklar GN. Salvage of sildenafil failures referred from primary care physicians. J Urol. 2003;170:2356.
17. Jiann BP, Yu CC, Su CC, et al. Rechallenge prior sildenafil nonresponders. Int J Impot Res. 2004;16:64.
18. Hatzichristou D, Moysidis K, Apostolidis A, et al. Sildenafil failures may be due to inadequate patient instructions and follow-up: a study on 100 non-responders. Eur Urol. 2005;47:518.
19. Gruenwald I, Shenfeld O, Chen J, et al. Positive effect of counseling and dose adjustment in patients with erectile dysfunction who failed treatment with sildenafil. Eur Urol. 2006;50:134.
20. Derogatis LR, Melisaratos N. The DSFI: a multidimensional measure of sexual functioning. J Sex Marital Ther. 1979;5:244.
21. Rust J, Golombok S. The GRISS: a psychometric instrument for the assessment of sexual dysfunction. Arch Sex Behav. 1986;15:157.
22. Rosen RC, Riley A, Wagner G, et al. The international index of erectile function (IIEF): a multidimensional scale for assessment of erectile dysfunction. Urology. 1997;49:822.
23. O'Leary MP, Fowler FJ, Lenderking WR, et al. A brief male sexual function inventory for urology. Urology. 1995;46:697.
24. Mulhall JP, Goldstein I, Bushmakin AG, et al. Validation of the erection hardness score. J Sex Med. 2007;4:1626.
25. Rosen RC, Catania J, Pollack L, et al. Male Sexual Health Questionnaire (MSHQ): scale development and psychometric validation. Urology. 2004;64:777.
26. Rosen RC, Cappelleri JC, Smith MD, et al. Development and evaluation of an abridged, 5-item version of the International Index of Erectile Function (IIEF-5) as a diagnostic tool for erectile dysfunction. Int J Impot Res. 1999;11:319.
27. Burnett AL, Nehra A, Breau RH, et al. Erectile dysfunction: AUA guideline. J Urol. 2018;200:633.
28. Wu FC, Tajar A, Beynon JM, et al. Identification of late-onset hypogonadism in middle-aged and elderly men. N Engl J Med. 2010;363:123.

29. Brambilla DJ, Matsumoto AM, Araujo AB, et al. The effect of diurnal variation on clinical measurement of serum testosterone and other sex hormone levels in men. J Clin Endocrinol Metab. 2009;94:907.
30. Corona G, Rastrelli G, Monami M, et al. Body weight loss reverts obesity-associated hypogonadotropic hypogonadism: a systematic review and meta-analysis. Eur J Endocrinol. 2013;168:829.
31. La J, Roberts NH, Yafi FA. Diet and Men's sexual health. Sex Med Rev. 2018;6:54.
32. Salas-Salvado J, Bullo M, Babio N, et al. Reduction in the incidence of type 2 diabetes with the Mediterranean diet: results of the PREDIMED-Reus nutrition intervention randomized trial. Diabetes Care. 2011;34:14.
33. Trichopoulou A, Costacou T, Bamia C, et al. Adherence to a Mediterranean diet and survival in a Greek population. N Engl J Med. 2003;348:2599.
34. Eleazu C, Obianuju N, Eleazu K, et al. The role of dietary polyphenols in the management of erectile dysfunction-mechanisms of action. Biomed Pharmacother. 2017;88:644.
35. Althof SE, Leiblum SR, Chevret-Measson M, et al. Psychological and interpersonal dimensions of sexual function and dysfunction. J Sex Med. 2005;2:793.
36. Stravynski A, Gaudette G, Lesage A, et al. The treatment of sexually dysfunctional men without partners: a controlled study of three behavioural group approaches. Br J Psychiatry. 1997;170:338.
37. Althof SE. When an erection alone is not enough: biopsychosocial obstacles to lovemaking. Int J Impot Res. 2002;14 Suppl 1:S99.
38. Hawton K. Integration of treatments for male erectile dysfunction. Lancet. 1998;351:7.
39. Rajfer J, Aronson WJ, Bush PA, et al. Nitric oxide as a mediator of relaxation of the corpus cavernosum in response to nonadrenergic, noncholinergic neurotransmission. N Engl J Med. 1992;326:90.
40. Kim N, Azadzoi KM, Goldstein I, et al. A nitric oxide-like factor mediates nonadrenergic-noncholinergic neurogenic relaxation of penile corpus cavernosum smooth muscle. J Clin Invest. 1991;88:112.
41. Burnett AL. Phosphodiesterase 5 mechanisms and therapeutic applications. Am J Cardiol. 2005;96:29M.
42. Carson CC, Lue TF. Phosphodiesterase type 5 inhibitors for erectile dysfunction. BJU Int. 2005;96:257.
43. Hellstrom WJ. Current safety and tolerability issues in men with erectile dysfunction receiving PDE5 inhibitors. Int J Clin Pract. 2007;61:1547.
44. Bruzziches R, Francomano D, Gareri P, et al. An update on pharmacological treatment of erectile dysfunction with phosphodiesterase type 5 inhibitors. Expert Opin Pharmacother. 2013;14:1333.
45. Guay AT. Optimizing response to phosphodiesterase therapy: impact of risk-factor management. J Androl. 2003;24:S59.
46. Kedia GT, Uckert S, Assadi-Pour F, et al. Avanafil for the treatment of erectile dysfunction: initial data and clinical key properties. Ther Adv Urol. 2013;5:35.
47. Mittleman MA, Maclure M, Glasser DB. Evaluation of acute risk for myocardial infarction in men treated with sildenafil citrate. Am J Cardiol. 2005;96:443.
48. Cheitlin MD, Hutter AM Jr, Brindis RG, et al. ACC/AHA expert consensus document. Use of sildenafil (Viagra) in patients with cardiovascular disease. American College of Cardiology/American Heart Association. J Am Coll Cardiol. 1999;33:273.
49. Liu W, Antonelli PJ, Dahm P, et al. Risk of sudden sensorineural hearing loss in adults using phosphodiesterase type 5 inhibitors: population-based cohort study. Pharmacoepidemiol Drug Saf. 2018;27:587.
50. Porst H, Burnett A, Brock G, et al. SOP conservative (medical and mechanical) treatment of erectile dysfunction. J Sex Med. 2013;10:130.
51. Kloner RA, Jackson G, Emmick JT, et al. Interaction between the phosphodiesterase 5 inhibitor, tadalafil and 2 alpha-blockers, doxazosin and tamsulosin in healthy normotensive men. J Urol. 2004;172:1935.

52. MacDiarmid SA, Hill LA, Volinn W, et al. Lack of pharmacodynamic interaction of silodosin, a highly selective alpha1a-adrenoceptor antagonist, with the phosphodiesterase-5 inhibitors sildenafil and tadalafil in healthy men. Urology. 2010;75:520.
53. Snyder PJ, Bhasin S, Cunningham GR, et al. Effects of testosterone treatment in older men. N Engl J Med. 2016;374:611.
54. Buvat J, Montorsi F, Maggi M, et al. Hypogonadal men nonresponders to the PDE5 inhibitor tadalafil benefit from normalization of testosterone levels with a 1% hydroalcoholic testosterone gel in the treatment of erectile dysfunction (TADTEST study). J Sex Med. 2011;8:284.
55. Ernst E, Pittler MH. Yohimbine for erectile dysfunction: a systematic review and meta-analysis of randomized clinical trials. J Urol. 1998;159:433.
56. Teloken C, Rhoden EL, Sogari P, et al. Therapeutic effects of high dose yohimbine hydrochloride on organic erectile dysfunction. J Urol. 1998;159:122.
57. Montorsi F, Strambi LF, Guazzoni G, et al. Effect of yohimbine-trazodone on psychogenic impotence: a randomized, double-blind, placebo-controlled study. Urology. 1994;44:732.
58. Krzastek SC, Bopp J, Smith RP, et al. Recent advances in the understanding and management of erectile dysfunction [version 1; peer reviewL 2 approved]. F1000Res. 2019;8:102.
59. Ribe N, Rajmil O, Bassas L, et al. Response to intracavernous administration of 3 different drugs in the same group of patients with erectile dysfunction. Arch Esp Urol. 2001;54:355.
60. Sharlip ID. Evaluation and nonsurgical management of erectile dysfunction. Urol Clin North Am. 1998;25:647.
61. Wolfson B, Pickett S, Scott NE, et al. Intraurethral prostaglandin E-2 cream: a possible alternative treatment for erectile dysfunction. Urology. 1993;42:73.
62. Williams G, Abbou CC, Amar ET, et al. Efficacy and safety of transurethral alprostadil therapy in men with erectile dysfunction. MUSE Study Group. Br J Urol. 1998;81:889.
63. Padma-Nathan H, Hellstrom WJ, Kaiser FE, et al. Treatment of men with erectile dysfunction with transurethral alprostadil. Medicated Urethral System for Erection (MUSE) Study Group. N Engl J Med. 1997;336:1.
64. Shokeir AA, Alserafi MA, Mutabagani H. Intracavernosal versus intraurethral alprostadil: a prospective randomized study. BJU Int. 1999;83:812.
65. Shabsigh R, Padma-Nathan H, Gittleman M, et al. Intracavernous alprostadil alfadex is more efficacious, better tolerated, and preferred over intraurethral alprostadil plus optional actis: a comparative, randomized, crossover, multicenter study. Urology. 2000;55:109.
66. McVary KT, McVary KT. Contemporary treatment of erectile dysfunction: a clinical guide. New York: Humana Press; 2011.
67. Small RG, Reed J. Bleeding during dacryocystorhinostomy: the importance of the suction cautery. Arch Ophthalmol. 1990;108:638.
68. Hellstrom WJ, Montague DK, Moncada I, et al. Implants, mechanical devices, and vascular surgery for erectile dysfunction. J Sex Med. 2010;7:501.
69. Canguven O, Bailen J, Fredriksson W, et al. Combination of vacuum erection device and PDE5 inhibitors as salvage therapy in PDE5 inhibitor nonresponders with erectile dysfunction. J Sex Med. 2009;6:2561.
70. Chen J, Sofer M, Kaver I, et al. Concomitant use of sildenafil and a vacuum entrapment device for the treatment of erectile dysfunction. J Urol. 2004;171:292.
71. Sun L, Peng FL, Yu ZL, et al. Combined sildenafil with vacuum erection device therapy in the management of diabetic men with erectile dysfunction after failure of first-line sildenafil monotherapy. Int J Urol. 2014;21:1263.
72. Chen J, Godschalk MF, Katz PG, et al. Combining intracavernous injection and external vacuum as treatment for erectile dysfunction. J Urol. 1995;153:1476.
73. John H, Lehmann K, Hauri D. Intraurethral prostaglandin improves quality of vacuum erection therapy. Eur Urol. 1996;29:224.
74. Marmar JL, DeBenedictis TJ, Praiss DE. The use of a vacuum constrictor device to augment a partial erection following an intracavernous injection. J Urol. 1988;140:975.

75. Limoge JP, Olins E, Henderson D, et al. Minimally invasive therapies in the treatment of erectile dysfunction in anticoagulated cases: a study of satisfaction and safety. J Urol. 1996;155:1276.
76. Owen JA, Saunders F, Harris C, et al. Topical nitroglycerin: a potential treatment for impotence. J Urol. 1989;141:546.
77. Sonksen J, Biering-Sorensen F. Transcutaneous nitroglycerin in the treatment of erectile dysfunction in spinal cord injured. Paraplegia. 1992;30:554.
78. Kim ED, el-Rashidy R, McVary KT. Papaverine topical gel for treatment of erectile dysfunction. J Urol. 1995;153:361.
79. Goldstein I, Payton TR, Schechter PJ. A double-blind, placebo-controlled, efficacy and safety study of topical gel formulation of 1% alprostadil (Topiglan) for the in-office treatment of erectile dysfunction. Urology. 2001;57:301.
80. Padma-Nathan H, Steidle C, Salem S, et al. The efficacy and safety of a topical alprostadil cream, Alprox-TD, for the treatment of erectile dysfunction: two phase 2 studies in mild-to-moderate and severe ED. Int J Impot Res. 2003;15:10.
81. Rooney M, Pfister W, Mahoney M, et al. Long-term, multicenter study of the safety and efficacy of topical alprostadil cream in male patients with erectile dysfunction. J Sex Med. 2009;6:520.
82. Schanz S, Hauck EW, Schmelz HU, et al. Topical treatment of erectile dysfunction with prostaglandin E(1) ethyl ester. J Dtsch Dermatol Ges. 2009;7:1055.
83. Le B, Burnett AL. Evolution of penile prosthetic devices. Korean J Urol. 2015;56:179.
84. Garber BB. Inflatable penile prostheses for the treatment of erectile dysfunction: an update. Expert Rev Med Devices. 2008;5:133.
85. Jarow JP, Nana-Sinkam P, Sabbagh M, et al. Outcome analysis of goal directed therapy for impotence. J Urol. 1996;155:1609.
86. Nehra A, Alterowitz R, Culkin DJ, et al. Peyronie's disease: AUA guideline. J Urol. 2015;194:745.
87. Jain S, Terry TR. Penile prosthetic surgery and its role in the treatment of end-stage erectile dysfunction – an update. Ann R Coll Surg Engl. 2006;88:343.
88. Mulcahy JJ, Wilson SK. Current use of penile implants in erectile dysfunction. Curr Urol Rep. 2006;7:485.
89. Bettocchi C, Palumbo F, Spilotros M, et al. Penile prostheses. Ther Adv Urol. 2010;2:35.
90. Anderson PC, Jain S, Summerton DJ, et al. Surgical atlas. Insertion of an inflatable penile prosthesis. BJU Int. 2007;99:467.
91. Wang R, Howard GE, Hoang A, et al. Prospective and long-term evaluation of erect penile length obtained with inflatable penile prosthesis to that induced by intracavernosal injection. Asian J Androl. 2009;11:411.
92. Wosnitzer MS, Greenfield JM. Antibiotic patterns with inflatable penile prosthesis insertion. J Sex Med. 2011;8:1521.
93. Jarow JP. Risk factors for penile prosthetic infection. J Urol. 1996;156:402.
94. Wilson SK, Carson CC, Cleves MA, et al. Quantifying risk of penile prosthesis infection with elevated glycosylated hemoglobin. J Urol. 1998;159:1537.
95. Montague DK, Angermeier KW. Penile prosthesis implantation. Urol Clin North Am. 2001;28:355.
96. Carson CC, Mulcahy JJ, Govier FE. Efficacy, safety and patient satisfaction outcomes of the AMS 700CX inflatable penile prosthesis: results of a long-term multicenter study. AMS 700CX study group. J Urol. 2000;164:376.
97. Michal V, Kramar R, Pospichal J, et al. Direct arterial anastomosis on corpora cavernosa penis in the therapy of erective impotence. Rozhl Chir. 1973;52:587.
98. Molodysky E, Liu SP, Huang SJ, et al. Penile vascular surgery for treating erectile dysfunction: current role and future direction. Arab J Urol. 2013;11:254.
99. Kawanishi Y, Kimura K, Nakanishi R, et al. Penile revascularization surgery for arteriogenic erectile dysfunction: the long-term efficacy rate calculated by survival analysis. BJU Int. 2004;94:361.

100. Munarriz R, Uberoi J, Fantini G, et al. Microvascular arterial bypass surgery: long-term outcomes using validated instruments. J Urol. 2009;182:643.
101. Kayigil O, Okulu E, Aldemir M, et al. Penile revascularization in vasculogenic erectile dysfunction (ED): long-term follow-up. BJU Int. 2012;109:109.
102. Wespes E, Schulman CC. Venous leakage: surgical treatment of a curable cause of impotence. J Urol. 1985;133:796.
103. Vale JA, Feneley MR, Lees WR, et al. Venous leak surgery: long-term follow-up of patients undergoing excision and ligation of the deep dorsal vein of the penis. Br J Urol. 1995;76:192.
104. Cakan M, Yalcinkaya F, Demirel F, et al. Is dorsale penile vein ligation (dpvl) still a treatment option in veno-occlusive dysfunction? Int Urol Nephrol. 2004;36:381.
105. Hsu GL, Chen HS, Hsieh CH, et al. Clinical experience of a refined penile venous stripping surgery procedure for patients with erectile dysfunction: is it a viable option? J Androl. 2010;31:271.
106. Hsu GL, Chen HS, Hsieh CH, et al. Salvaging penile venous stripping surgery. J Androl. 2010;31:250.
107. Hsu GL, Chen HS, Hsieh CH, et al. Insufficient response to venous stripping surgery: is the penile vein recurrent or residual? J Androl. 2006;27:700.
108. Hwang TI, Yang CR. Penile vein ligation for venogenic impotence. Eur Urol. 1994;26:46.
109. Xu JK, Chen HJ, Li XD, et al. Optimal intensity shock wave promotes the adhesion and migration of rat osteoblasts via integrin beta1-mediated expression of phosphorylated focal adhesion kinase. J Biol Chem. 2012;287:26200.
110. Liu T, Shindel AW, Lin G, et al. Cellular signaling pathways modulated by low-intensity extracorporeal shock wave therapy. Int J Impot Res. 2019;31:170.
111. Rassweiler JJ, Knoll T, Kohrmann KU, et al. Shock wave technology and application: an update. Eur Urol. 2011;59:784.
112. Wang CJ. An overview of shock wave therapy in musculoskeletal disorders. Chang Gung Med J. 2003;26:220.
113. Vardi Y, Appel B, Kilchevsky A, et al. Does low intensity extracorporeal shock wave therapy have a physiological effect on erectile function? Short-term results of a randomized, double-blind, sham controlled study. J Urol. 2012;187:1769.
114. Olsen AB, Persiani M, Boie S, et al. Can low-intensity extracorporeal shockwave therapy improve erectile dysfunction? A prospective, randomized, double-blind, placebo-controlled study. Scand J Urol. 2015;49:329.
115. Srini VS, Reddy RK, Shultz T, et al. Low intensity extracorporeal shockwave therapy for erectile dysfunction: a study in an Indian population. Can J Urol. 2015;22:7614.
116. Kalyvianakis D, Hatzichristou D. Low-intensity shockwave therapy improves hemodynamic parameters in patients with vasculogenic erectile dysfunction: a triplex ultrasonography-based sham-controlled trial. J Sex Med. 2017;14:891.
117. Sekiguchi H, Ii M, Losordo DW. The relative potency and safety of endothelial progenitor cells and unselected mononuclear cells for recovery from myocardial infarction and ischemia. J Cell Physiol. 2009;219:235.
118. Takeuchi H, Natsume A, Wakabayashi T, et al. Intravenously transplanted human neural stem cells migrate to the injured spinal cord in adult mice in an SDF-1- and HGF-dependent manner. Neurosci Lett. 2007;426:69.
119. Bahk JY, Jung JH, Han H, et al. Treatment of diabetic impotence with umbilical cord blood stem cell intracavernosal transplant: preliminary report of 7 cases. Exp Clin Transplant. 2010;8:150.
120. Yiou R, Hamidou L, Birebent B, et al. Safety of intracavernous bone marrow-mononuclear cells for postradical prostatectomy erectile dysfunction: an open dose-escalation pilot study. Eur Urol. 2016;69:988.
121. Haahr MK, Jensen CH, Toyserkani NM, et al. Safety and potential effect of a single intracavernous injection of autologous adipose-derived regenerative cells in patients with erectile dysfunction following radical prostatectomy: an open-label phase I clinical trial. EBioMedicine. 2016;5:204.

122. Levy JA, Marchand M, Iorio L, et al. Determining the feasibility of managing erectile dysfunction in humans with placental-derived stem cells. J Am Osteopath Assoc. 2016;116:e1.
123. Hall MP, Band PA, Meislin RJ, et al. Platelet-rich plasma: current concepts and application in sports medicine. J Am Acad Orthop Surg. 2009;17:602.
124. Ding XG, Li SW, Zheng XM, et al. The effect of platelet-rich plasma on cavernous nerve regeneration in a rat model. Asian J Androl. 2009;11:215.
125. Wu CC, Wu YN, Ho HO, et al. The neuroprotective effect of platelet-rich plasma on erectile function in bilateral cavernous nerve injury rat model. J Sex Med. 2012;9:2838.
126. Scott S, Roberts M, Chung E. Platelet-rich plasma and treatment of erectile dysfunction: critical review of literature and global trends in platelet-rich plasma clinics. Sex Med Rev. 2019;7:306.

Chapter 7
Management of BPH and LUTS

Benjamin Brucker, Matthew Katz, and Michael Siev

Introduction

Benign prostatic hyperplasia (BPH) is the pathologic process of nonmalignant enlargement of the prostate gland. BPH is one of the common causes of lower urinary tract symptoms (LUTS) seen in aging men. Historically, the clinical symptoms associated with LUTS in men were referred to as "prostatism" and thought to be due to obstruction of the bladder by an enlarged prostate. It is now clear that LUTS are related to multiple pathologic processes and BPH is just one of the possible contributors. Recently, there has been increased emphasis on the symptoms of LUTS rather than the perceived causative role of any specific organ. The clinical symptoms described by LUTS can also be due to detrusor dysfunction, polyuria, sleep disorders, and systemic medical conditions such as diabetes mellitus, spine disease, Parkinson's disease, or cerebrovascular disease.

LUTS can be broadly organized into two symptom groups, characterized by either storage (related to bladder filling) symptoms or voiding (related to bladder emptying) symptoms. Storage symptoms include frequency, urgency, nocturia, and incontinence. Voiding symptoms include hesitancy, decreased flow, intermittency, straining, terminal dribbling, and incomplete bladder emptying.

BPH and LUTS are highly prevalent in men, and severity typically increases with age. Among men over 50 years old, 50–75% experience BPH/LUTS, and among men over 70 years old, 80% on average are impacted by BPH/LUTS [1]. Although LUTS is not a life-threatening condition, the symptoms can have a significant impact on quality of life. The diagnosis and management of LUTS is therefore an integral aspect in the healthcare of male patients. To provide appropriate treatment of LUTS, it is important to have a basic understanding of the pathophysiology involved. Multiple pharmacologic classes are available to treat patients, and

B. Brucker (✉) · M. Katz · M. Siev
NYU, Department of Urology, New York, NY, USA
e-mail: Benjamin.brucker@nyumc.org; matthew.katz@nyumc.org; Michael.siev@nyumc.org

© Springer Nature Switzerland AG 2021   127
J. P. Alukal et al. (eds.), *Design and Implementation of the Modern Men's Health Center*, https://doi.org/10.1007/978-3-030-54482-9_7

choosing the correct medical treatment can be complex. When medical treatment fails, various surgical options are available. The goal of this chapter is to provide a foundation on the causes of LUTS and help guide a provider at a men's center on the appropriate workup and treatment of BPH/LUTS that encompasses the symptoms' wide range of etiologies.

Pathophysiology

BPH is a histological diagnosis and is characterized by increased number of epithelial and stromal cells typically within the periurethral area of the prostate. The molecular mechanism of hyperplasia is incompletely understood. The increased number of cells in the prostate may be due to increased proliferation or decreased cell death. Multiple pathways have been implicated in the development of hyperplasia including the influence of androgens, estrogens, growth factors, and neurotransmitters. Prostatic hyperplasia ultimately leads to increased urethral resistance and possible secondary upstream compensation by the bladder.

Androgens

The exact mechanism of androgen-induced hyperplasia of the prostate has not been fully elucidated; however, it is known that androgens are required for normal cell proliferation of the prostate gland and also act to inhibit cell death [2]. It is believed that both testosterone and the more metabolically active dihydrotestosterone (DHT) influence prostate growth by binding to androgen receptors which result in increased transcription of androgen-dependent genes and downstream protein synthesis. There is conflicting evidence on the importance of circulating testosterone and DHT. In a large BPH study, there was no relationship between serum testosterone and prostate size [3]. In contrast, in a 20-year prospective study, higher baseline DHT levels were associated with increased risk of BPH [4]. In the prostate, type 2 5α-reductase converts testosterone into DHT. There is also a type 1 5α-reductase that is primarily located outside the prostate. Type 2 5α-reductase plays a crucial role in both the normal development of the prostate and the hyperplastic process within the prostate. While the mechanism of androgen-induced hyperplasia remains incompletely studied, it is known that androgens are needed to develop BPH and therefore remain an important target in treatment of BPH.

Anatomic Features

BPH develops in the periurethral transition zone of the prostate as shown by McNeal in 1978 [5]. The transition zone consists of the two lateral glands just proximal to the verumontanum which marks the preprostatic sphincter. All BPH nodules develop in the transition zone. It is important to note that the actual size of the prostate does not necessarily correlate with the degree of obstruction or symptoms [6]. Patients with small prostates can potentially develop hyperplasia in the transition zone leading to significant LUTS. In some cases, there is predominant growth at the bladder neck that results in a median lobe. The median lobe is not considered part of the transition zone but can form a "ball valve" to obstruct the bladder. Growth of the prostate and nodules can lead to increased outlet resistance.

The bladder's response to obstruction can lead to physiological changes that result in pathological remodeling. In animal models, bladder obstruction leads to smooth muscle hypertrophy in the detrusor muscle [7]. This adaptive response can lead to changes in the bladder muscle that result in detrusor instability (or overactivity) and decreased contractility (detrusor underactivity). Detrusor instability can then result in symptoms of urinary frequency and urgency. In addition, decreased detrusor contractility can further worsen the force of the urinary stream, leading to hesitancy, and increased post-void residuals. In one study, approximately one third of men who had elective prostatectomy continued to have significant voiding dysfunction with storage symptoms after relief of obstruction [8]. These residual symptoms are possibly due to bladder remodeling.

Epidemiology/Natural History/Complications

As discussed previously, BPH is a histological diagnosis. The clinical significance of BPH is dependent on the development of LUTS. Patients can have benign prostatic enlargement (BPE) with or without evidence of BPH on histology and with or without symptoms of obstruction. Some literature uses the term benign prostatic obstruction (BPO), which describes patients with symptoms of obstruction. There have been multiple studies to assess the prevalence of BPH. Many of the epidemiological studies are based on autopsy assessment of histologic hyperplasia. A landmark study by Berry and colleagues found that virtually no men under the age of 30 had evidence of BPH; however, by the age of 50, half of the males studied had BPH. The prevalence of BPH increased in an age-dependent manner, reaching nearly 100% by the ninth decade of life [9].

Many studies have been performed to better elucidate the prevalence of clinically significant LUTS, as not all men with histologic hyperplasia will develop symptoms. The difficulty in assessing clinical BPH is that the clinical definition of BPH varies widely. Various tools have been used to assess the impact of LUTS including standardized questionnaires such as the International Prostate Symptom Score (IPSS) – which is also known as the American Urological Association symptom score (AUASS) (Fig. 7.1). Other tools used to define or categorize BPH are prostate gland size and measurements of bladder outlet obstruction.

In a very large international study of LUTS in Asian men, it was found that 18%, 29%, 40%, and 56% of men in their 40s, 50s, 60s, and 70s, respectively, have moderate to severe LUTS [10]. In this study, men were considered to be symptomatic if they had an IPSS >8. Other studies in different populations have been published

Question	Not at All	Less Than 1 Time in 5	Less Than Half the Time	About Half the Time	More Than Half the Time	Almost Always
1. During the last month or so, how often have you had a sensation of not emptying your bladder completely after you finished urinating?	0	1	2	3	4	5
2. During the last month or so, how often have you had to urinate again less than 2 hours after you finished urinating?	0	1	2	3	4	5
3. During the last month or so, how often have you found you stopped and started sgain several times when you urinated?	0	1	2	3	4	5
4. During the last month or so, how often have you found it dissicult to postpone urination?	0	1	2	3	4	5
5. During the last month or so, how often have you had a week urinary stream?	0	1	2	3	4	5
6. During the last month or so, how often have you had to push or strain to begin urination?	0	1	2	3	4	5
	None	1 Time	2 Times	3 Times	4 Times	5 or More times
7. During the last month, how many times did you most typically get up to urinate from the time you went to bed at night until the time you got up in the morning?	0	1	2	3	4	5

AUA symptom score = sum of questions 1 to 7.

Fig. 7.1 The AUA symptom index

with similar findings [11, 12]. Though there is some variation in prevalence rates, there is a general trend toward increasing symptom scores with increasing age.

Prostate size has also been used as a surrogate for LUTS. While size can be estimated by digital rectal exam (DRE), ultrasound and MRI are much more reliable. DRE tends to underestimate size. In general, prostate volume has been found to increase steadily with advancing age [13, 14]. Increasing size has been found to be associated with worsening LUTS. In a study of Norwegian men, the median prostate volume increased from 29.5 mL for men with mild LUTS to 37.0 mL for men with severe symptoms based on IPSS [13].

Definitive diagnosis of bladder obstruction is made by pressure flow studies, urodynamics. Pressure flow studies require a catheter to be placed in the bladder transurethrally and a pressure transducer transrectally. Noninvasive flow studies can be performed as well to characterize urinary velocity and flow pattern and suggest the presence or absence of obstruction. Generally, maximum flow rate (Qmax) greater than 15 mL/s is considered normal, and a flow rate less than 10 mL/s indicates high probability of obstruction. A flow rate between 10 and 15 mL/s is equivocal. In the Olmsted County Study, the median flow rate decreased to 11.3 mL/s for men in their 70s from 20.3 mL/s for men in their 40s [12]. While flow rates can help diagnose obstruction, patients who have poor bladder contractility will also have low flow rates. Thus, a flow rate cannot definitively diagnose BPH/LUTS. Further, even if obstruction is found on invasive urodynamics, the location of the obstruction may need to be confirmed. This can be done with direct visualization (cystoscopy) or fluoroscopy (i.e., video urodynamics).

The symptoms associated with BPH/LUTS tend to increase with time and if left untreated can result in complications. In a study by Djavan and colleagues (2004), 397 men were followed after presenting to a urology clinic with mild LUTS, and the cumulative incidence of clinical progression to moderate/severe symptoms was calculated. The likelihood of progressing was found to be 6%, 13%, 15%, 24%, 28%, and 31% at 6, 12, 18, 24, 36, and 48 months, respectively [15]. In the Medical Therapy of Prostatic Symptoms (MTOPS) study, 14% of placebo-treated patients experienced a 4-point or more worsening of symptoms on IPSS over the course of the study, which had a mean follow-up of 4.5 years [16].

Aside from the symptoms of BPH and impact on quality of life, there are multiple serious complications from BPH. These complications are usually secondary to the bladder outlet obstruction that can exist from BPH. BPH is a chronic progressive condition. Monitoring and treating men with BPH aims to identify and avoid these complications.

Bladder stones are eight times more common in men with BPH compared to controls, though the risk is still relatively small [17, 18]. Advanced age, decreased urinary flow, and intravesical protrusion of the prostate have all been shown to be associated with the presence of bladder stones [19].

Bladder decompensation can result from long-term obstruction. The bladder becomes progressively more fibrotic and trabeculated [20]. Contractility worsens and patients can develop detrusor instability, incomplete emptying, and eventually detrusor muscle failure and urinary retention [21, 22].

Urinary incontinence can develop in patients with BPH and may be due to over-distention of the bladder secondary to retention or due to detrusor instability [23]. Patients with BPH may be at increased risk of urinary tract infections (UTI) [24]. One study found a self-reported rate of 5.2% of UTI in men with BPH [18]. UTIs have historically been one of the most common indications for surgical intervention in patients with BPH [25].

Urinary retention is one of the most significant complications of BPH. Rates of urinary retention have been quite variable in the literature. In the Health Professionals Follow-Up Study, 82 men reported an episode of acute retention resulting in an incidence rate of 4.5 per 1000 person-years [26]. In the Olmsted County Study, 57 subjects had a first episode of retention which resulted in an incidence rate of 6.8 per 1000 person-years [27].

Though rare now, injury to the upper tracts can result from chronic obstruction. This can result in renal failure in some patients. The pathophysiologic mechanism is thought to be due to increased pressure secondary to obstruction and urinary retention. Rates of significant renal damage have been reported from 0.4% to 1.7% [28, 29]. It is important to note that men can develop renal damage even if their LUTS are not very significant. Treatment of the patient's obstruction can result in improvement of renal function [28].

Hematuria is commonly seen in BPH and is thought to be caused by increased prostatic vascular density due to the upregulation of VEG-F expression in BPH tissue [30, 31]. Finasteride and dutasteride have been suggested as possible therapeutic options for hematuria due to BPH, as they counteract the angiogenic effects of androgen stimulation, though evidence of their efficacy is mixed [32]. Management of hematuria is dependent on the clinical presentation and can vary from watchful waiting to operative intervention.

Diagnosis and Evaluation

History

In the initial evaluation of a patient with LUTS, a detailed medical history should be obtained with a focus on the patient's urinary symptoms. This should include the time course that the symptoms developed. The symptoms should be documented as well as how the symptoms are impacting the patients' day-to-day routines. It is crucial to obtain a thorough past medical history including comorbid conditions and previous surgeries. The medical history should include any other etiologies of bladder dysfunction including cerebrovascular disease or neurologic disease. Medical conditions like diabetes can also impact LUTS. Prior trauma to the urethra or pelvis may suggest that other etiologies such as urethral stricture may be the cause of the symptoms. It is important to assess for sleep apnea if patients have complaints of nocturia. The history should also include all prescription and over-the-counter medications, as diuretics, over-the-counter nasal decongestants, and antihistamines may all exacerbate urinary symptoms. In addition, it is important to ask patients about their fluid intake. Dietary factors such as water, caffeine, and alcohol consumption may be contributors to the overall clinical symptoms and are often easily modifiable. To fully assess the severity of urinary symptoms, a provider should use the AUASS/IPSS. Symptoms are classified based on the score as mild (0–7), moderate [8–19], or severe [20–35]. The symptom score can then be used on follow-up visits to assess the effectiveness of medical/surgical interventions.

Physical Exam

A general physical exam should be performed in all patients. On abdominal exam, the suprapubic area should be assessed for a palpable bladder. A digital rectal exam should be performed to assess sphincter tone and the prostate gland. The prostate size, shape, and consistency should be fully assessed, and any tenderness noted. Assessing the phallus and urethral meatus can also help identify abnormalities that may contribute to urinary symptoms. The testicles and inguinal canals should also be assessed. A focused neurological exam may be performed to help rule out any neurological causes for urinary symptoms if there is suspicion based on the history above.

Laboratory

A urinalysis should be performed in all patients. The urinalysis is necessary to rule out hematuria or evidence of a UTI. It is also useful to assess for glucosuria, which may affect patient management. A discussion on PSA testing should take place, with a shared decision after the risks and benefits of PSA testing are discussed. In this population presenting with urinary symptoms, PSA can be considered a diagnostic test rather than a screening test.

Optional Tests

The following diagnostic tests are considered optional but may be useful in patients with more bothersome symptoms.

Flow Rate (Uroflow)

Urine flow rate can be recorded via noninvasive testing. The maximal flow rate (Qmax) is considered the most useful parameter in identifying patients with bladder outlet obstruction. Rates less than 10 mL/s are associated with significant risk of obstruction. Ideally, the voided volume should be greater than 150 mL when determining flow rates.

Post-void Residual (PVR)

Measurements of post-void residual can be obtained by catheterization or by ultrasound. Elevated post-void residuals indicate decreased ability to fully empty and put patients at increased risk of retention. The MTOPS study showed that 7% of men with a post-void residual greater than 39 mL required surgical intervention over the study period [16].

Voiding Diary

A voiding diary is a record of voided volumes and fluid intake. This can be done for various periods of time from 24 h to a week. The patient records the volume of each void and fluid intake as well as the time of the event. Additionally, urgency leaks or pad changes can be recorded. The diary can help identify patients with nocturnal polyuria and excessive fluid intake. Frequency volume charts are used as well but record just the frequency and volume of voids.

Prostate Imaging

Transabdominal or transrectal ultrasonography of the prostate can be used to better assess prostate size, shape, and configuration. Imaging may be useful to assess these key characteristics of the prostate, which may affect the success rates or appropriateness of approach of certain surgical treatments. There is also data about mediation success that can be gained on prostate volume. 3T MRI is used now more commonly in the workup of elevated PSA and evaluation of prostate cancer. This imaging modality can give information about size configuration and likelihood of clinically significant prostate cancer.

Endoscopy of the Lower Urinary Tract

Endoscopy is not recommended for routine evaluation of BPH. It may be useful in certain patients to better assess prostate configuration when planning a surgical intervention. When the diagnosis of LUTS is not clearly related to the prostate, cystoscopy may have more value. For example, if there is a concern about irritative symptoms, or a patient has hematuria, then cystoscopy has an important role. In addition to detecting bladder cancer and/or carcinoma in situ, the cystoscopy is also useful to assess for bladder stones, bladder trabeculations, etc.

Upper Urinary Tract Imaging

Routine imaging of the upper tract with ultrasonography or CT urography is not typically indicated unless there is a concern for other urinary pathology, such as nephrolithiasis, or for workup of hematuria.

Differential Diagnosis

There are many conditions aside from BPH that can result in LUTS. One of the important etiologies that should be assessed is prostate cancer. A digital rectal exam (DRE) and PSA test can be helpful in differentiating between BPH and prostate cancer. It is important to note that low-risk early-stage prostate cancer can present asymptomatically and that patients can present with both BPH and prostate cancer concurrently. There is ongoing controversy regarding PSA screening, and it is important to note that patients with LUTS may not have been screened. A discussion of the risks and benefits of PSA testing should be performed, and a shared decision should be made on whether to check a PSA. The most recent US Preventative Task Force guideline on PSA testing does allow for prostate cancer screening in patients aged 55–69 years old [33]. In patients with risk factors for prostate cancer, including a strong family history, it is very important to at least discuss PSA testing with the patient. When first assessing patients with LUTS, it is important to consider prostate cancer in the differential diagnosis.

Another condition that should be considered in assessing patients with LUTS is prostatitis. Inflammation of the prostate may be secondary to a bacterial infection or a noninfectious inflammatory process. Many of the symptoms of LUTS will overlap with prostatitis. Acute bacterial prostatitis typically presents with fevers, pelvic pain, and a very tender prostate on exam. Chronic bacterial and nonbacterial prostatitis are more indolent in presentation, and patients may have dysuria, pelvic pain, and obstructive voiding symptoms.

Urethral stricture disease can present with symptoms similar to BPH. Patients with stricture may complain of decreased flow of stream, post-void dribbling, and dysuria. History of urethritis or trauma should increase provider suspicion for stricture disease.

Bladder cancer can present with a variety of symptoms including hematuria and irritative voiding symptoms. If patients have hematuria, an appropriate hematuria workup should be conducted. In those patients with bladder cancer risk factors including strong family history or smoking history, a referral to a urologist can be considered. Another common urologic diagnosis that should be considered in patients with LUTS is overactive bladder (OAB). The symptoms of OAB can overlap with BPH/LUTS and treatment may differ.

As stated previously, many systemic medical conditions can present with urinary symptoms. Patients should be assessed for diabetes, polydipsia, neurologic disease, kidney stones, and cerebrovascular disease. In addition, all medications should be reviewed as medications with anticholinergic side effects can cause LUTS.

Management

Primary care providers can perform the initial evaluation in patients with LUTS/ BPH and may feel comfortable providing counseling on therapy options. Certainly, if primary care is going to consider evaluating patients, an understanding of the differential diagnosis and attention to a focused exam are important. Additionally, if empiric treatment is considered, providers should be able to discuss the risks and benefits of the treatment option. After explaining the natural history of LUTS/BPH, the patient and doctor may discuss watchful waiting conservative management and/ or medical therapy. An understanding of the procedural and surgical intervention is also important to have an understanding about when a referral is needed.

Patients who choose to proceed with observation, conservative, or medical therapy should be followed to assess for changes in symptoms. After initiation of medical therapy, timing of treatment effect may vary based on the pharmacological agent. A follow-up visit should be arranged to assess symptoms. The use of the IPSS questionnaire is a helpful objective measure of symptoms. If treatment is successful, follow-up should be repeated on a yearly basis to assess for symptom progression. If treatment fails as manifested by worsening symptoms, changes in medical therapy may be indicated. If the diagnosis is uncertain and the observation or medical therapy has been suboptimal or inadequate, the providers should consider referral to a urologist for further evaluation.

Watchful Waiting/Conservative Treatment

When patients are screened for or present with LUTS, it is important to assess the degree of bother. In patients who are not significantly bothered by the symptoms, it is reasonable to provide no treatment – watchful waiting. This does assume no concomitant issues like UTIs, hematuria, and/or concern about renal insufficiency. A patient that has an enlarged prostate and is suspected of having LUTS secondary to BPH can be reassured that the symptoms are not dangerous and treatment would only be needed if the symptoms became bothersome or if they developed complications as described previously. Watchful waiting is a safe option as most patients with non-bothersome LUTS will not experience any detrimental health effects. Certain symptoms can affect quality of life and thus may indicate a need for treatment.

Lifestyle modification may improve symptoms in patients who choose conservative therapy. Patients should avoid a sedentary lifestyle. Weight loss should be recommended in those who are overweight. Patients should also be counseled on dietary advice and avoidance of bladder irritants. Decreasing caffeine and alcohol intake can improve storage symptoms. Decreasing fluid intake before sleeping may improve nocturia. Avoidance of bladder irritants such as spicy foods, chocolate, acidic fruit, and carbonated drinks may also improve symptoms.

Medical Management

Medical management became a mainstay of therapy for men with LUTS in the 1990s with the advent of several classes of medication to target the physiologic and mechanical causes of LUTS in men with BPH [34]. The proper selection of medications depends on the patient's symptomatology and side effect tolerance. Not every medication will work for every patient, and concurrent use of several agents may be needed to optimize symptom management. Just as LUTS can be subdivided into storage or voiding symptoms, medications can be thought of as being aimed at treating one or the other.

α-Blockers

α-blockers are very commonly used for treatment of LUTS due to BPH. Noradrenergic sympathetic nerve stimulation has been shown to cause contraction of the prostatic smooth muscle [35], mostly in the prostatic stroma [36], which results in constriction of the prostatic urethra and obstructive symptoms. Blockade of the noradrenergic receptors relaxes the smooth muscle of the prostate and relieves obstruction [36].

There are currently five α-blockers approved for treatment of LUTS – terazosin, doxazosin, tamsulosin, alfuzosin, and silodosin. Over time, drug development has evolved toward subtype-selective agents with longer half-lives, resulting in decreased side effects and simplified dosing regimens without compromising effectiveness [37]. Clinical efficacy of these medications is usually considered fairly equal with subtle pharmacological differences. With more modern α-blockers that do not require dose titration, initial agent selection may be dictated by external factors such as insurance coverage and provider preference or drug interaction and sensitivities.

Tamsulosin, alfuzosin, and silodosin are all single strength formulations designed to be taken daily, though taking two doses per day is a relatively common clinical practice in cases with significant symptom burden. Doxazosin and terazosin are available in multiple concentrations, and dose strength can be increased for greater symptom relief. Common side effects from α-blockers include symptomatic hypotension, dizziness, increased risk of falls, and retrograde ejaculation due to the relaxation of the prostatic urethra resulting in decreased resistance along the retrograde pathway. However, these medications are generally well tolerated with minimal adverse effects [37]. Patients should be counseled to take α-blockers just prior to bedtime to minimize the risk of symptomatic hypotension. Patients must also be counseled that doubling a dose increases their risk of side effects and may be an "off-label" use.

It is important to note that a significant complication of α-blockers is an increased risk of intraoperative floppy iris syndrome (IFIS) in cataract correction surgery. Some studies have cited risks ranging from 43% to 90%, though a recent study in JAMA noted a number needed to harm of 255 specifically for tamsulosin [38–50]. It is unclear what dose or duration of α-blocker exposure increases the risk of IFIS, and it is not known whether stopping the α-blockers prior to surgery mitigates the risk.

As such, an AUA guideline panel recommended withholding initiation of α-blocker therapy in patients with LUTS until after any planned cataract surgery. In patients without planned cataract surgery, the AUA panel noted that there was insufficient data to recommend withholding α-blocker therapy. Patients should be counseled to inform their ophthalmologist that they are taking α-blockers prior to considering any cataract corrective procedure [51].

5-α Reductase Inhibitors

5-α reductase inhibitors (5-ARIs) inhibit 5-α reductase, which converts testosterone into DHT. DHT is thought to be an "amplified" form of testosterone and has been shown to cause prostatic hyperplasia [52]. Finasteride and dutasteride are the two 5-ARIs approved by the FDA for BPH/LUTS. Finasteride selectively inhibits the 5-AR type II isoenzyme and decreases serum DHT levels by 70%, while dutasteride inhibits both types I and II and decreases serum DHT by 95% [53]. However, the prostate overwhelmingly contains the 5-AR type II isoenzyme, especially in the hyperplastic tissue [52]. As such, the decrease in DHT in the prostate has been measured as approximately 80% with finasteride [54] and approximately 94% with dutasteride [55]. Decrease in DHT results in a decrease in prostate size, though this is a slow process, and those patients with significantly enlarged prostates are the ones who are most likely to experience a clinical benefit. In general practice, 5-α reductase inhibitors are reserved for use in patients who have documented enlarged prostates, usually larger than 40 g.

Indeed, there have been multiple trials showing the superiority of α-blockers, as compared to 5-ARIs, in significantly improving IPSS scores in patients with small prostates over a relatively short period of time [56, 57]. Quick improvement in LUTS is not the strength of the 5-ARIs. Instead, they excel in preventing disease progression and, when used in combination with an α-blocker, provide greater symptomatic relief than monotherapy alone. This has been demonstrated by two well-known, large multicenter trials.

The Medical Therapy of Prostatic Symptoms (MTOPS) trial compared doxazosin, finasteride, and combination therapy to placebo [16]. 3047 men were enrolled and followed for a mean of 4.5 years. The study was double blinded. The primary endpoint was BPH progression, defined as a 4-point increase in baseline

AUASS. While doxazosin and finasteride both significantly reduced the relative risk of progression (39% and 34%, respectively), combination therapy resulted in a 66% decrease and was significantly more effective than either doxazosin or finasteride monotherapy.

The Combination of Avodart and Tamsulosin (CombAT) trial was a multicenter, randomized, double-blind, parallel-group study, which followed 4844 men over 4 years and compared daily tamsulosin, dutasteride, or combination therapy [58]. It showed that combination therapy was superior to both monotherapies at reducing the relative risk of BPH progression and provided a significantly greater symptom benefit at 4 years. Combination therapy was also significantly superior to tamsulosin monotherapy, but tellingly not dutasteride monotherapy, at reducing the risk of acute urinary retention of urologic surgery.

Given the results of the studies above, 5-ARIs can be used as primary therapy for LUTS, though they are most often used in combination with α-blockers. Combining these medications results in fast relief of LUTS as well as prevention of disease progression. Both the 5-ARI and α-blocker are usually continued indefinitely, as long as the patient tolerates the regimen. Side effects of 5-ARIs include decreased libido, ejaculatory disorders, orgasmic disorders, and gynecomastia. There is concern that the sexual side effects continue past the cessation of therapy [59]. However, these medications are overall very well tolerated.

It is important to note that the FDA placed a black box warning on 5-ARIs due to concerns that they increase the risk of high-grade prostate cancer based on the results of the Prostate Cancer Prevention Trial (PCPT) [60]. However, several studies have called this conclusion into question for multiple reasons [61], most recently a study from Sweden examining 23,442 men on 5-ARIs, which showed no increased risk of high-grade or low-grade prostate cancer as compared to the general population [62]. Patients should be counseled about the black box warning, as well as the most recent data, when electing to initiate 5-ARI therapy. In addition, it is important to note that 5-α reductase inhibitors will reduce PSA values. Patients who get yearly PSAs should have the PSA adjusted for the reduction effect of 5-α reductase inhibitor. The PSA will typically be halved, so the PSA should be doubled to determine the true value.

Phosphodiesterase Type 5 (PDE-5) Inhibitors

PDE-5 inhibitors are primarily used to treat erectile dysfunction (ED), but they have been shown to be effective in treating LUTS in four large, randomized, placebo-controlled clinical trials [63–65]. This action is usually attributed to the relaxation of prostate smooth muscle, which is mediated by nitric oxide, though other theories include endothelin inactivation, decrease in autonomic hyperactivity, or reduction of pelvic ischemia [66, 67]. A multinational survey published in 2003 showed that men with ED tended to have more significant LUTS [68]. As such, PDE-5 inhibitors can be used as monotherapy for two common complaints.

The PDE-5 inhibitors available currently are sildenafil, tadalafil, vardenafil, and avanafil. However, sildenafil and vardenafil have short durations of action (4 h) as opposed to tadalafil which has a half-life of 17.5 h and a duration of action of up to 36 h [34]. As such, 5 mg daily of tadalafil is approved by the FDA for treatment of both ED and LUTS [64, 69]. It is important to note that PDE-5 inhibitors do not affect objective measurements of outlet obstruction, such as uroflow parameters or post-void residual volume [34].

Common side effects of PDE-5 inhibitors include hypotension, dizziness, headache, flushing, nasal congestion, nasopharyngitis, and dyspepsia. Though rare, patients should be warned of the risk of priapism and counseled to present to their physician's office or the emergency department for a painful erection lasting longer than 4 h [69].

Anticholinergics

In patients with LUTS that are primarily storage, anticholinergic therapy is a good option for providing symptomatic relief. Anticholinergic agents competitively inhibit the pro-contractility effects of acetylcholine signaling on the muscarinic receptors of the bladder. There are five classes of muscarinic receptor in the bladder muscle (M1–M5). M2 receptors are the predominant receptor class in bladder muscle; however, M3 receptors are responsible for bladder muscle contraction [70].

The available anticholinergic agents commonly used in urologic practice to treat overactive bladder include tolterodine, oxybutynin, trospium, solifenacin, darifenacin, and fesoterodine. Though each agent has a unique side effect profile, common side effects include dry eyes, dry mouth, constipation, vision changes, and cognitive impairment [71]. Patients should be counseled regarding these side effects, and care should be taken when prescribing anticholinergic medication to the elderly. Trospium is a quaternary amine and is thought to poorly penetrate the blood-brain barrier due to its size, making it an attractive choice in older patients [72].

All patients should be counseled that anticholinergic medications can increase the risk of urinary retention [71]. Intermittent monitoring of the post-void residual with in-office bladder scan can be considered if there is suspicion for incomplete emptying to ensure that patients on anticholinergic therapy do not develop chronic retention as their BPH progresses.

Desmopressin

Desmopressin has been used to treat patients with a primary complaint of nocturia. Desmopressin is a synthetic analog of vasopressin and works by binding receptors in the renal collecting system, increasing reabsorption of water which results in concentrating the urine, and decreasing the volume of urine excreted. Many different formulations of desmopressin have been studied. In one randomized controlled trial, 46% of patients treated with desmopressin were found to have 50% or greater reduction in nocturnal voids compared with 7% in the placebo group ($P < 0.001$) [73]. The problem with desmopressin is the unfavorable side effect profile which includes headaches, hyponatremia, nausea, and reported episodes of death. Noctiva is a newly FDA-approved nasal spray which consists of desmopressin acetate and has been approved for treatment of nocturia. A randomized controlled phase 3 study which did not exclude men who had concomitant BPH (about 30%) showed that desmopressin acetate was well tolerated and resulted in significant efficacy in treatment of nocturia compared to placebo [74]. Nocdurna is another form of desmopressin recently approved for treatment of nocturia in the majority of EU countries. In a phase 3 randomized study, Nocdurna was found to significantly reduce the number of nocturnal voids and increased the odds of a 33% or greater response compared with placebo [75].

Surgical Management

In patients who have been inadequately treated by, or are intolerant of, or not willing to chronicly take medical therapy, surgery for LUTS is an excellent therapeutic option. For decades surgery was the gold standard in managment of male LUTS. At its core, surgery seeks to debulk the prostate tissue causing obstruction. How this is achieved is what differentiates the different treatment modalities. Currently, there exist a multitude of different procedural options for management of BPH/LUTS, and there are often several different options with variable efficacy and side effect profiles. Operator expertise, availability of technology, patient preference, and insurance coverage may guide treatment selection in these cases, and there can often be several "right answers."

Endoscopic Management

Endoscopic management is extremely popular due to its minimally invasive nature, as well as its decreased risk of complications. Several new technologies have been developed over the past several decades, increasing the options available to patients and providers.

Transurethral Resection of Prostate (TURP)

The mainstay of traditional endoscopic management of LUTS due to BPH is the TURP. TURP can be safely performed on prostates of various sizes, though the risk of intraoperative complication does increase with larger glands, and operator preference will often play a role in dictating procedure choice. In general, TURP is appropriate for patients with moderately enlarged prostates (30–80 g).

TURP is performed using a rigid resectoscope through the penis to resect prostate adenoma, thus opening the channel for urination and decreasing outlet obstruction. All instrumentation is done through the urethral meatus and no incisions are made.

Risks of TURP include infection, hematuria, retrograde ejaculation or anejaculation, incontinence, urethral stricture, or bladder neck contracture [76, 77]. Patients usually require a catheter for 1–2 days and are admitted for observation and bladder irrigation after the procedure. Length of stay is usually 1–2 days. As tissue is sent to pathology after TURP, there is again a possibility of incidentally discovering prostate cancer of approximately 10% [77].

Transurethral Electrovaporization of Prostate (TUVP)

TUVP is similar to TURP in that an electrode is used to remove prostatic tissue. However, the tissue is vaporized, not resected. Thus, tissue is not submitted to pathology. TUVP has less bleeding, a shorter hospital stay, and a shorter duration of catheterization. However, reoperation rates due to AUR within the first year of surgery are higher for TUVP than TURP; this effect disappears at 5 years. There is no significant difference in clinical efficacy between TURP and TUVP, and the risks of TUVP are similar to that of TURP. Given that tissue is being resected, there is still a risk of incontinence, urethral stricture, and retrograde ejaculation with TUVP [78, 79].

Photoselective Vaporization of the Prostate (PVP)

PVP is performed using a 532 nm laser (the GreenLight laser system) to energize oxyhemoglobin in the prostate tissue, resulting in tissue vaporization with a low depth of penetration. The laser fiber is passed through a rigid cystoscope, and this procedure too is performed under general anesthesia. PVP has been shown to have similar functional outcomes to TURP, with a shorter length of stay and less immediate postoperative hematuria [80–82]. The risks of PVP are similar to TUVP and TURP.

Laser Enucleation of the Prostate (LEP)

LEP can be best thought of as a hybrid between TURP and simple prostatectomy. An energy source is used to separate the prostate adenoma from the capsule and deposit it in the bladder via a transurethral approach. The adenoma is then morcellated and extracted. Common energy sources used are holmium or thulium:YAG lasers. LEP is a technically complex operation with a significant learning curve; as such, finding a clinician proficient in the technique can be difficult.

LEP has less bleeding, a shorter hospital stay, and less catheterization time than open prostatectomy [83]. It has also been shown to have significantly more improvement in IPSS and postoperative Qmax than TURP; additionally, LEP has a higher volume of tissue resected as compared to TURP, with less bleeding and a shorter hospital stay [83]. Literature reports successful LEP in glands as large as 376 g in the hands of experts [84]. Risks include gross hematuria, anejaculation or retrograde ejaculation, urethral stricture, bladder neck contracture, and incontinence. It remains an excellent therapeutic option, if available.

Transurethral Microwave Thermotherapy (TUMT)

TUMT is a minimally invasive outpatient procedure with minimal instrumentation. A microwave catheter is inserted into the urethra under local anesthesia, and microwave energy is emitted into the prostate to induce coagulative necrosis in the prostatic tissue, relieving obstruction. A rectal catheter is also placed to ensure that the surrounding tissues are not injured. TUMT is a good procedural option for those patients who are too sick to undergo surgery [85]. Risks include gross hematuria, irritative voiding symptoms, incontinence, or infection. Patients usually require a catheter for several days after the procedure due to post-procedure swelling, and it can take several weeks for patients to notice a change in urinary symptoms.

A Cochrane review concluded that TUMT is an effective alternative to TURP or medical therapy; however, TURP provides greater symptomatic relief and improvements in QMax, while patients who undergo TUMT are less likely to have retrograde ejaculation, gross hematuria, or urethral strictures but are more likely to require subsequent treatments for BPH. TUMT does cause a significant improvement in symptoms and Qmax as compared to α-blockers [86].

Convective Radiofrequency Water Vapor Thermal Therapy (Rezum)

Rezum is a relatively new outpatient transurethral therapy designed to relieve obstruction. Sterile water vapor is injected into the periurethral prostatic tissue using a specialized cystoscope, causing tissue death and eventual atrophy. Given the surgical tissue planes of the prostate, this effect is limited to the transition zone. Resorption of the atrophied tissue reduces urethral obstruction and eases LUTS [87, 88].

It takes approximately 3 months for maximal efficacy to occur. Rezum has been shown to improve Qmax and IPSS scores without sexual side effects at 3 and 12 months in a small randomized control trial [88–91]. When Rezum patient data was compared to data from the MTOPS trial over a 3-year time period, it was shown that Rezum has equivalent symptomatic control to combination medical therapy, though it is superior to monotherapy. Patients on medical therapy were five times as likely to have clinical progression of BPH as compared to patients who underwent Rezum [92].

Waterjet Ablation Therapy (Aquablation)

Aquablation is an ablative therapy that combines intraoperative ultrasound, cystoscopy, and computer guidance to ablate the prostate. Procedures are done under general anesthesia. The surgeon programs a robotic system with a set of ablation parameters using both cystoscopy and ultrasound guidance. The robotic system then proceeds to use high-velocity saline beams to ablate the selected regions of the prostate. It is indicated for glands 30–80 g. In the small cohort of patients who have undergone aquablation, there have been no reported cases of erectile dysfunction, retrograde ejaculation, or urinary incontinence [93, 94]. Aquablation was found to have equivalent symptomatic improvement to TURP at 1 year in a double-blinded, multicenter prospective randomized controlled trial, with fewer adverse events or sexual side effects [95]. Given the novelty of this treatment modality, it is not widely accessible, and more long-term data is needed to better assess the long-term outcomes of this modality.

Prostatic Urethral Lift (Urolift)

Urolift is an endoscopic procedure that uses implants to retract prostatic tissue and relieve LUTS. It can be performed in the office under local anesthesia and has been shown to improve symptoms and urinary flow as compared to placebo while preserving sexual function [96]. Though it was initially indicated in prostates 30–80 g, it can be used successfully in larger prostates as well, depending on the anatomy [97]. When compared to TURP, Urolift has a quicker recovery, with shorter hospital stays and less time of catheterization, as well as fewer adverse events, but TURP resulted in significantly greater improvement in IPSS, PVR, and Qmax as compared to Urolift [98]. Overall, Urolift is superior to medical therapy but inferior to traditional surgical therapies, though with a better complication profile, and is a good option in the carefully selected patient [99].

Prostatectomy

Simple prostatectomy removes the vast majority of the prostate adenoma while leaving the prostate capsule and seminal vesicles intact. It can be performed using an open, laparoscopic, or robotic approach [100]. Given the technical skill required for laparoscopic prostatectomy, most primary care physicians will interact with urologists who perform either open or robotic-assisted simple prostatectomy (RASP), and these shall be the focus of this text. For large glands (i.e., >80 g), simple prostatectomy remains the gold standard [51], though there are specialists who manage significantly larger glands endoscopically. Patients must be healthy enough to undergo abdominal or laparoscopic surgery.

Given the excellent visualization and access during simple prostatectomy, resection of the vast majority of the adenoma is often achieved. As such, simple prostatectomy is very effective at improving IPSS or AUASS and quality of life scores. It also results in significantly improved Qmax and decreases in post-void residual [101–109]. Several studies have shown an increase in sexual desire, satisfaction, and erectile function after simple prostatectomy [103, 110].

Risks include pain, bleeding, infection, bladder neck contraction (3–6%), and urinary incontinence (0.5–8%). Hospital stay for open prostatectomy was traditionally between 5 and 7 days, though length of stay is less in more recent series (4 days) [101–109]. Length of stay and blood loss are significantly less for RASP, though mean operative time is increased. There is no significant difference in symptom relief and objective measurements of obstruction between RASP and open simple prostatectomy [111, 112].

Patients should be counseled that they will have a catheter postoperatively for 1–2 weeks. Patients will have to be admitted postoperatively for continuous bladder irrigation and monitoring. Many urologists perform a cystogram prior to catheter removal. Given that the prostate is responsible for a large proportion of ejaculate volume, it is important to counsel patients that their ejaculatory volume will significantly decrease after prostatectomy and that many patients develop anejaculatory orgasm or retrograde ejaculation after surgery.

Given that the prostatic capsule is left in situ, this is not an oncologic operation. It is important to counsel patients regarding this, as incidentally discovered prostate cancer has been reported at rates ranging from 2% to 17% [101, 102, 104, 107, 113].

Prostatic Stent

Prostatic stenting is done in the outpatient setting in those patients who are too ill to undergo a procedure and would be otherwise relegated to indwelling or intermittent catheterization. Stents can reduce urinary symptoms by greater than 50% and relieve obstruction, allowing patients in retention to spontaneously void. Risks include stent occlusion, migration, stent failure, irritative voiding symptoms, infection, incontinence, stone formation, and gross hematuria. Stents are easily removable and are a good therapeutic option in a carefully selected cohort of patients [114–116].

Prostatic Artery Embolization (PAE)

Embolization of the prostatic arteries is something that has been explored in the past and has more recently been evaluated. This should only be suggested by a urologist that is able to evaluate patients that might be appropriate for fluoroscopic guidance of a selective embolization. This results in prostatic tissue death and atrophy of the prostate, relieving obstruction [117]. The data is still very limited and immature. Exclusion criteria have not been rigidly defined but are generally considered to include prostate cancer, pronounced arteriosclerosis, renal insufficiency, a neurogenic bladder, bladder stones, significant UTIs, or urethral strictures [117, 118]. Proper patient selection is key.

PAE results in improved IPSS, PVR, and QMax, though TURP has been shown to be significantly more effective at relieving LUTS and improving objective measurements than PAE. In some studies, PAE has also been shown to have more adverse events and complications than TURP, specifically when considering postprocedure retention and treatment failure rates [119, 120]. A "post-PAE syndrome" has also been described, consisting of perineal pain, nausea, vomiting, and dysuria. This can occur in 9–11% of patients and responds well to NSAIDs. Other risks include hematuria, UTI, and puncture site hematomas [121].

Conclusions

BPH/LUTS are very prevalent in the general population and are an important aspect in the evaluation of male patients in the primary care setting. The etiology of symptoms can vary and may not solely be due to an enlarged prostate. Thus, treatment should be focused on symptom relief rather than any causative process. The management of BPH/LUTS has shifted from a primary surgical approach to medical therapy. In turn, primary care physicians have become the principle care takers of patients with BPH/LUTS. Primary care providers can be actively involved in the initial management of patients and can be key in understanding when referral to a specialist is needed. When medical management is insufficient, not tolerated, or not desired, urologists can provide advanced management and surgical intervention. There are many new and innovative technologies to successfully treat patients in a minimally invasive fashion.

Bibliography

1. Egan KB. The epidemiology of benign prostatic hyperplasia associated with lower urinary tract symptoms: prevalence and incident rates. Urol Clin North Am. 2016;43(3):289–97.
2. Isaacs JT. Antagonistic effect of androgen on prostatic cell death. Prostate. 1984;5(5):545–57.
3. Marberger M, Roehrborn CG, Marks LS, Wilson T, Rittmaster RS. Relationship among serum testosterone, sexual function, and response to treatment in men receiving dutasteride for benign prostatic hyperplasia. J Clin Endocrinol Metab. 2006;91(4):1323–8.
4. Parsons JK, Palazzi-Churas K, Bergstrom J, Barrett-Connor E. Prospective study of serum dihydrotestosterone and subsequent risk of benign prostatic hyperplasia in community dwelling men: the Rancho Bernardo Study. J Urol. 2010;184(3):1040–4.
5. McNeal JE. Origin and evolution of benign prostatic enlargement. Investig Urol. 1978;15(4):340–5.
6. Roehrborn CG. Male lower urinary tract symptoms (LUTS) and benign prostatic hyperplasia (BPH). Med Clin N Am. 2011;95(1):87–100.

7. Levin RM, Haugaard N, O'Connor L, Buttyan R, Das A, Dixon JS, et al. Obstructive response of human bladder to BPH vs. rabbit bladder response to partial outlet obstruction: a direct comparison. Neurourol Urodyn. 2000;19(5):609–29.
8. Abrams PH, Farrar DJ, Turner-Warwick RT, Whiteside CG, Feneley RC. The results of prostatectomy: a symptomatic and urodynamic analysis of 152 patients. J Urol. 1979;121(5):640–2.
9. Berry SJ, Coffey DS, Walsh PC, Ewing LL. The development of human benign prostatic hyperplasia with age. J Urol. 1984;132(3):474–9.
10. Homma Y, Kawabe K, Tsukamoto T, Yamanaka H, Okada K, Okajima E, et al. Epidemiologic survey of lower urinary tract symptoms in Asia and Australia using the international prostate symptom score. Int J Urol. 1997;4(1):40–6.
11. Nacey JN, Morum P, Delahunt B. Analysis of the prevalence of voiding symptoms in Maori, Pacific Island, and Caucasian New Zealand men. Urology. 1995;46(4):506–11.
12. Girman CJ, Epstein RS, Jacobsen SJ, Guess HA, Panser LA, Oesterling JE, et al. Natural history of prostatism: impact of urinary symptoms on quality of life in 2115 randomly selected community men. Urology. 1994;44(6):825–31.
13. Overland GB, Vatten L, Rhodes T, DeMuro C, Jacobsen G, Vada K, et al. Lower urinary tract symptoms, prostate volume and uroflow in norwegian community men. Eur Urol. 2001;39(1):36–41.
14. Bosch JL, Hop WC, Niemer AQ, Bangma CH, Kirkels WJ, Schroder FH. Parameters of prostate volume and shape in a community based population of men 55 to 74 years old. J Urol. 1994;152(5 Pt 1):1501–5.
15. Djavan B, Fong YK, Harik M, Milani S, Reissigl A, Chaudry A, et al. Longitudinal study of men with mild symptoms of bladder outlet obstruction treated with watchful waiting for four years. Urology. 2004;64(6):1144–8.
16. McConnell JD, Roehrborn CG, Bautista OM, Andriole GL, Dixon CM, Kusek JW, et al. The long-term effect of doxazosin, finasteride, and combination therapy on the clinical progression of benign prostatic hyperplasia. N Engl J Med. 2003;349(25):2387–98.
17. Grosse H. Frequency, localization and associated disorders in urinary calculi. Analysis of 1671 autopsies in urolithiasis. Z Urol Nephrol. 1990;83(9):469–74.
18. Hunter DJ, Berra-Unamuno A, Martin-Gordo A. Prevalence of urinary symptoms and other urological conditions in Spanish men 50 years old or older. J Urol. 1996;155(6):1965–70.
19. Kim JW, Oh MM, Park HS, Cheon J, Lee JG, Kim JJ, et al. Intravesical prostatic protrusion is a risk factor for bladder stone in patients with benign prostatic hyperplasia. Urology. 2014;84(5):1026–9.
20. Gosling JA, Dixon JS. Structure of trabeculated detrusor smooth muscle in cases of prostatic hypertrophy. Urol Int. 1980;35(5):351–5.
21. Lepor H. Pathophysiology, epidemiology, and natural history of benign prostatic hyperplasia. Rev Urol. 2004;6(Suppl 9):S3–s10.
22. Fusco F, Creta M, De Nunzio C, Iacovelli V, Mangiapia F, Li Marzi V, et al. Progressive bladder remodeling due to bladder outlet obstruction: a systematic review of morphological and molecular evidences in humans. BMC Urol. 2018;18(1):15.
23. McConnell JD, Barry MJ, Bruskewitz RC. Benign prostatic hyperplasia: diagnosis and treatment. Agency for Health Care Policy and Research. Clin Pract Guide Quick Ref Guide Clin. 1994;8:1–17.
24. Heyns CF. Urinary tract infection associated with conditions causing urinary tract obstruction and stasis, excluding urolithiasis and neuropathic bladder. World J Urol. 2012;30(1):77–83.
25. Holtgrewe HL, Mebust WK, Dowd JB, Cockett AT, Peters PC, Proctor C. Transurethral prostatectomy: practice aspects of the dominant operation in American urology. J Urol. 1989;141(2):248–53.
26. Meigs JB, Barry MJ, Giovannucci E, Rimm EB, Stampfer MJ, Kawachi I. Incidence rates and risk factors for acute urinary retention: the health professionals follow-up study. J Urol. 1999;162(2):376–82.

27. Jacobsen SJ, Jacobson DJ, Girman CJ, Roberts RO, Rhodes T, Guess HA, et al. Natural history of prostatism: risk factors for acute urinary retention. J Urol. 1997;158(9):481–7.
28. Mukamel E, Nissenkorn I, Boner G, Servadio C. Occult progressive renal damage in the elderly male due to benign prostatic hypertrophy. J Am Geriatr Soc. 1979;27(9):403–6.
29. Wasson JH, Reda DJ, Bruskewitz RC, Elinson J, Keller AM, Henderson WG. A comparison of transurethral surgery with watchful waiting for moderate symptoms of benign prostatic hyperplasia. The Veterans Affairs Cooperative Study Group on Transurethral Resection of the Prostate. N Engl J Med. 1995;332(2):75–9.
30. Ravindranath N, Wion D, Brachet P, Djakiew D. Epidermal growth factor modulates the expression of vascular endothelial growth factor in the human prostate. J Androl. 2001;22(3):432–43.
31. Pareek G, Shevchuk M, Armenakas NA, Vasjovic L, Hochberg DA, Basillote JB, et al. The effect of finasteride on the expression of vascular endothelial growth factor and microvessel density: a possible mechanism for decreased prostatic bleeding in treated patients. J Urol. 2003;169(1):20–3.
32. Bruha M, Welliver C. Is there a role for preoperative 5 alpha reductase inhibitors in reducing prostate vascularity and blood loss? Curr Urol Rep. 2017;18(10):75.
33. Grossman DC, Curry SJ, Owens DK, Bibbins-Domingo K, Caughey AB, Davidson KW, et al. Screening for prostate cancer: US Preventive Services Task Force recommendation statement. JAMA. 2018;319(18):1901–13.
34. Lepor H. Medical treatment of benign prostatic hyperplasia. Rev Urol. 2011;13(1):20–33.
35. Kobayashi S, Tang R, Shapiro E, Lepor H. Characterization and localization of prostatic alpha 1 adrenoceptors using radioligand receptor binding on slide-mounted tissue section. J Urol. 1993;150(6):2002–6.
36. Lepor H. Alpha blockade for the treatment of benign prostatic hyperplasia. Urol Clin North Am. 1995;22(2):375–86.
37. Lepor H. The evolution of alpha-blockers for the treatment of benign prostatic hyperplasia. Rev Urol. 2006;8(Suppl 4):S3–9.
38. Srinivasan S, Radomski S, Chung J, Plazker T, Singer S, Slomovic AR. Intraoperative floppy-iris syndrome during cataract surgery in men using alpha-blockers for benign prostatic hypertrophy. J Cataract Refract Surg. 2007;33(10):1826–7.
39. Chadha V, Borooah S, Tey A, Styles C, Singh J. Floppy iris behaviour during cataract surgery: associations and variations. Br J Ophthalmol. 2007;91(1):40–2.
40. Abdel-Aziz S, Mamalis N. Intraoperative floppy iris syndrome. Curr Opin Ophthalmol. 2009;20(1):37–41.
41. Amin K, Fong K, Horgan SE. Incidence of intra-operative floppy iris syndrome in a U.K. district general hospital and implications for future workload. Surg. 2008;6(4):207–9.
42. Bell CM, Hatch WV, Fischer HD, Cernat G, Paterson JM, Gruneir A, et al. Association between tamsulosin and serious ophthalmic adverse events in older men following cataract surgery. JAMA. 2009;301(19):1991–6.
43. Blouin MC, Blouin J, Perreault S, Lapointe A, Dragomir A. Intraoperative floppy-iris syndrome associated with alpha1-adrenoreceptors: comparison of tamsulosin and alfuzosin. J Cataract Refract Surg. 2007;33(7):1227–34.
44. Cantrell MA, Bream-Rouwenhorst HR, Steffensmeier A, Hemerson P, Rogers M, Stamper B. Intraoperative floppy iris syndrome associated with alpha1-adrenergic receptor antagonists. Ann Pharmacother. 2008;42(4):558–63.
45. Chang DF, Campbell JR. Intraoperative floppy iris syndrome associated with tamsulosin. J Cataract Refract Surg. 2005;31(4):664–73.
46. Chang DF, Osher RH, Wang L, Koch DD. Prospective multicenter evaluation of cataract surgery in patients taking tamsulosin (Flomax). Ophthalmology. 2007;114(5):957–64.
47. Cheung CM, Awan MA, Sandramouli S. Prevalence and clinical findings of tamsulosin-associated intraoperative floppy-iris syndrome. J Cataract Refract Surg. 2006;32(8):1336–9.
48. Keklikci U, Isen K, Unlu K, Celik Y, Karahan M. Incidence, clinical findings and management of intraoperative floppy iris syndrome associated with tamsulosin. Acta Ophthalmol. 2009;87(3):306–9.

49. Oshika T, Ohashi Y, Inamura M, Ohki K, Okamoto S, Koyama T, et al. Incidence of intraoperative floppy iris syndrome in patients on either systemic or topical alpha(1)-adrenoceptor antagonist. Am J Ophthalmol. 2007;143(1):150–1.
50. Takmaz T, Can I. Clinical features, complications, and incidence of intraoperative floppy iris syndrome in patients taking tamsulosin. Eur J Ophthalmol. 2007;17(6):909–13.
51. McVary KT, Roehrborn CG, Avins Al, Barry MJ, Bruskewitz RC, Donell RF, et al. Update on AUA guidline on the management of benign prostatic hyperplasia. J Urol. 2011;185(5):1793–03.
52. Andriole G, Bruchovsky N, Chung LW, Matsumoto AM, Rittmaster R, Roehrborn C, et al. Dihydrotestosterone and the prostate: the scientific rationale for 5alpha-reductase inhibitors in the treatment of benign prostatic hyperplasia. J Urol. 2004;172(4 Pt 1):1399–403.
53. Clark RV, Hermann DJ, Cunningham GR, Wilson TH, Morrill BB, Hobbs S. Marked suppression of dihydrotestosterone in men with benign prostatic hyperplasia by dutasteride, a dual 5alpha-reductase inhibitor. J Clin Endocrinol Metab. 2004;89(5):2179–84.
54. McConnell JD, Wilson JD, George FW, Geller J, Pappas F, Stoner E. Finasteride, an inhibitor of 5 alpha-reductase, suppresses prostatic dihydrotestosterone in men with benign prostatic hyperplasia. J Clin Endocrinol Metab. 1992;74(3):505–8.
55. Wurzel R, Ray P, Major-Walker K, Shannon J, Rittmaster R. The effect of dutasteride on intraprostatic dihydrotestosterone concentrations in men with benign prostatic hyperplasia. Prostate Cancer Prostatic Dis. 2007;10(2):149–54.
56. Lepor H, Williford WO, Barry MJ, Brawer MK, Dixon CM, Gormley G, et al. The efficacy of terazosin, finasteride, or both in benign prostatic hyperplasia. Veterans Affairs Cooperative Studies Benign Prostatic Hyperplasia Study Group. N Engl J Med. 1996;335(8):533–9.
57. Kirby RS, Roehrborn C, Boyle P, Bartsch G, Jardin A, Cary MM, et al. Efficacy and tolerability of doxazosin and finasteride, alone or in combination, in treatment of symptomatic benign prostatic hyperplasia: the Prospective European Doxazosin and Combination Therapy (PREDICT) trial. Urology. 2003;61(1):119–26.
58. Roehrborn CG, Siami P, Barkin J, Damiao R, Major-Walker K, Nandy I, et al. The effects of combination therapy with dutasteride and tamsulosin on clinical outcomes in men with symptomatic benign prostatic hyperplasia: 4-year results from the CombAT study. Eur Urol. 2010;57(1):123–31.
59. Fertig RM, Gamret AC, Darwin E, Gaudi S. Sexual side effects of 5-alpha-reductase inhibitors finasteride and dutasteride: a comprehensive review. Dermatol Online. J. 2017;23(11).
60. Thompson IM, Goodman PJ, Tangen CM, Lucia MS, Miller GJ, Ford LG, et al. The influence of finasteride on the development of prostate cancer. N Engl J Med. 2003;349(3):215–24.
61. Chau CH, Price DK, Till C, Goodman PJ, Chen X, Leach RJ, et al. Finasteride concentrations and prostate cancer risk: results from the Prostate Cancer Prevention Trial. PLoS One. 2015;10(5):e0126672.
62. Wallerstedt A, Strom P, Gronberg H, Nordstrom T, Eklund M. Risk of prostate cancer in men treated with 5alpha-reductase inhibitors-a large population-based prospective study. J Natl Cancer Inst. 2018;110:1216–21.
63. McVary KT, Monnig W, Camps JL Jr, Young JM, Tseng LJ, van den Ende G. Sildenafil citrate improves erectile function and urinary symptoms in men with erectile dysfunction and lower urinary tract symptoms associated with benign prostatic hyperplasia: a randomized, double-blind trial. J Urol. 2007;177(3):1071–7.
64. Roehrborn CG, McVary KT, Elion-Mboussa A, Viktrup L. Tadalafil administered once daily for lower urinary tract symptoms secondary to benign prostatic hyperplasia: a dose finding study. J Urol. 2008;180(4):1228–34.
65. Stief CG, Porst H, Neuser D, Beneke M, Ulbrich E. A randomised, placebo-controlled study to assess the efficacy of twice-daily vardenafil in the treatment of lower urinary tract symptoms secondary to benign prostatic hyperplasia. Eur Urol. 2008;53(6):1236–44.
66. Liu L, Zheng S, Han P, Wei Q. Phosphodiesterase-5 inhibitors for lower urinary tract symptoms secondary to benign prostatic hyperplasia: a systematic review and meta-analysis. Urology. 2011;77(1):123–9.

67. Takeda M, Tang R, Shapiro E, Burnett AL, Lepor H. Effects of nitric oxide on human and canine prostates. Urology. 1995;45(3):440–6.
68. Rosen R, Altwein J, Boyle P, Kirby RS, Lukacs B, Meuleman E, et al. Lower urinary tract symptoms and male sexual dysfunction: the multinational survey of the aging male (MSAM-7). Eur Urol. 2003;44(6):637–49.
69. Huang SA, Lie JD. Phosphodiesterase-5 (PDE(5)) inhibitors in the management of erectile dysfunction. Pharm Therap. 2013;38(7):407–19.
70. Caulfield MP, Birdsall NJM. International Union of Pharmacology. XVII. Classification of muscarinic acetylcholine receptors. Pharmacol Rev. 1998;50(2):279–90.
71. Yamada S, Ito Y, Nishijima S, Kadekawa K, Sugaya K. Basic and clinical aspects of antimuscarinic agents used to treat overactive bladder. Pharmacol Ther. 2018;189:130–48.
72. Staskin DR, Zoltan E. Anticholinergics and central nervous system effects: are we confused? Rev Urol. 2007;9(4):191–6.
73. Lose G, Lalos O, Freeman RM, van Kerrebroeck P. Efficacy of desmopressin (Minirin) in the treatment of nocturia: a double-blind placebo-controlled study in women. Am J Obstet Gynecol. 2003;189(4):1106–13.
74. Kaminetsky J, Wein A, Dmochowski R, Herschkowitz S, Cheng M, Abrams S, et al. MP74-01 A randomized, double-blind, placebo controlled study of 2 doses of SER120 (low dose desmopressin) nasal spray in patients with nocturia. J Urol. 2016;195(4):e969.
75. Weiss JP, Herschorn S, Albei CD, van der Meulen EA. Efficacy and safety of low dose desmopressin orally disintegrating tablet in men with nocturia: results of a multicenter, randomized, double-blind, placebo controlled, parallel group study. J Urol. 2013;190(3):965–72.
76. Rassweiler J, Teber D, Kuntz R, Hofmann R. Complications of transurethral resection of the prostate (TURP)--incidence, management, and prevention. Eur Urol. 2006;50(5):969–79; discussion 80.
77. Reich O, Gratzke C, Bachmann A, Seitz M, Schlenker B, Hermanek P, et al. Morbidity, mortality and early outcome of transurethral resection of the prostate: a prospective multicenter evaluation of 10,654 patients. J Urol. 2008;180(1):246–9.
78. Ekengren J, Haendler L, Hahn RG. Clinical outcome 1 year after transurethral vaporization and resection of the prostate. Urology. 2000;55(2):231–5.
79. Hammadeh MY, Madaan S, Singh M, Philp T. A 3-year follow-up of a prospective randomized trial comparing transurethral electrovaporization of the prostate with standard transurethral prostatectomy. BJU Int. 2000;86(6):648–51.
80. Mordasini L, Di Bona C, Klein J, Mattei A, Wirth GJ, Iselin CE. 80-W GreenLight laser vaporization versus transurethral resection of the prostate for treatment of benign prostatic obstruction: 5-year outcomes of a single-center prospective randomized trial. Urology. 2018;116:144–9.
81. Brunken C, Seitz C, Woo HH. A systematic review of experience of 180-W XPS GreenLight laser vaporisation of the prostate in 1640 men. BJU Int. 2015;116(4):531–7.
82. Lukacs B, Loeffler J, Bruyere F, Blanchet P, Gelet A, Coloby P, et al. Photoselective vaporization of the prostate with GreenLight 120-W laser compared with monopolar transurethral resection of the prostate: a multicenter randomized controlled trial. Eur Urol. 2012;61(6):1165–73.
83. Michalak J, Tzou D, Funk J. HoLEP: the gold standard for the surgical management of BPH in the 21(st) century. Am J Clin Exp Urol. 2015;3(1):36–42.
84. Kuo RL, Paterson RF, Kim SC, Siqueira TM Jr, Elhilali MM, Lingeman JE. Holmium laser enucleation of the prostate (HoLEP): a technical update. World J Surg Oncol. 2003;1:6.
85. Aagaard MF, Niebuhr MH, Jacobsen JD, Kroyer Nielsen K. Transurethral microwave thermotherapy treatment of chronic urinary retention in patients unsuitable for surgery. Scand J Urol. 2014;48(3):290-4. 2168–1813 (Electronic).
86. Hoffman RM, Monga M, Elliott SP, Macdonald R, Langsjoen J, Tacklind J, Wilt TJ, et al. Microwave thermotherapy for benign prostatic hyperplasia. Cochrane Database Syst Rev. 2012;(9):CD004135. 1469–493X (Electronic).

87. Dixon CM, Rijo Cedano E, Mynderse LA, Larson TR. Transurethral convective water vapor as a treatment for lower urinary tract symptomatology due to benign prostatic hyperplasia using the Rezum((R)) system: evaluation of acute ablative capabilities in the human prostate. Res Rep Urol. 2015;7:13–8.

88. Helo S, Holland B, McVary KT. Convective radiofrequency water vapor thermal therapy with Rezum system. Curr Urol Rep. 2017;18(10):78.

89. Dixon C, Cedano ER, Pacik D, Vit V, Varga G, Wagrell L, et al. Efficacy and safety of Rezum system water vapor treatment for lower urinary tract symptoms secondary to benign prostatic hyperplasia. Urology. 2015;86(5):1042–7.

90. McVary KT, Gange SN, Gittelman MC, Goldberg KA, Patel K, Shore ND, et al. Minimally invasive prostate convective water vapor energy ablation: a multicenter, randomized, controlled study for the treatment of lower urinary tract symptoms secondary to benign prostatic hyperplasia. J Urol. 2016;195(5):1529–38.

91. McVary K, Mynderse L, Gange S, Gittelman M, Goldberg K, Patel K, et al. PII-LBA1 using the thermal energy of convectively delivered water vapor for the treatment of lower urinary tract symptoms due to benign prostatic hyperplasia: the rezum II study. J Urol. 2015;193(4):e495.

92. Gupta N, Rogers T, Holland B, Helo S, Dynda D, McVary KT. Three-year treatment outcomes of water vapor thermal therapy compared to doxazosin, finasteride and combination drug therapy in men with benign prostatic hyperplasia: cohort data from the MTOPS trial. J Urol. 2018;200:405–13.

93. Gilling P, Reuther R, Kahokehr A, Fraundorfer M. Aquablation – image-guided robot-assisted waterjet ablation of the prostate: initial clinical experience. BJU Int. 2016;117(6):923–9.

94. Yassaie O, Silverman JA, Gilling PJ. Aquablation of the prostate for symptomatic benign prostatic hyperplasia: early results. Curr Urol Rep. 2017;18(12):91.

95. Kasivisvanathan V, Hussain M. Aquablation versus transurethral resection of the prostate: 1 year United States – cohort outcomes. Can J Urol. 2018;25(3):9317–22.

96. Roehrborn CG, Gange SN, Shore ND, Giddens JL, Bolton DM, Cowan BE, et al. The prostatic urethral lift for the treatment of lower urinary tract symptoms associated with prostate enlargement due to benign prostatic hyperplasia: the L.I.F.T. Study. J Urol. 2013;190(6):2161–7.

97. Shah BB, Tayon K, Madiraju S, Carrion RE, Perito P. Prostatic urethral lift: does size matter? J Endourol. 2018;32(7):635–8.

98. Sonksen J, Barber NJ, Speakman MJ, Berges R, Wetterauer U, Greene D, et al. Prospective, randomized, multinational study of prostatic urethral lift versus transurethral resection of the prostate: 12-month results from the BPH6 study. Eur Urol. 2015;68(4):643–52.

99. Larcher A, Broglia L, Lughezzani G, Mistretta F, Abrate A, Lista G, et al. Urethral lift for benign prostatic hyperplasia: a comprehensive review of the literature. Curr Urol Rep. 2013;14(6):620–7.

100. Ferretti M, Phillips J. Prostatectomy for benign prostate disease: open, laparoscopic and robotic techniques. Can J Urol. 2015;22 Suppl 1:60–6.

101. Adam C, Hofstetter A, Deubner J, Zaak D, Weitkunat R, Seitz M, et al. Retropubic transvesical prostatectomy for significant prostatic enlargement must remain a standard part of urology training. Scand J Urol Nephrol. 2004;38(6):472–6.

102. Condie JD Jr, Cutherell L, Mian A. Suprapubic prostatectomy for benign prostatic hyperplasia in rural Asia: 200 consecutive cases. Urology. 1999;54(6):1012–6.

103. Gacci M, Bartoletti R, Figlioli S, Sarti E, Eisner B, Boddi V, et al. Urinary symptoms, quality of life and sexual function in patients with benign prostatic hypertrophy before and after prostatectomy: a prospective study. BJU Int. 2003;91(3):196–200.

104. Gratzke C, Schlenker B, Seitz M, Karl A, Hermanek P, Lack N, et al. Complications and early postoperative outcome after open prostatectomy in patients with benign prostatic enlargement: results of a prospective multicenter study. J Urol. 2007;177(4):1419–22.

152

105. Helfand B, Mouli S, Dedhia R, McVary KT. Management of lower urinary tract symptoms secondary to benign prostatic hyperplasia with open prostatectomy: results of a contemporary series. J Urol. 2006;176(6 Pt 1):2557–61; discussion 61.
106. Serretta V, Morgia G, Fondacaro L, Curto G, Lo bianco A, Pirritano D, et al. Open prostatectomy for benign prostatic enlargement in southern Europe in the late 1990s: a contemporary series of 1800 interventions. Urology. 2002;60(4):623–7.
107. Shaheen A, Quinlan D. Feasibility of open simple prostatectomy with early vascular control. BJU Int. 2004;93(3):349–52.
108. Tubaro A, Carter S, Hind A, Vicentini C, Miano L. A prospective study of the safety and efficacy of suprapubic transvesical prostatectomy in patients with benign prostatic hyperplasia. J Urol. 2001;166(1):172–6.
109. Varkarakis I, Kyriakakis Z, Delis A, Protogerou V, Deliveliotis C. Long-term results of open transvesical prostatectomy from a contemporary series of patients. Urology. 2004;64(2):306–10.
110. Li Z, Chen P, Wang J, Mao Q, Xiang H, Wang X, et al. The impact of surgical treatments for lower urinary tract symptoms/benign prostatic hyperplasia on male erectile function: a systematic review and network meta-analysis. Medicine. 2016;95(24):e3862.
111. Sorokin I, Sundaram V, Singla N, Walker J, Margulis V, Roehrborn C, et al. Robot-assisted versus open simple prostatectomy for benign prostatic hyperplasia in large glands: a propensity score-matched comparison of perioperative and short-term outcomes. J Endourol. 2017;31(11):1164–9.
112. Holden M, Parsons JK. Robotic-assisted simple prostatectomy: an overview. Urol Clin North Am. 2016;4(3):385–91.
113. Hill AG, Njoroge P. Suprapubic transvesical prostatectomy in a rural Kenyan hospital. East Afr Med J. 2002;79(2):65–7.
114. Chiou RK, Chen WS, Akbari A, Foley S, Lynch B, Taylor RJ. Long-term outcome of prostatic stent treatment for benign prostatic hyperplasia. Urology. 1996;48(4):589–93.
115. Sethi K, Bozin M, Jabane T, McMullin R, Cook D, Forsyth R, et al. Thermo-expandable prostatic stents for bladder outlet obstruction in the frail and elderly population: an underutilized procedure? Investig Clin Urol. 2017;58(6):447–52.
116. Skydsgaard Schou-Jensen K, Dahl C, Azawi NH. Prostate stent is an option for selected patients who are unsuitable for transurethral resection of the prostate. Dan Med J. 2014;61(10):A4937.
117. McWilliams JP, Kuo MD, Rose SC, Bagla S, Caplin DM, Cohen EI, et al. Society of Interventional Radiology position statement: prostate artery embolization for treatment of benign disease of the prostate. J Vasc Interv Radiol. 2014;25(9):1349–51.
118. Teichgraber U, Aschenbach R, Diamantis I, von Rundstedt FC, Grimm MO, Franiel T. Prostate artery embolization: indication, technique and clinical results. RoFo. 2018;190(9):847–55.
119. Gao YA, Huang Y, Zhang R, Yang YD, Zhang Q, Hou M, et al. Benign prostatic hyperplasia: prostatic arterial embolization versus transurethral resection of the prostate--a prospective, randomized, and controlled clinical trial. Radiology. 2014;270(3):920–8.
120. Petrillo M, Pesapane F, Fumarola EM, Emili I, Acquasanta M, Patella F, et al. State of the art of prostatic arterial embolization for benign prostatic hyperplasia. Gland Surg. 2018;7(2):188–99.
121. Maclean D, Maher B, Modi S, Harris M, Dyer J, Somani B, et al. Prostate artery embolization: a new, minimally invasive treatment for lower urinary tract symptoms secondary to prostate enlargement. Ther Adv Urol. 2017;9(8):209–16.

Chapter 8
Management of Testosterone Deficiency in the Aging Male

Patricia Freitas Corradi, Renato B. Corradi, and Loren Wissner Greene

Serum testosterone concentrations decrease as men age. The age-related decline in testosterone levels, confirmed in several studies, results from defects in both testicular and hypothalamic-pituitary function [1]. In some cases, it is unclear whether coexisting nonspecific signs and symptoms, such as decreases in energy and muscle mass, are a consequence of the age-related decline in endogenous testosterone or whether they are a result of other factors, such as coexisting conditions, concomitant medications, or perhaps aging itself [2]. There is a widespread belief that undesirable changes in body composition and sexual dysfunction in men with hypogonadism are due to androgen deficiency. However, studies have shown that the amount of testosterone required to maintain lean mass, fat mass, strength, and sexual function varies widely in men [3]. Therefore, benefits of raising testosterone levels in older men have not been established [4]. In addition, metabolic and cardiovascular benefits or risks from testosterone therapy are still being debated.

Serum testosterone levels vary significantly as a result of circadian and circannual rhythms, episodic secretion, and measurement variations. A feature of testosterone with increasing age is a loss of circadian rhythmicity. Whereas young men exhibit a prominent morning peak, older men show only a minor increase in testosterone secretion. The threshold testosterone level below which symptoms of androgen deficiency and adverse health outcomes occur is not known and may be age-dependent. Furthermore, the testosterone concentration below which testosterone administration improves outcomes is unknown and may vary among individuals and among target organs [5]. Thus, before considering hormone replacement,

P. F. Corradi (✉)
Rede Mater Dei de Saúde, Department of Endocrinology, Belo Horizonte, Minas Gerais, Brazil

R. B. Corradi
Rede Mater Dei de Saúde, Department of Urology, Belo Horizonte, Minas Gerais, Brazil

L. W. Greene
New York University School of Medicine, New York, NY, USA

© Springer Nature Switzerland AG 2021   153
J. P. Alukal et al. (eds.), *Design and Implementation of the Modern Men's Health Center*, https://doi.org/10.1007/978-3-030-54482-9_8

even in the presence of symptoms or signs suggesting deficiency, low testosterone levels should be confirmed by two total testosterone measurements taken on two different early mornings. According to the latest American Urological Association's guidelines, a total testosterone level below 300 ng/dL is a reasonable cutoff in support of the diagnosis of low testosterone [6].

Serum total testosterone concentrations, representing the sum of the unbound and protein bound testosterone in circulation, are measured by radioimmunoassays or by immunometric assays. Total testosterone is 58% loosely bound to albumin, 40% tightly bound to sex hormone-binding globulin (SHBG), and the remaining 0.5–2.0% circulates in free form, which is the fraction taken to be biologically active. SHBG can be found to be *increased* with aging process itself, but also in illnesses such as hepatic cirrhosis and hepatitis, hyperthyroidism, HIV infection, and with concomitant use of anticonvulsants and estrogens. The conditions often associated with *decreased* SHBG are obesity, diabetes mellitus, hypothyroidism, acromegaly, decreased albumin states such as chronic illness and nephrotic syndrome, and drugs such as glucocorticoids, progestins, and androgenic steroids. If abnormalities in concentrations of SHBG are suspected, measurement of free or bioavailable testosterone is indicated [7, 8].

After the initial diagnosis of low testosterone, measurement of gonadotropins will determine if this is primary gonadal deficiency or secondary (pituitary or hypothalamic) hypogonadism, as raised gonadotropin concentrations suggest primary testicular failure. In primary hypogonadism, impairment of spermatogenesis is generally greater than that of testosterone production, whereas in secondary hypogonadism both functions are affected to the same degree [8]. Occasionally patients may notice reduced testicular size or asymmetry or decreased pubic hair. A thorough physical exam with measurement of testicular volume and consistency should be performed. Wooden beads of different sizes are useful to estimate the testicular volume. Also, testicular ultrasound may give additional information about testicular dimensions and contents.

Secondary causes of low testosterone, such as diabetes mellitus, anorexia nervosa, obesity, sleep apnea, chronic systemic illness, use of steroids, glucocorticoids or opiates, must be ruled out. It is important to point out that many hypogonadal men are sick and/or obese, and weight reduction, lifestyle modification, and good treatment of comorbidities are essential before considering testosterone replacement therapy (TRT).

Because impeccable coordination of the hypothalamic-pituitary-gonadal axis is required for normal testicular function in the male, including normal testosterone production and male fertility [9], pituitary or higher causes of hypogonadism must be excluded if luteinizing hormone levels are low. The measurement of serum prolactin and iron saturation can help determine the presence of hyperprolactinemia and hemochromatosis, respectively. Hyperprolactinemia leads to secondary hypogonadism through suppression of GnRH synthesis and secretion. Hemochromatosis is implicated in both primary and secondary hypogonadism. Assessment of anterior pituitary function, if clinically indicated or in the presence of severe secondary hypogonadism (testosterone level < 150 ng/dL), can uncover other pituitary hormone deficiencies. Pituitary imaging (MRI with gadolinium) might be necessary. Tumors, radiation, infiltrative diseases, pituitary apoplexy, surgery, head trauma, and subarachnoid hemorrhage may cause gonadotropin deficiency. When there are concomitant elevated prolactin levels, unless gonadotrophs are damaged by mass effect from a pituitary adenoma, the gonadal axis generally recovers after normalization of prolactin concentrations. Dopamine agonists are used to treat prolactinomas and idiopathic hyperprolactinemia.

In the absence of further abnormalities, treatment with testosterone to restore serum concentrations in young men with classic hypogonadism has long been considered the standard of care. The goal of treatment is to induce and maintain secondary sex characteristics and improve sexual function, sense of well-being, and bone mineral density. The Endocrine Society suggests aiming at achieving serum testosterone levels during treatment in the mid-normal range for healthy young men [10]. However, the standards for treating older men remain more contentious.

Testosterone therapy can be initiated with any of the suggested regimens, in accord with considerations of patient's preference, pharmacokinetics of testosterone formulation, treatment burden, and cost. The currently available testosterone formulations are oral preparations, intramuscular injections, transdermal gel and patches, subcutaneous implants, and buccal testosterone. Short-acting preparations are preferred to long-acting depot administration in the initial treatment phase, so that any adverse events that may develop can be observed early and treatment can be discontinued if needed.

The short-action preparations such as transdermal gels and patches are recommended to be applied daily over dry intact skin of upper arms, back, stomach, or thighs and are generally well tolerated. Among their potential benefits, they can mimic the normal diurnal rhythm of testosterone secretion and cause a lesser increase in hemoglobin when compared with injectable formulations. However, there might occur skin transfer and serum testosterone levels in some androgen-deficient men, maybe in the low normal range, demanding dose adjustments [11].

An oral testosterone is not available in the USA. It is a highly lipophilic oral formulation of testosterone undecanoate that is absorbed almost exclusively via the intestinal lymphatics thereby bypassing hepatic metabolism. For reasons of the dependence on lymphatic absorption, oral testosterone must be ingested with a meal containing some fat to allow for its optimal absorption. However, gastrointestinal side effects are a disadvantage often related to this formulation and can worsen compliance [12].

Pharmacokinetic testing with buccal testosterone formulations shows peak serum hormone levels at 30 min, with levels returning to baseline in 4–6 h. It is recommended to be taken twice daily. However, it has been associated with a less sustained effect and poor adherence because of gum or mouth irritation [13].

Subcutaneous testosterone pellets are also a viable treatment modality for testosterone deficiency. Incision is required for insertion and it can last for 3–6 months. Optimal dosing, frequency of reimplantation, and long-term safety of T pellets remain incompletely elucidated parameters [14].

Intramuscular long-acting injections include testosterone enanthate, testosterone cypionate, and mixture of testosterone esters of propionate, phenylpropionate, isocaproate, and decanoate. Dose is usually fixed and injections are either weekly or every other week, depending on testosterone plasma levels and symptoms. Because they are depot drugs, testosterone levels frequently fluctuate, and adverse effects such as development of polycythemia, changes in serum lipids, and increased serum PSA can happen and take longer to resolve [15].

Testosterone undecanoate is an extra-long-acting injectable with safety profile that can be administered only four times annually, and so it is recommended for long-term use after initial trial with a shorter-acting testosterone formulation. Long-term studies have validated the clinical efficacy of testosterone undecanoate in maintaining stable therapeutic levels of testosterone. Patient preference for the convenient dosing schedule might also lead to better compliance [16].

However testosterone should not be automatically prescribed; the risk:benefit ratio should be considered and discussed with the patient. In addition, proper patient follow-up is necessary for optimal safety [17]. Though current guidelines are not consistent concerning follow-up intervals and the parameters to be evaluated, it is probably advisable to see the patient following initiation of treatment after 3, 6, and 12 months and then annually, [10, 18] to assess whether symptoms have responded to treatment and whether the patient is suffering any adverse effects and to check compliance.

TRT is generally considered a safe and effective treatment for testosterone deficiency in younger and middle-aged men, but the same may not be true for older hypogonadal men. Aging men may experience exaggerated treatment side effects due to reduced capacity to metabolize testosterone and higher burden of comorbid disease [19].

Studies have reported positive effects of TRT compared with placebo on quality of life, depression, and some aspects of sexual function, such as libido and erectile function. However, the results of individual trials have been mixed, and there is variation in testosterone formulations and doses. A recent published meta-analysis has shown that compared with placebo, TRT was associated with a small but significant increase in sexual desire or libido, erectile function, and sexual satisfaction, but had no effect on energy or mood. TRT was associated with an increased risk of developing erythrocytosis compared with placebo but had no significant effect on lower urinary tract symptoms including those related to benign prostatic hypertrophy [20].

Men with low testosterone levels usually have a correspondingly low baseline PSA level that rises predictively on testosterone therapy. As part of monitoring plan for men under TRT, it is recommended that PSA levels are measured every 3–6 months. In men for whom sequential PSA measurements are available for >2 years, PSA velocity may identify men at higher risk for prostate cancer [21]. In a systematic review, the average PSA increase after initiation of testosterone therapy was 0.3 ng/mL in young, hypogonadal men and 0.44 ng/mL in older men. An increase of more than 0.4 ng/mL/year should warrant a urological evaluation and more intensive future surveillance for prostate cancer [22].

The relationship between testosterone therapy and prostate cancer has been debated. Although there is recent evidence against a link between testosterone therapy and prostate cancer development [4, 23], the US Food and Drug Administration retains a warning regarding the potential risks of growth promotion of microscopic or subclinical prostate cancer in patients who are prescribed testosterone therapy. Some clinicians have advocated testosterone use to treat the hypogonadism that often follows treatment for prostate cancer, but there is no good evidence for the safety of this approach. Clinicians should inform their patients that testosterone replacement therapy is still contraindicated in men with hormone-responsive tumors, such as prostate or breast cancers. Men with PSA > 4 ng/mL, prostate abnormalities on digital rectal examination, or abnormal prostate-specific antigen concentrations should be assessed further before testosterone replacement therapy is started [24].

Testosterone replacement therapy in androgen-deficient men has been shown to have beneficial effects on metabolic profiles with increased insulin sensitivity, lower blood glucose levels, and lower hemoglobin A1c values [25]. In addition, TRT has been associated with reductions in total body weight, increases in lean body mass, and decreased body mass index [26].

Recent studies have described a relationship between low levels of endogenous testosterone and atherosclerosis, coronary artery disease, or CV events [27, 28]. There are also reports on an inverse relationship between serum testosterone and carotid intima thickness [29]. So far, it is unclear if this is a causal association or due to low testosterone itself being a biomarker of poor health. However, there is also concern about the cardiovascular safety of TRT replacement therapy in all men, as men younger and older than 65 years of age with pre-existing cardiovascular disease had an increased risk of myocardial infarction when treated with testosterone. The US Veterans Affairs observational study of older men with a low testosterone also found a 30% increased risk of stroke myocardial infarction and death in the men treated with testosterone [30, 31]. There is evidence that testosterone may cause salt and water retention, particularly in older men [32], and this could contribute to edema, hypertension, and congestive heart failure. Also, as testosterone is converted to estradiol, the associated increase in estradiol may promote inflammation, coagulation, and platelet aggregation [33]. Also the use of anabolic steroids has been associated with left ventricular hypertrophy and systolic and diastolic dysfunction [34].

The Testosterone Trials (TTrials), a group of seven placebo-controlled, coordinated trials, designed to determine the efficacy of testosterone treatment of men aged 65 years or older with low testosterone concentrations for no apparent reason other than age, showed positive results of TRT in most of the evaluated variables [4], such as sexual function, walking, mood, depressive symptoms, anemia, and bone density, all to modest degrees. However, testosterone treatment did not improve vitality or cognitive function, and in the Cardiovascular Trial, testosterone increased the coronary artery noncalcified plaque volume as assessed using computed tomographic angiography [35]. This has led the Food and Drug Administration requiring that manufacturers of testosterone products add information to the labeling about this possible increase in cardiovascular risk. The European Medicines Agency, American Association of Clinical Endocrinologists, and American College of Endocrinology have agreed that there is no consistent evidence that testosterone therapy either increases or decreases cardiovascular risk. Meta-analyses of clinical trials have shown no association between testosterone treatment and cardiovascular adverse events, but none of the individual trials included in the meta-analyses were designed to assess these events prospectively [36]. Thus, the Endocrine Society suggests that large-scale, controlled studies are needed to resolve this controversy, since even a small potential risk is unwarranted, when balanced against a small potential benefit [37].

Frail elderly men with limitations in mobility are more likely to have clinical and subclinical cardiovascular disease than are those who do not have limitations in mobility. In a population of older men with limitations in mobility and a high prevalence of chronic disease, TRT was associated with an increased risk of cardiovascular adverse events [38]. Prior hypogonadism raises the risk of osteoporotic hip fractures with high morbidity including immobility and mortality. The risk of venous thrombosis and pulmonary emboli might be compounded by the use of testosterone and its conversion to estradiol.

Symptoms of sleep apnea, such as snoring and daytime somnolence, should be assessed because testosterone replacement therapy can worsen untreated obstructive sleep apnea. On the other hand, low testosterone has been associated with fatigue, sleep disturbance, and sleepiness.

Erythrocytosis is the most frequent adverse event related to testosterone replacement therapy. Testosterone replacement therapy generally leads to a mean increase in hematocrit of 3.18% [39]. Testosterone promotes erythropoiesis via erythropoietin production, bone marrow stimulation, and suppression of hepcidin, a regulatory protein whose inhibition increases iron availability. The potential significance of this adverse effect is that in the Framingham Heart Study, men who had the highest hematocrit levels (46–70 percent) had greater overall mortality and cardiovascular mortality [40]. Prior to commencing testosterone therapy, all patients should undergo a baseline measurement of hemoglobin/hematocrit. If the hematocrit exceeds 50%, clinicians should consider withholding testosterone therapy until the etiology is formally investigated. While on testosterone therapy, a hematocrit $\geq$54% warrants intervention, such as dose reduction or temporary discontinuation [41].

One of the most common complications of testosterone treatment is a decrease in testicular size with changes in consistency, predicting a decrease in sperm production. This might be only cosmetic concern for an older man; however this is an important issue if he still hopes to have reproductive success as exogenous testosterone lowers endogenous testosterone and decreases the sperm count significantly.

For those who are *not* seeking fertility, testosterone alone is considered first-line therapy, once it can reduce gonadotropin pulses through a negative feedback, though there are recent trials using clomiphene to increase gonadotropin stimulation of testosterone in men with hypogonadotropic hypogonadism (or hypogonadism due to hypothalamic disease).

Recently older men are attempting to have biological children, even as their testosterone and sperm count and quality declines with age. The first-line recommended fertility treatment for men with hypogonadotropic hypogonadism (or hypogonadism due to pituitary or hypothalamic disease) is hCG (human chorionic gonadotropin) as it acts dually to increase production of intratesticular testosterone and stimulate spermatogenesis. With its structure and function similar to LH, hCG is cheaper than LH and has a longer half-life. Through modern techniques of assisted reproductive technology, including ICSI (intracytoplasmic sperm insertion into an egg for fertilization), only a few good sperm need to be produced. However, after a course of hCG, hMG might need to be added if sperm production is still insufficient. By competitively binding to estrogen receptors of the pituitary and hypothalamus, serum estrogen receptor modulators (SERMs), such as clomiphene, increase pituitary production of LH in men with hypogonadotropic hypogonadism, to improve testicular production of testosterone and increase spermatogenesis. This approach is popular as it avoids the costly and painful injections of gonadotropins. SERMs improve libido and sense of well-being in secondary hypogonadism, but SERMS do not help in treating most primary hypogonadism. This is still considered to be an off-label use of clomiphene, and SERMs may have additional risks including venous thrombosis as estrogen levels may increase. A new trans-isomer of clomiphene, Androxal, has been used in clinical trials specifically for secondary hypogonadism [20, 21]. Another approach is to use the nonsteroidal aromatase inhibitors, anastrozole or letrozole, which do not block adrenal hormone synthesis. These aromatase inhibitors partially block the conversion of testosterone to estrogen, thereby decreasing estrogen levels reaching the pituitary and hypothalamus, so negative feedback should increase LH secretion, thereby increasing native testosterone production and simultaneously improving spermatogenesis. However, there is increasing concern about the health of the offspring of older fathers including an increase in schizophrenia, autism, depression, congenital malformations, and genetic mutations. Furthermore variabilities in telomere length in older men's spermatozoa might even predict increased risk of cardiovascular disease and decreased life spans for their children [42–44].

Bone density declines with age in men as well as women, and hypogonadal men may have osteoporosis at an earlier age than their peers. Bone mineral density of the lumbar spine and hip including the femoral neck should be measured every 1–2 years in hypogonadal men with osteopenia or osteoporosis. In addition, bone density should be obtained before consideration of aromatase inhibitors, as these drugs that blocks estrogen production estrogen usually hasten bone loss. Although testosterone stimulates bone formation and inhibits bone resorption through multiple mechanisms that involve both androgen and estrogen receptor-mediated processes [45] in men, the effects of testosterone on the bone are considered to be predominantly indirect, since estradiol is the major regulator of the bone. Low testosterone is known as a risk factor for osteoporosis largely because less substrate is available for conversion to estradiol [46]. Although testosterone therapy is not recommended for treatment of male osteoporosis, testosterone plays a role in bone remodeling either directly or via aromatization to estradiol by activating sex steroid receptors in bone cells, and studies have shown that testosterone treatment leads to improvements in areal and volumetric BMD at the spine and hip [47]. Nevertheless, to date, there are no trials reporting the effect of testosterone on bone fractures. Low testosterone is associated with low muscle mass, and this may have indirect effects to lower bone mass. As sarcopenia has been associated with increased falls and fracture risk in older men, and testosterone increases muscle mass, perhaps testosterone therapy might also help to reduce osteoporosis morbidity and mortality, by increasing muscle, though again this is unproven [48, 49].

In conclusion, aging itself is a risk factor for a variety of morbidities. Many of the symptoms attributed to male hypogonadism are commonly seen in normal male aging or in the presence of comorbid conditions. Also, low testosterone is often a marker for chronic disease. Before considering starting testosterone therapy, it is important to rule out secondary causes of low testosterone and to confirm the clinical suspicion of hypogonadism with biochemical testing. TRT should be offered only to individuals in whom a combination of symptoms of testosterone deficiency with careful documentation of low serum testosterone. Many testosterone studies are observational, and the effects on such findings as improved mood or cognition and even sexual function might sometimes represent a placebo effect. Patients receiving TRT may note positive effects on objective parameters including obesity, metabolic syndrome, type 2 diabetes mellitus, muscle function, and bone health, but should undergo scheduled regular testing for adverse events. Potential effects of TRT on cardiovascular disease, prostate cancer, and sleep apnea in older male are yet unclear and remain to be investigated in large-scale prospective studies.

References

1. Elliott J, et al. Testosterone therapy in hypogonadal men: a systematic review and network meta-analysis. BMJ Open. 2017;7(11):e015284.
2. Nguyen CP, et al. Testosterone and "age-related hypogonadism"– FDA concerns. N Engl J Med. 2015;373(8):689–91.
3. Finkelstein JS, et al. Gonadal steroids and body composition, strength, and sexual function in men. N Engl J Med. 2013;369(11):1011–22.
4. Snyder PJ, et al. Effects of testosterone treatment in older men. N Engl J Med. 2016;374(7):611–24.
5. Kelleher S, Conway AJ, Handelsman DJ. Blood testosterone threshold for androgen deficiency symptoms. J Clin Endocrinol Metab. 2004;89(8):3813–7.
6. Mulhall JP, et al. Evaluation and management of testosterone deficiency: AUA guideline. J Urol. 2018;200(2):423–32.
7. Dhindsa SS, Irwig MS, Wyne K. Gonadopenia and aging in men. Endocr Pract. 2018;24(4):375–85.
8. Basaria S. Male hypogonadism. Lancet. 2014;383(9924):1250–63.
9. Corradi PF, Corradi RB, Greene LW. Physiology of the hypothalamic pituitary gonadal axis in the male. Urol Clin North Am. 2016;43(2):151–62.
10. Bhasin S, et al. Testosterone therapy in men with androgen deficiency syndromes: an Endocrine Society clinical practice guideline. J Clin Endocrinol Metab. 2010;95(6):2536–59.

11. Hadgraft J, Lane ME. Transdermal delivery of testosterone. Eur J Pharm Biopharm. 2015;92:42–8.
12. Roth MY, et al. Steady-state pharmacokinetics of oral testosterone undecanoate with concomitant inhibition of 5alpha-reductase by finasteride. Int J Androl. 2011;34(6 Pt 1):541–7.
13. Dobs AS, et al. Pharmacokinetic characteristics, efficacy, and safety of buccal testosterone in hypogonadal males: a pilot study. J Clin Endocrinol Metab. 1998;83(1):33–9.
14. Pastuszak AW, et al. Pharmacokinetic evaluation and dosing of subcutaneous testosterone pellets. J Androl. 2012;33(5):927–37.
15. Behre HM, et al. Intramuscular injection of testosterone undecanoate for the treatment of male hypogonadism: phase I studies. Eur J Endocrinol. 1999;140(5):414–9.
16. Edelstein D, Basaria S. Testosterone undecanoate in the treatment of male hypogonadism. Expert Opin Pharmacother. 2010;11(12):2095–106.
17. Layton JB, et al. Testosterone lab testing and initiation in the United Kingdom and the United States, 2000 to 2011. J Clin Endocrinol Metab. 2014;99(3):835–42.
18. Nieschlag E. Current topics in testosterone replacement of hypogonadal men. Best Pract Res Clin Endocrinol Metab. 2015;29(1):77–90.
19. Tyagi V, et al. Revisiting the role of testosterone: are we missing something? Rev Urol. 2017;19(1):16–24.
20. Ponce OJ, et al. The efficacy and adverse events of testosterone replacement therapy in hypogonadal men: a systematic review and meta-analysis of randomized, placebo-controlled trials. J Clin Endocrinol Metab. 2018;103:1745–54.
21. Carter HB. PSA variability versus velocity. Urology. 1997;49(2):305.
22. Bhasin S, et al. Managing the risks of prostate disease during testosterone replacement therapy in older men: recommendations for a standardized monitoring plan. J Androl. 2003;24(3):299–311.
23. Brock G, et al. Effect of testosterone solution 2% on testosterone concentration, sex drive and energy in hypogonadal men: results of a placebo controlled study. J Urol. 2016;195(3):699–705.
24. Calof OM, et al. Adverse events associated with testosterone replacement in middle-aged and older men: a meta-analysis of randomized, placebo-controlled trials. J Gerontol A Biol Sci Med Sci. 2005;60(11):1451–7.
25. Jones TH, et al. Testosterone replacement in hypogonadal men with type 2 diabetes and/or metabolic syndrome (the TIMES2 study). Diabetes Care. 2011;34(4):828–37.
26. Srinivas-Shankar U, et al. Effects of testosterone on muscle strength, physical function, body composition, and quality of life in intermediate-frail and frail elderly men: a randomized, double-blind, placebo-controlled study. J Clin Endocrinol Metab. 2010;95(2):639–50.
27. Oskui PM, et al. Testosterone and the cardiovascular system: a comprehensive review of the clinical literature. J Am Heart Assoc. 2013;2(6):e000272.
28. Cheetham TC, et al. Association of testosterone replacement with cardiovascular outcomes among men with androgen deficiency. JAMA Intern Med. 2017;177(4):491–9.
29. Soisson V, et al. Low plasma testosterone and elevated carotid intima-media thickness: importance of low-grade inflammation in elderly men. Atherosclerosis. 2012;223(1):244–9.
30. Vigen R, et al. Association of testosterone therapy with mortality, myocardial infarction, and stroke in men with low testosterone levels. JAMA. 2013;310(17):1829–36.
31. Finkle WD, et al. Increased risk of non-fatal myocardial infarction following testosterone therapy prescription in men. PLoS One. 2014;9(1):e85805.
32. Bhasin S, et al. Older men are as responsive as young men to the anabolic effects of graded doses of testosterone on the skeletal muscle. J Clin Endocrinol Metab. 2005;90(2):678–88.
33. Ajayi AA, Mathur R, Halushka PV. Testosterone increases human platelet thromboxane A2 receptor density and aggregation responses. Circulation. 1995;91(11):2742–7.
34. D'Andrea A, et al. Left ventricular early myocardial dysfunction after chronic misuse of anabolic androgenic steroids: a Doppler myocardial and strain imaging analysis. Br J Sports Med. 2007;41(3):149–55.
35. Snyder PJ, et al. Lessons from the testosterone trials. Endocr Rev. 2018;39(3):369–86.

36. Budoff MJ, et al. Testosterone treatment and coronary artery plaque volume in older men with low testosterone. JAMA. 2017;317(7):708–16.
37. Dimopoulou C, et al. EMAS position statement: testosterone replacement therapy in the aging male. Maturitas. 2016;84:94–9.
38. Basaria S, et al. Adverse events associated with testosterone administration. N Engl J Med. 2010;363(2):109–22.
39. Bachman E, et al. Testosterone induces erythrocytosis via increased erythropoietin and suppressed hepcidin: evidence for a new erythropoietin/hemoglobin set point. J Gerontol A Biol Sci Med Sci. 2014;69(6):725–35.
40. Gagnon DR, et al. Hematocrit and the risk of cardiovascular disease--the Framingham study: a 34-year follow-up. Am Heart J. 1994;127(3):674–82.
41. Wheeler KM, et al. A comparison of secondary polycythemia in hypogonadal men treated with clomiphene citrate versus testosterone replacement: a multi-institutional study. J Urol. 2017;197(4):1127–31.
42. Bray I, Gunnell D, Davey Smith G. Advanced paternal age: how old is too old? J Epidemiol Community Health. 2006;60(10):851–3.
43. Antunes DM, et al. A single-cell assay for telomere DNA content shows increasing telomere length heterogeneity, as well as increasing mean telomere length in human spermatozoa with advancing age. J Assist Reprod Genet. 2015;32(11):1685–90.
44. Zhu JL, et al. Paternal age and mortality in children. Eur J Epidemiol. 2008;23(7):443–7.
45. Riggs BL, Khosla S, Melton LJ III. Sex steroids and the construction and conservation of the adult skeleton. Endocr Rev. 2002;23(3):279–302.
46. Ng Tang Fui M, et al. Effect of testosterone treatment on bone remodelling markers and mineral density in obese dieting men in a randomized clinical trial. Sci Rep. 2018;8(1):9099.
47. Snyder PJ, et al. Effect of testosterone treatment on volumetric bone density and strength in older men with low testosterone: a controlled clinical trial. JAMA Intern Med. 2017;177(4):471–9.
48. Scott D, et al. Sarcopenic obesity and its temporal associations with changes in bone mineral density, incident falls, and fractures in older men: the Concord health and ageing in men project. J Bone Miner Res. 2017;32(3):575–83.
49. Bhasin S, et al. Drug insight: testosterone and selective androgen receptor modulators as anabolic therapies for chronic illness and aging. Nat Clin Pract Endocrinol Metab. 2006;2(3):146–59.

Chapter 9
Controversies in Prostate Cancer Diagnosis and Management

Benjamin H. Press, Samir S. Taneja, and Marc A. Bjurlin

Introduction

The American Cancer Society (ACS) estimates that 164,690 new cases of prostate cancer will be diagnosed in the United States in 2018 alone, accounting for 19% of all new cancer diagnoses. The ACS also estimates 29,430 deaths related to prostate cancer [1]. Other than advanced age, common risk factors for the development of prostate cancer include a first-degree relative with prostate cancer and African-American race [1]. Prostate cancer is a disease of aging men; the average age of diagnosis is 66 years. A landmark study of autopsy results among men having died of causes unrelated to prostate cancer detected occult prostate cancer in 2%, 29%, 55%, and 64% in men in their 20s, 30s, 40s, 50s, and 60s, respectively [2].

Prostate cancer is largely an indolent malignancy, with diagnosis frequently preceding risk of mortality by decades, resulting in a 5-year relative survival rate in the United States for all stages of >99%. The 5-year survival rate for local metastatic disease is also >99%; however, patients with distant metastatic disease have a 5-year survival rate of only 30% [1]. The contemporary challenge for urologists assessing men at risk of prostate cancer is to consider the goal of early detection of potentially lethal prostate cancers while also avoiding the incidental over-detection of indolent disease.

B. H. Press
Department of Urology, Yale School of Medicine, New Haven, CT, USA

S. S. Taneja
Division of Urologic Oncology, Department of Urology, NYU Langone Health, New York, NY, USA

M. A. Bjurlin (✉)
Department of Urology, Lineberger Comprehensive Cancer Center, University of North Carolina at Chapel Hill, Chapel Hill, NC, USA

© Springer Nature Switzerland AG 2021
J. P. Alukal et al. (eds.), *Design and Implementation of the Modern Men's Health Center*, https://doi.org/10.1007/978-3-030-54482-9_9

The current prostate cancer grading system was developed between 1966 and 1974 by Donald Gleason and the Veterans Administration Cooperative Urological Research Group [3]. It has since been modified to better apply to prostate cancer as it is diagnosed and treated today [4–6]. The Gleason grading system is used to describe the microscopic appearance of prostate cancer. A higher Gleason score represents a more aggressive and more poorly differentiated cancer. A total score is calculated based on cell morphology patterns of the tumor specimen (graded from 1 to 5). Combining the two dominant patterns of morphology creates a Gleason score (i.e., Gleason 3 + 4 = 7). Gleason score has been recently grouped into simplified grade groups: Grade Group 1 = Gleason 6, Grade Group 2 = Gleason 3 + 4 = 7, Grade Group 3 = Gleason 4 + 3 = 7, Grade Group 4 = Gleason 8, and Grade Group 5 = Gleason 9 or 10. The National Comprehensive Cancer Network (NCCN) developed six risk group categories based on PSA level, prostate size, needle biopsy findings, and the stage of cancer outlined in Table 9.1 [7].

The difficulty in the diagnosis and management of prostate cancer is to determine whether or not a patient's disease is indolent and clinically insignificant, which may never impact a man's longevity and may not need treatment, or clinically significant and requiring curative action. While there is no universally accepted

Table 9.1 NCCN risk stratification

Risk group	Criteria
Very low risk	T1c Gleason score ≤ 6 PSA <10 ng/mL Fewer than three prostate biopsy cores positive, ≤50% cancer in any core PSA density < 0.15 ng/mL/g
Low risk	Stage T1c or T2a Gleason score ≤ 6 PSA less than 10 ng/mL
Favorable intermediate risk	T2b-T2c OR Gleason score 3 + 4 = 7 OR PSA 10–20 ng/mL AND Percentage of positive biopsy cores <50%
Unfavorable intermediate risk	T2b-T2c OR Gleason score 3 + 4 = 7 or Gleason score 4 + 3 = 7 OR PSA 10–20 ng/mL
High risk	T3a OR Gleason score 8 or Gleason score 4 + 5 = 9 OR PSA > 20 ng/mL
Very high	T3b-T4 OR Primary Gleason pattern 5 or >4 cores with Gleason score 8–10

Adapted from [7]

definition of clinically insignificant vs. significant prostate cancer disease, it is generally accepted that Gleason 6 prostate cancer is indolent, and Gleason ≥ 7 is clinically significant [8, 9]. This is supported by the American Urological Association (AUA)/American Society for Radiation Oncology (ASTRO)/Society of Urologic Oncology (SUO) recommendation for active surveillance for men with Gleason 6 prostate cancer [10, 11].

PSA Screening

Mortality rates for prostate cancer have decreased significantly over the last few decades. Five-year survival rates for all stages of disease have risen from 68% to 83% to 99% for the years 1975–1977, 1987–1989, and 2007–2013, respectively [1]. It has been estimated that the prostate cancer death rate has decreased 3% per year since 2009 [12]. While improved surgical technique and increased public awareness deserve recognition for this decline in mortality, a considerable amount of credit can be attributed to the early detection of prostate cancer utilizing community-based screening with prostate-specific antigen (PSA), an enzyme specifically secreted by the epithelial cells of the prostate gland [13–15]. The use of PSA in prostate cancer screening began in the late 1980s following Food and Drug Administration approval of PSA in 1986 for use as a serum marker for monitoring treatment response and recurrence [16]. The widespread use of PSA screening has caused a stage migration to an increased lower-grade, non-metastatic disease diagnosis [17, 18]. The utility of PSA-based screening is limited by the fact that PSA is not a cancer-specific marker. In fact, many nonneoplastic conditions such as benign prostatic hyperplasia (BPH), urinary tract infection (UTI), and prostatitis may lead to an elevated PSA in men [19]. Nonetheless, PSA detection has attained an important role in the screening and diagnosis of prostate cancer.

The European Randomized Study of Screening for Prostate Cancer (ERSPC) randomly assigned 162,243 men between the ages of 55 and 69 years to receive a screening approximately every 4 years or to not receive screening. The results demonstrated an approximate 20% reduction in prostate cancer mortality among those who underwent annual PSA screening [20–22]. Beyond the mortality reduction observed, the number needed to treat was shown to decline with increasing follow-up, illustrating the importance of prolonged survival to benefit from prostate cancer screening.

The Prostate, Lung, Colorectal, and Ovarian (PLCO) Cancer Screening Trial carried out in the United States randomly assigned 76,693 patients between the ages of 55 and 74 years to either annual screening with PSA and digital rectal exam or "usual care," which could also include screening [23]. This trial found no difference in prostate cancer mortality between those who received annual screening and those who received "usual care" [24, 25]. The PLCO outcomes have been subsequently questioned given the high rate of contamination in the control arm, as nearly as many men received the PSA testing as the screened arm [26].

The Göteborg Randomized Prostate Cancer Screening Trial analyzed 20,000 men born between 1920 and 1944 and randomized to either a screening arm of biennial PSA screening or to a control arm. Death from prostate cancer was reduced by 40% in the screening arm when compared to the control arm [13]. This trial also highlighted the stage migration in PSA screening. Almost twice as many incidences of prostate cancer were diagnosed in the screening arm, but the absolute number of advanced cases was lower in the screening arm than in the control arm.

Reconciling USPSTF Recommendations

The US Preventive Services Task Force (USPSTF) issued a grade D recommendation against population-based PSA screening for men over the age of 75 in 2008 and then again for all men in 2012 (Table 9.2), meaning, "there is moderate or high certainty that the service has no net benefit or that the harms outweigh the benefits" [27]. The USPSTF recommendation was largely based on the conflicting results of the ERSPC and PLCO trials [28]. These guidelines differ from recommendations of the American Urological Association (AUA), the NCCN, and the European Association of Urology (EAU), which all recommend shared decision-making about PSA screening [7, 29, 30].

The intense debate regarding PSA screening is based on the desire to limit the excessive diagnosis and treatment of indolent, low-grade, prostate cancer. One of the key components contributing to the controversy of screening and diagnosis of prostate cancer is what follows an elevated PSA measurement in clinical practice [31]. Over 1 million men undergo transrectal ultrasound-guided biopsy in Europe and the United States every year [32]. Indications for biopsy include an abnormal digital rectal exam (DRE) and elevated PSA, with a cutoff of >3 (NCCN) or >4

Table 9.2 Outline of USPSTF recommendations

Year	Population	Recommendation	Grade
2008	Men <75 years old	The USPSTF concludes that the current evidence is insufficient to assess the balance of benefits and harms of prostate cancer screening	I
2008	Men ≥75 years old	The USPSTF recommends against screening for prostate cancer	D
2012	Men	The US Preventive Services Task Force (USPSTF) recommends against prostate-specific antigen (PSA)-based screening for prostate cancer	D
Current (not final)	Men 55–69 years old	The USPSTF recommends that clinicians inform men ages 55–69 years about the potential benefits and harms of prostate-specific antigen (PSA)-based screening for prostate cancer	C
	Men ≥70 years old	The USPSTF recommends against PSA-based screening for prostate cancer in men age 70 years and older	D

Adapted from https://www.uspreventiveservicestaskforce.org

(AUA) ng/mL commonly used in contemporary practice. This procedure is not without risk of complications, of which include hematuria, rectal bleeding, hematospermia urinary tract infections, urinary retention, and sepsis [33–35].

The goal of a prostate biopsy is to detect actionable disease while avoiding the detection of clinically insignificant disease. Overdiagnosis predictions of indolent prostate cancer have been estimated to be as low as 1.7% and as high as 67% [36]. Detection of indolent and clinically insignificant prostate cancer may lead to unnecessary treatment and future biopsies on surveillance. These additional procedures incur a financial burden onto the patient and can result in unnecessarily escalated patient anxiety as a result of the cancer diagnosis, ultimately further contributing to the controversy of prostate cancer screening and diagnosis.

Since the 2012 recommendation, the USPSTF has revised their guidelines on PSA screening for men between the ages of 55 and 69. Physicians are now advised to have individualized discussion of screening with patients in this age group. However, the USPSTF still advises against PSA-based screening for men aged 70 and older [27]. While they have reconsidered their position on PSA screening, the message appears to be that vigilant assessment of competing risks for mortality is an essential first consideration, particularly before biopsy, rather than before treatment.

Improvement of Prostate Cancer Detection and Risk Stratification: Biomarkers

Several PSA derivatives, secondary urine and blood biomarkers, and imaging techniques have been appraised for their ability to refine risk assessment in men with elevated PSA. A summary of new biomarker screening can be found in Table 9.3.

PSA Derivatives

Due to the limitations of PSA, considerable attempts have been made to improve its use as a diagnostic tool. Such attempts include stratifying PSA levels by age [37], PSA velocity [38, 39], the ratio of PSA to the prostate volume (PSAD) [40], and isoforms of PSA [41]. Among these tools, PSA velocity and PSAD are mechanisms most frequently used in clinical practice. PSA velocity has demonstrated a significant association with high-risk cancer [42]. However, accurate measurement requires multiple evaluations and stringent follow-up. PSAD has been shown to be a valuable predictive marker for disease progression [43, 44]. One limitation of PSAD is that it requires an ultrasound in order to properly establish prostate volume [45], and ultrasound accuracy is operator dependent. This appears to be somewhat attenuated in the era of prostate MRI. It has been consistently documented that PSA is correlated with age and prostate volume [37]. Current literature differs on the

Table 9.3 Summary of biomarkers in detection of prostate cancer

Biomarker	Sample	Method	Regulation	Study findings
Prostate Health Index	Serum	Isomer of precursor PSA found in higher concentrations in men with prostate cancer	FDA approved for men with PSA 4–10 ng/mL CE-IVD	Improved predictive accuracy for overall prostate cancer AND clinically significant prostate cancer when compared to %fPSA, [−2]pPSA, and tPSA
4Kscore	Serum	Panel of kallikrein markers + clinical data	CAP accreditation	Improved Gleason ≥7 detection compared to modified PCPTRC Addition of kallikrein panel improved high-grade cancer detection compared with models based on clinical data
PCA3	Urine	Noncoding mRNA overexpressed in neoplastic prostatic tissue	FDA approved for men > 50 years old with at least one prior negative biopsy	Reduction in the burden of prostate biopsies among men undergoing repeat biopsy, but no consensus on cutoff
TMPRSS2:ERG	Urine	Fusion protein	CLIA accreditation	Improved predictive accuracy for prostate cancer detection when compared to tPSA
MiPS	Urine	PCA3 + TMPRSS2:ERG + tPSA		Addition to models improved predictive ability for high-grade prostate cancer detection
SelectMDx	Urine	mRNA levels of DLX1 and HOXC6 biomarkers	CAP accreditation CLIA accreditation	Greater prediction of high-grade prostate cancer when compared to PCPTRC
ExoDx Prostate IntelliScore	Urine	Exosomal RNA or PCA3, TMPRSS2:ERG, SPDEF	CLIA accreditation	Improved ability to discriminate between low- and high-grade cancers when compared to clinical variables

utility of age-stratified PSA ranges for biopsy indication, with some studies advocating for its use [46, 47] and other studies highlighting its limited utility [48, 49].

Free PSA

PSA exists in both bound and unbound forms. Men with prostate cancer have a lower percentage of the unbound form (%fPSA) than men without prostate cancer [50, 51]. The US Food and Drug Administration (FDA) has approved the use of

%fPSA in men with PSA between 4 and 10 ng/mL. In a multicenter study of 773 men with PSA between 4 and 10 ng/mL, Catalona et al. found that the use of a 25% fPSA cutoff detected 95% of prostate cancer and avoided 20% of unnecessary biopsies [52]. Ankerst et al. demonstrated that %fPSA was an early indicator of prostate cancer. Using thresholds of 25% and 15%, fPSA detected prostate cancer earlier than PSA in 71% and 34% of cases, respectively [53].

Prostate Health Index

Prostate Heath Index (phi) incorporates PSA, fPSA, and (−2) proPSA, an isoform of fPSA. The PDA has approved phi for men with PSA levels between 4 and 10 ng/mL. In a multicenter prospective trial, Loeb et al. discovered that, for men over 50 with PSA between 4 and 10 ng/mL, phi was a superior predictor of prostate cancer than any of the other individual components of the index [54]. At a cutoff of 28.6 for phi, 30.1% of patients with either benign or clinically insignificant prostate cancer could have avoided an unnecessary biopsy, compared to only 21.7% of patients using %fPSA alone [50]. A multicenter study with two independent prospective cohorts determined that phi had a higher specificity for prostate cancer than PSA and %fPSA at 95% sensitivity. The authors also found that a phi cutoff of 24 avoided unnecessary biopsies at 41% and 36% in the two cohorts [55].

4Kscore

The 4Kscore is a panel of kallikrein markers (tPSA, fPSA, intact PSA, human kallikrein 2) integrated with age, DRE, and prior prostate biopsy results to predict the probability of a high-grade prostate cancer biopsy result. Although not FDA approved, the 4Kscore is certified by the Clinical Laboratory Improvement Amendments (CLIA) program of the Centers for Medicare and Medicaid Services. The 4Kscore was validated in a prospective study of 1012 patients across 26 centers in the United States. The study found that in regard to detection of Gleason ≥7, the 4Kscore demonstrated superior predictive ability when compared to a modified Prostate Cancer Prevention Trial Prostate Cancer Risk Calculator (AUC 0.82 vs. 0.74). At a cutoff of 4K ≥ 9%, the 4Kscore revealed an avoidance of 43% of biopsies while only missing 2.4% of high-grade disease [56]. In another validation study, Vickers et al. found that the addition of the kallikrein panel enhanced high-grade cancer detection compared with a model based only on PSA, age, and DRE (AUC 0.78 vs. 0.70) and a model based only on PSA and age (AUC 0.76 vs. 0.64). Using a 4K ≥ 20% cutoff, this study indicated the number of biopsies would reduce by over 50% while missing 12% of high-grade disease [57]. The ability of the 4Kscore to properly detect high-grade prostate cancer on biopsy has been further established in a number of studies [58–61]. The 4Kscore has also exhibited a significant association with [62] and improved estimation [63] of higher pathologic grades in radical prostatectomy specimens.

Prostate Cancer Antigen 3

Prostate cancer antigen 3 (PCA3) is noncoding mRNA that is overexpressed in prostatic tumors when compared to nonneoplastic prostate tissue [64, 65]. It is detectable in urine after a digital rectal exam. The FDA has approved the use of PCA3 with a cutoff of 25 in men older the age of 50 who have had at least one prior negative biopsy. The National Cancer Comprehensive Network (NCCN) recommends a PCA3 cutoff of 35 in patients with PSA >3 ng/mL considering a repeat biopsy, who have had a previous negative biopsy [66]. The superiority of PCA3 in predicting outcomes of prostate biopsy when compared to PSA [67] and %fPSA [68] has been well-documented in published studies. Despite this, evidence frames PCA3 as a supplementary tool, rather than a sole predictor of prostate cancer. In a multicenter trial of 859 men, Wei et al. demonstrated that utilizing a PCA3 cutoff of 20 would avoid a repeat biopsy in 46% of patients. However, this cutoff failed to diagnose prostate cancer in 12% of patients and high-grade cancer in 3% of patients. When applying the same cutoff to the initial biopsy, an aggressive cancer diagnosis is missed in 13% of patients [69].

MiPS

The Mi-Prostate Score (MiPS) combines these two urinary biomarkers (PCA3 + TMPRSS2:ERG) with serum tPSA in order to predict the risk of any prostate cancer and high-grade prostate cancer on biopsy [34]. Tomlins et al. validated this diagnostic tool in a study of 1244 men undergoing prostate biopsy. They found that the predictive ability of MiPS to detect any prostate cancer (AUC 0.751) was significantly higher than that of PSA + PCA3 (0.726) PSA + TMPRSS2:ERG (0.693) and PSA (0.585). The authors also found the predictive ability of MiPS to detect Gleason >6 prostate cancer (AUC 0.772) was significantly higher than of PSA + PCA3 (0.729) PSA + TMPRSS2:ERG (0.747) and PSA (0.651). They concluded that utilizing MiPS can reduce unnecessary biopsies [70].

SelectMDx

SelectMDx is a urine-based molecular test that measures the mRNA levels of DLX1 and HOXC6 biomarkers (Fig. 9.1). Leyten et al. found that a panel of DLX1, HOXC6, and a third biomarker TDRD1 had greater accuracy in predicting Gleason ≥7 prostate

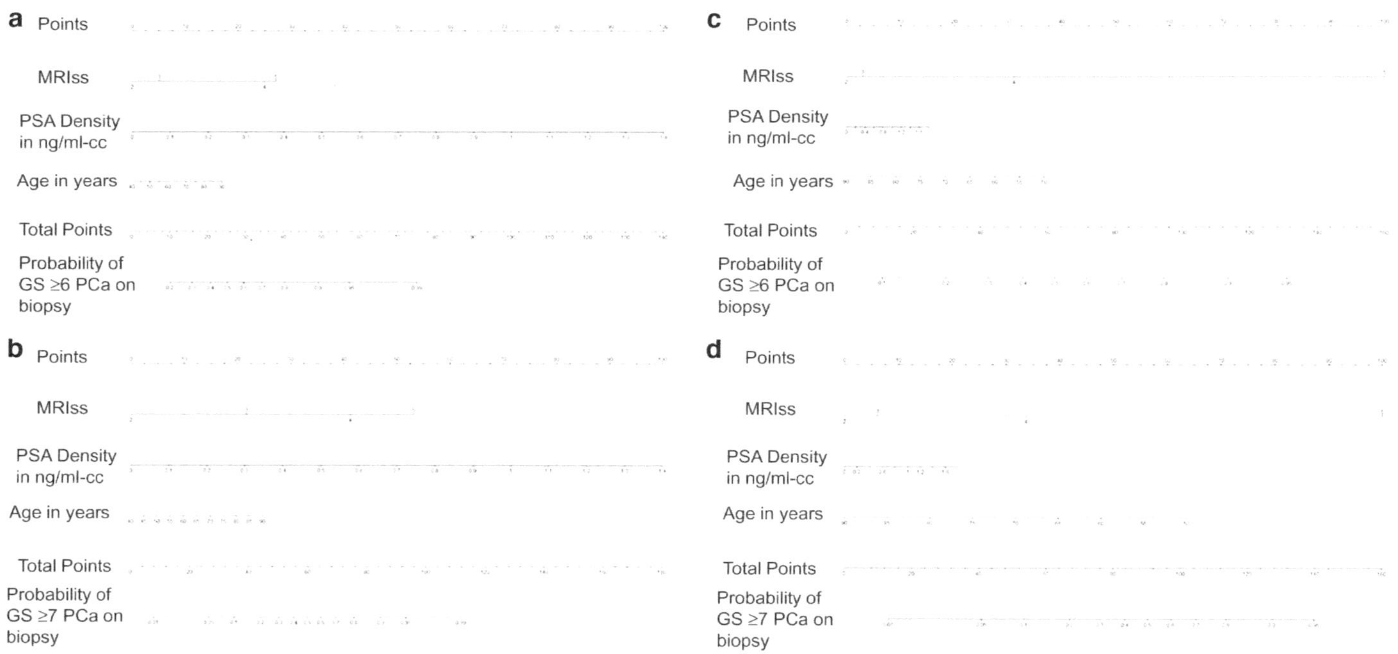

Fig. 9.1 Nomogram prediction model for predicting overall (**a**) and Gleason ≥7 PCa (**b**) in men without a prior biopsy and with a prior negative biopsy (**c, d**), respectively. The nomogram is used by first locating a patient's position for each variable on its horizontal scale, and then a point value is assigned according to the points' scale (top axis) and summed for all variables. Total points correspond to a probability value for having PCa or Gleason score ≥ 7. GS, Gleason score; MRIss, magnetic resonance suspicion score; PCa, prostate cancer; PSA, prostate-specific antigen. (Reprinted from Bjulrin et al. [97], with permission from Elsevier)

cancer when compared with PCA3 and PSA (Table 9.1) [71]. Van Neste et al. subsequently developed the SelectMDx tool in an initial cohort of 519 patients. The superiority of the SelectMDx tool in predicting high-grade prostate cancer when compared to PCPTRC was validated in a cohort of 386 men [72]. Though not FDA approved, a recent British cost-effectiveness study determined that at a diagnostic sensitivity cut-off of 95.7% for high-grade prostate cancer, SelectMDx demonstrated a savings of €128($143) and a gain of 0.025 quality-of-life years compared with using only PSA to select for prostate biopsy [73]. These data are encouraging and may portend future approval, which would facilitate more extensive use of this biomarker.

Improvement in Prostate Cancer Detection and Risk Stratification: MRI

Prostate magnetic resonance imaging (MRI) is increasingly utilized in clinical practice as the diagnostic pathway for prostate cancer [74]. MTI has utility as both a pre-biopsy risk assessment tool that may influence the decision as to whether to perform a biopsy and a noninvasive technique for tumor localization in direct targeted biopsy [75]. The prostate MRI and the MRI suspicion score (Prostate Imaging Reporting and Data System [PI-RADS]) have demonstrated the potential for improved individualized risk stratification. For example, several studies have indicated an association between the pre-biopsy MRI level of suspicion and biopsy outcomes [76–78]. In particular, the MRI suspicion score has dependably served as a strong predictor of the likelihood of significant prostate cancer on a subsequent biopsy, even in the context of other clinical risk factors [79–81]. Our institutional experience has revealed that clinically significant cancer ($\geq$Gleason score 7) is found on MRI targeted biopsy of PI-RADS 2, 3, 4, and 5 lesions in 5%, 14%, 49%, and 82%, respectively [82]. Other studies have shown results equivalent to our experience [83]. PI-RADS v2 scores have revealed predictive indications of cancer aggressiveness on radical prostatectomy, as well [84]. A recent pooled data meta-analysis measuring the performance of prostate MRI in prostate cancer detection exhibited a specificity of 88% and sensitivity of 74%, with a negative predictive value of 65% to 94% [85].

Quantitative metrics of diffusion-weighted MRI, such as apparent diffusion coefficient (ADC), correlate well with disease aggressiveness [86]. ADC has been shown to predict Gleason score, progression on active surveillance [86–88, 89], risk of adverse surgical pathology [87, 90], and biochemical relapse after surgery [91–93]. Despite the strong correlation of ADC with Gleason score, the confidence intervals for low, intermediate, and high risk widely overlap [94], ensuring Gleason score prediction impossible if solely based on the diffusion-weighted imaging.

Nomograms and risk calculators have been developed to assist in identifying patients at risk for prostate cancer prior to biopsy, providing an opportunity for counseling on both cancer risk and the need for biopsy. Historically, nomogram variables have included PSA, percentage of free-PSA, prostate volume, and digital rectal examination, but recently nomogram enhancement has occurred via assimilation of MRI findings in predicting both overall and clinically significant cancer risk in the pre-biopsy setting as well as after a negative biopsy [95–98] (Figs. 9.1 and 9.2). These predictive nomograms may potentially reduce unnecessary prostate biopsies and overdiagnosis while refining risk stratification counseling. In addition to the capacity to aid in clinically significant cancer prediction, the MRI can provide valuable information regarding disease volume and local advancement. An example of multiparametric prostate MRI is depicted in Fig. 9.3.

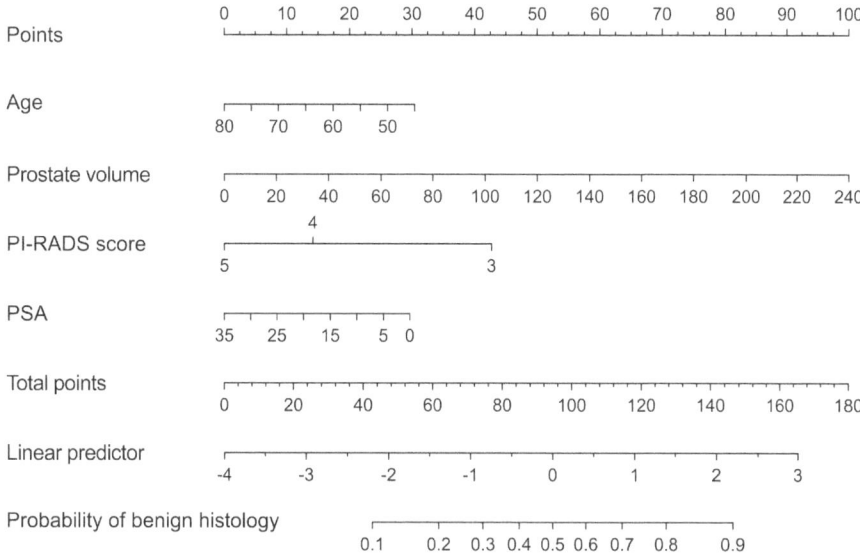

Fig. 9.2 Nomogram to predict benign pathology in patients with prior negative systematic biopsy findings and PI-RADS scores of 3–5. PI-RADS Prostate Imaging Reporting and Data System, PSA prostate-specific antigen. (Reprinted from Bjurlin et al. [98]. [Epub ahead of print], with permission from Elsevier)

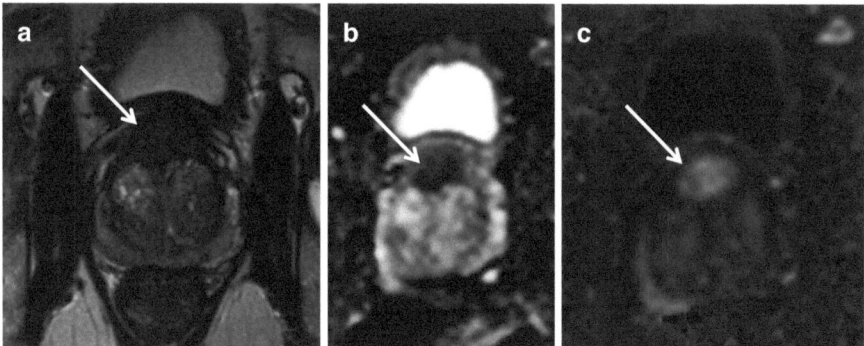

Fig. 9.3 Patient is a 67-year-old male with a PSA of 8.8 and two prior negative 12-core systematic biopsies at outside facility. Multiparametric MRI demonstrated PI-RADS 5 lesion in the midline anterior base-to-apex transition zone on (**a**) T2-weighted, (**b**) apparent diffusion coefficient and (**c**) early dynamic contrast-enhanced acquisition imaging. Patient MRI-ultrasound fusion targeted biopsy, revealing Gleason 4 + 3 = 7 prostate cancer in 4/4 targeted cores with maximum core length of 17 mm. All 12 cores from systematic biopsy were negative for prostate cancer

Management Options for Prostate Cancer Treatment

Whole Gland Therapy

Two common definitive whole gland treatments for prostate cancer include radical prostatectomy and radiation therapy. These treatment modalities are reserved for non-metastatic intermediate- and high-grade disease [7, 99] due to their gastrointestinal and genitourinary side-effect profiles [100–106]. In addition there is no evidence supporting the use of whole gland therapy for men with low-grade disease.

Two large-scale clinical trials compared observation versus intervention: Prostate Testing for Cancer and Treatment (ProtecT) and the Prostate Cancer Intervention Versus Observation Trial (PIVOT). The results of the ProtecT trial revealed that both all-cause and prostate cancer-specific mortality were not significantly dissimilar between patients under active monitoring, patients who underwent surgery, and patients who were treated with radiation. However, there was a significant increase in metastases and disease progression in men who did not undergo treatment with curative intent [107]. However, because the trial was randomized following detection, the majority of men in both treatment and observation arms harbored low-risk cancers, with likely long lead times to cancer mortality. The benefits of therapy are not well defined by the study in the scope of men with more advanced and higher risk cancer at presentation. Treatment of cancers with shorter lead time to treatment may offer greater benefit.

The results of the PIVOT trial revealed similar results, but the study has been greatly criticized for several aspects. The investigators found that there was a nonsignificant difference in all-cause mortality between patients on observation and patients who underwent radical prostatectomy. There was an increase in disease progression and additional treatment in patients on observation versus patients who underwent surgery [108]. It was noted in the first report of the study, published in 2012, that the inclusion criteria of the trial were expanded to include older men, and men with greater comorbidity, due to poor accrual by the original, intended criteria. As a result, men in this study most often died of competing risks long before prostate cancer would have caused harm. In an updated 20-year follow-up report, at a median follow-up of 12.7 years, the PIVOT study continued to demonstrate no improvement in survival among men treated [109]. At 19.5 years of follow-up, 65% of enrolled men died, with 20%, 40%, and 50% having died at 5, 10, and 12 years, respectively. Less than 10% of men died of prostate cancer, but two thirds died overall [109]. The high early death rate resulted in too few men alive at prolonged follow-up points to demonstrate benefit of treatment, despite longer lead time. Despite its shortcomings, the PIVOT trial clearly demonstrates the importance of carefully selecting men for prostate cancer evaluation who have adequate anticipated longevity and may benefit from prostate cancer treatment.

Active Surveillance

Active surveillance (AS) has been increasingly used in the current management of low-grade localized prostate cancer [110, 111]. Current guidelines approved by the American Society of Clinical Oncology recommend AS as the preferred treatment option for most patients with Gleason 6 prostate cancer and select patients with low-volume Gleason 7(3 + 4) disease [112]. The use of active surveillance for low-risk prostate cancer may reduce the overtreatment of indolent, clinically insignificant prostate cancer, sustaining curative treatment for patients whose cancer progresses to higher-risk disease. The selection criteria of most AS protocols were based upon the D'Amico or National Comprehensive Cancer Network (NCCN) classification of low-risk cancer ($\leq$cT2a, PSA < 10 ng/mL, GS $\leq$ 6) [7, 10, 113, 114]. Despite this, some AS protocols have made exceptions for intermediate-risk (Gleason 7 (3 + 4)) cancer in certain circumstances [7, 10, 114–116].

When evaluating major active surveillance cohorts at $\geq$5 years of follow-up, the 5-year treatment rates range from 24% to 40% [115–119]. Three studies reported 10-year treatment rates ranging from 36% to 55% [115, 116, 118]. Overall prostate cancer-specific mortality ranged from 0% to 1.5%. The Johns Hopkins active surveillance cohort reported both 10- and 15-year prostate cancer-specific mortality as 0.1% [118]. The Sunnybrook active surveillance cohort reported 10- and 15-year prostate cancer-specific mortality as 1.9% and 5.7%, respectively [116]. The results of these studies demonstrate that active surveillance for favorable-risk and select early intermediate-risk prostate cancer is feasible and seems to be safe over 15 years. While a portion of men on active surveillance will progress to treatment due to increased grade group, cancer volume, or stage, adherence to an active surveillance protocol still allows a window of opportunity to provide curative treatment for those men who require it.

Focal Therapy

In order to cure and control cancer in patients with localized prostate cancer, the concept of focal therapy has emerged. Focal destruction of cancer, with simultaneous preservation of the surrounding organ, exists as a feasible treatment option in the kidney, bladder, breast, and brain. Given the potential sexual and urinary side effects of radical prostate surgery and radiation, focal therapy for prostate cancer exhibits the distinct benefit of avoiding those side effects. In prostate cancer, the vast majority of metastases find their origin in the same prostate cancer cell clone, derived from the dominant or "index" lesion [120, 121]. To date, limited clinical data exists regarding outcomes of focal therapy [122, 123].

Cryotherapy, the use of extreme cold temperatures to freeze and kill prostate tissue, was first evaluated by Onik et al. [124] and has been subsequently evaluated in the management of localized prostate cancer [125, 126]. Of upmost importance in the use of cryoablation is accurate mapping of the malignant tissue, as well as accurate placement of probes [127]. This maximizes the destruction of malignant tissue while sparing benign prostatic tissue. Reports from the largest study to evaluate cryosurgery for prostate cancer reveal a 3-year biochemical recurrence rate of 75.1%. Prostate biopsy in patients treated was positive for prostate cancer in only 3.7% of treated patients, although only 14.1% of patients were actually biopsied [128]. Updates from this same database revealed a 5-year biochemical recurrence rate of 59.1% for high-grade localized cancer [129].

High-intensity focused ultrasound (HIFU) works by ablating tissue via ultrasound-guided application of mechanical and thermal energy. There is limited data in the use of HIFU as a focal therapy, as much of the literature evaluates its efficacy as a whole-gland treatment. In spite of the paucity of evidence, the early results are promising, demonstrating substantial cancer control, as well as preserved urinary and sexual function [130, 131]. Muto et al. compared patients receiving whole-gland HIFU with focal HIFU and found no significant differences in both oncologic and functional outcomes at 12-month follow-up [132]. The effectiveness of focal HIFU has been shown in a large, multicenter study by Guillaumier et al. They identified failure-free survival (as avoidance of local salvage therapy, systemic therapy, metastases, and prostate cancer-specific death) of 99%, 92%, and 88% at 1, 3, and 5 years, respectively. Only 2% of patients required pad use for urinary incontinence [133].

Other modalities of focal therapy include focal laser ablation (FLA) and bipolar radiofrequency ablation (bRFA). FLA involves real-time use of MRI to locate and ablate suspicious lesions, theoretically improving precision of treatment. A phase I trial of 12 patients resulted in 50% disease-free and 67% disease-free at the ablation site after biopsies at 3 and 6 months posttreatment [134]. bRFA can be performed under transrectal guidance [135–137] and has been approved by the FDA for the treatment of prostate tissue (though the specific disease process has not been specified). Currently, no trials have reported on the outcomes of this treatment option.

Conclusion

The implementation of widespread PSA screening has undoubtedly advanced the diagnosis and treatment of prostate cancer. Since its introduction as a key screening tool, the development of additional diagnostic tools, such as imaging, biomarkers, and predictive nomograms, has allowed clinicians to diagnose more high-risk prostate cancer and reduce the overdiagnosis of indolent, low-risk disease. In order to reduce overdiagnosis and overtreatment of prostate cancer, physicians should use all tools available to them in order to efficiently risk-stratify patients. Careful consideration should be taken when determining the appropriate disease management option for patients diagnosed with prostate cancer.

References

1. Cancer Facts and Figures 2018. Available from: https://www.cancer.org/content/dam/cancer-org/research/cancer-facts-and-statistics/annual-cancer-facts-and-figures/2018/cancer-facts-and-figures-2018.pdf.
2. Sakr WA, Grignon D, Crissman J, Heilbrun L, Cassin B, Pontes JJE, Haas GP. High grade prostatic intraepithelial neoplasia (HGPIN) and prostatic adenocarcinoma between ages of 20-69: autopsy study of 249 cases. In Vivo. 1993;8:439–43.
3. Gleason DF, Mellinger GT. Prediction of prognosis for prostatic adenocarcinoma by combined histological grading and clinical staging. J Urol. 1974;111(1):58–64.
4. Epstein JI, Allsbrook WC Jr, Amin MB, Egevad LL. The 2005 International Society of Urological Pathology (ISUP) consensus conference on Gleason grading of prostatic carcinoma. Am J Surg Pathol. 2005;29(9):1228–42.
5. Epstein JI, Egevad L, Amin MB, Delahunt B, Srigley JR, Humphrey PA. The 2014 International Society of Urological Pathology (ISUP) consensus conference on Gleason grading of prostatic carcinoma: definition of grading patterns and proposal for a new grading system. Am J Surg Pathol. 2016;40(2):244–52.
6. Epstein JI, Zelefsky MJ, Sjoberg DD, Nelson JB, Egevad L, Magi-Galluzzi C, et al. A contemporary prostate cancer grading system: a validated alternative to the Gleason score. Eur Urol. 2016;69(3):428–35.
7. NCCN Guidelines Version 3.2018.
8. Epstein JI, Walsh PC, Carmichael M, Brendler CB. Pathologic and clinical findings to predict tumor extent of nonpalpable (stage T1c) prostate cancer. JAMA. 1994;271(5):368–74.
9. Arumainayagam N, Ahmed HU, Moore CM, Freeman A, Allen C, Sohaib SA, et al. Multiparametric MR imaging for detection of clinically significant prostate cancer: a validation cohort study with transperineal template prostate mapping as the reference standard. Radiology. 2013;268(3):761–9.
10. Sanda MG, Cadeddu JA, Kirkby E, Chen RC, Crispino T, Fontanarosa J, et al. Clinically localized prostate cancer: AUA/ASTRO/SUO guideline. Part II: recommended approaches and details of specific care options. J Urol. 2018;199(4):990–7.
11. Sanda MG, Cadeddu JA, Kirkby E, Chen RC, Crispino T, Fontanarosa J, et al. Clinically localized prostate cancer: AUA/ASTRO/SUO guideline. Part I: risk stratification, shared decision making, and care options. J Urol. 2018;199(3):683–90.
12. Fernandez EB, Moul JW, Foley JP, Colon E, McLeod DG. Retroperitoneal imaging with third and fourth generation computed axial tomography in clinical stage I nonseminomatous germ cell tumors. Urology. 1994;44(4):548–52.
13. Hugosson J, Carlsson S, Aus G, Bergdahl S, Khatami A, Lodding P, et al. Mortality results from the Goteborg randomised population-based prostate-cancer screening trial. Lancet Oncol. 2010;11(8):725–32.
14. Klotz L. Prostate cancer overdiagnosis and overtreatment. Curr Opin Endocrinol Diabetes Obes. 2013;20(3):204–9.
15. Schroder FH, Hugosson J, Roobol MJ, Tammela TL, Ciatto S, Nelen V, et al. Screening and prostate-cancer mortality in a randomized European study. N Engl J Med. 2009;360(13):1320–8.
16. Stamey TA, Yang N, Hay AR, McNeal JE, Freiha FS, Redwine E. Prostate-specific antigen as a serum marker for adenocarcinoma of the prostate. N Engl J Med. 1987;317(15):909–16.
17. Han M, Partin AW, Piantadosi S, Epstein JI, Walsh PC. Era specific biochemical recurrence-free survival following radical prostatectomy for clinically localized prostate cancer. J Urol. 2001;166(2):416–9.
18. Noldus J, Graefen M, Haese A, Henke RP, Hammerer P, Huland H. Stage migration in clinically localized prostate cancer. Eur Urol. 2000;38(1):74–8.

19. Morote Robles J, Ruibal Morell A, Palou Redorta J, de Torres Mateos JA, Soler Rosello A. Clinical behavior of prostatic specific antigen and prostatic acid phosphatase: a comparative study. Eur Urol. 1988;14(5):360–6.
20. Johansson JE, Holmberg L, Johansson S, Bergstrom R, Adami HO. Fifteen-year survival in prostate cancer. A prospective, population-based study in Sweden. JAMA. 1997;277(6):467–71.
21. Schroder FH, Hugosson J, Roobol MJ, Tammela TL, Ciatto S, Nelen V, et al. Prostate-cancer mortality at 11 years of follow-up. N Engl J Med. 2012;366(11):981–90.
22. Schroder FH, Hugosson J, Roobol MJ, Tammela TLJ, Zappa M, Nelen V, et al. Screening and prostate cancer mortality: results of the European Randomised Study of Screening for Prostate Cancer (ERSPC) at 13 years of follow-up. Lancet. 2014;384(9959):2027–35.
23. Andriole GL, Crawford ED, Grubb RL 3rd, Buys SS, Chia D, Church TR, et al. Mortality results from a randomized prostate-cancer screening trial. N Engl J Med. 2009;360(13):1310–9.
24. Andriole GL, Crawford ED, Grubb RL 3rd, Buys SS, Chia D, Church TR, et al. Prostate cancer screening in the randomized Prostate, Lung, Colorectal, and Ovarian Cancer Screening Trial: mortality results after 13 years of follow-up. J Natl Cancer Inst. 2012;104(2):125–32.
25. Pinsky PF, Parnes HL, Andriole G. Mortality and complications after prostate biopsy in the Prostate, Lung, Colorectal and Ovarian Cancer Screening (PLCO) trial. BJU Int. 2014;113(2):254–9.
26. Shoag JE, Mittal S, Hu JC. Reevaluating PSA testing rates in the PLCO trial. N Engl J Med. 2016;374(18):1795–6.
27. Available from: https://screeningforprostatecancer.org/.
28. Chou R, Croswell JM, Dana T, Bougatsos C, Blazina I, Fu R, et al. Screening for prostate cancer: a review of the evidence for the U.S. Preventive Services Task Force. Ann Intern Med. 2011;155(11):762–71.
29. Carter HB, Albertsen PC, Barry MJ, Etzioni R, Freedland SJ, Greene KL, et al. Early detection of prostate cancer: AUA guideline. J Urol. 2013;190(2):419–26.
30. Mottet N, Bellmunt J, Bolla M, Briers E, Cumberbatch MG, De Santis M, et al. EAU-ESTRO-SIOG guidelines on prostate cancer. Part 1: screening, diagnosis, and local treatment with curative intent. Eur Urol. 2017;71(4):618–29.
31. Johansson JE, Andren O, Andersson SO, Dickman PW, Holmberg L, Magnuson A, et al. Natural history of early, localized prostate cancer. JAMA. 2004;291(22):2713–9.
32. Loeb S, Walter D, Curnyn C, Gold HT, Lepor H, Makarov DV. How active is active surveillance? Intensity of follow-up during active surveillance for prostate cancer in the United States. J Urol. 2016;196(3):721–6.
33. Loeb S, Vellekoop A, Ahmed HU, Catto J, Emberton M, Nam R, et al. Systematic review of complications of prostate biopsy. Eur Urol. 2013;64(6):876–92.
34. Bjurlin MA, Wysock JS, Taneja SS. Optimization of prostate biopsy: review of technique and complications. Urol Clin North Am. 2014;41(2):299–313.
35. Loeb S, Carter HB, Berndt SI, Ricker W, Schaeffer EM. Complications after prostate biopsy: data from SEER-Medicare. J Urol. 2011;186(5):1830–4.
36. Loeb S, Bjurlin MA, Nicholson J, Tammela TL, Penson DF, Carter HB, et al. Overdiagnosis and overtreatment of prostate cancer. Eur Urol. 2014;65(6):1046–55.
37. Oesterling JE, Jacobsen SJ, Chute CG, Guess HA, Girman CJ, Panser LA, et al. Serum prostate-specific antigen in a community-based population of healthy men. Establishment of age-specific reference ranges. JAMA. 1993;270(7):860–4.
38. Carter HB, Pearson JD, Metter J, Brant LJ, Chan DW, Andres R, et al. Longitudinal evaluation of prostate-specific antigen levels in men with and without prostate disease. JAMA. 1992;267(16):2215–20.
39. Loughlin KR. PSA velocity: a systematic review of clinical applications. Urol Oncol. 2014;32(8):1116–25.
40. Verma A, St Onge J, Dhillon K, Chorneyko A. PSA density improves prediction of prostate cancer. Can J Urol. 2014;21(3):7312–21.

41. Guazzoni G, Nava L, Lazzeri M, Scattoni V, Lughezzani G, Maccagnano C, et al. Prostate-specific antigen (PSA) isoform p2PSA significantly improves the prediction of prostate cancer at initial extended prostate biopsies in patients with total PSA between 2.0 and 10 ng/ml: results of a prospective study in a clinical setting. Eur Urol. 2011;60(2):214–22.
42. Loeb S, Kettermann A, Ferrucci L, Landis P, Metter EJ, Carter HB. PSA doubling time versus PSA velocity to predict high-risk prostate cancer: data from the Baltimore Longitudinal Study of Aging. Eur Urol. 2008;54(5):1073–80.
43. Barayan GA, Brimo F, Begin LR, Hanley JA, Liu Z, Kassouf W, et al. Factors influencing disease progression of prostate cancer under active surveillance: a McGill University Health Center cohort. BJU Int. 2014;114(6b):E99–E104.
44. San Francisco IF, Werner L, Regan MM, Garnick MB, Bubley G, DeWolf WC. Risk stratification and validation of prostate specific antigen density as independent predictor of progression in men with low risk prostate cancer during active surveillance. J Urol. 2011;185(2):471–6.
45. Loeb S, Han M, Roehl KA, Antenor JA, Catalona WJ. Accuracy of prostate weight estimation by digital rectal examination versus transrectal ultrasonography. J Urol. 2005;173(1):63–5.
46. Oesterling JE, Jacobsen SJ, Cooner WH. The use of age-specific reference ranges for serum prostate specific antigen in men 60 years old or older. J Urol. 1995;153(4):1160–3.
47. Partin AW, Criley SR, Subong EN, Zincke H, Walsh PC, Oesterling JE. Standard versus age-specific prostate specific antigen reference ranges among men with clinically localized prostate cancer: a pathological analysis. J Urol. 1996;155(4):1336–9.
48. Borer JG, Sherman J, Solomon MC, Plawker MW, Macchia RJ. Age specific prostate specific antigen reference ranges: population specific. J Urol. 1998;159(2):444–8.
49. Crawford ED, Leewansangtong S, Goktas S, Holthaus K, Baier M. Efficiency of prostate-specific antigen and digital rectal examination in screening, using 4.0 ng/ml and age-specific reference range as a cutoff for abnormal values. Prostate. 1999;38(4):296–302.
50. Partin AW, Brawer MK, Subong EN, Kelley CA, Cox JL, Bruzek DJ, et al. Prospective evaluation of percent free-PSA and complexed-PSA for early detection of prostate cancer. Prostate Cancer Prostatic Dis. 1998;1(4):197–203.
51. Christensson A, Björk T, Nilsson O, Dahlén U, Matikainen M-T, Cockett ATK, et al. Serum prostate specific antigen complexed to α 1-antichymotrypsin as an indicator of prostate cancer. J Urol. 1993;150(1):100–5.
52. Catalona WJ, Partin AW, Slawin KM, Brawer MK, Flanigan RC, Patel A, et al. Use of the percentage of free prostate-specific antigen to enhance differentiation of prostate cancer from benign prostatic disease – a prospective multicenter clinical trial. JAMA. 1998;279(19):1542–7.
53. Ankerst DP, Gelfond J, Goros M, Herrera J, Strobl A, Thompson IM Jr, et al. Serial percent free prostate specific antigen in combination with prostate specific antigen for population based early detection of prostate cancer. J Urol. 2016;196(2):355–60.
54. Loeb S, Sanda MG, Broyles DL, Shin SS, Bangma CH, Wei JT, et al. The prostate health index selectively identifies clinically significant prostate cancer. J Urol. 2015;193(4):1163–9.
55. de la Calle C, Patil D, Wei JT, Scherr DS, Sokoll L, Chan DW, et al. Multicenter evaluation of the prostate health index to detect aggressive prostate cancer in biopsy naive men. J Urol. 2015;194(1):65–72.
56. Parekh DJ, Punnen S, Sjoberg DD, Asroff SW, Bailen JL, Cochran JS, et al. A multi-institutional prospective trial in the USA confirms that the 4Kscore accurately identifies men with high-grade prostate cancer. Eur Urol. 2015;68(3):464–70.
57. Vickers A, Cronin A, Roobol M, Savage C, Peltola M, Pettersson K, et al. Reducing unnecessary biopsy during prostate cancer screening using a four-kallikrein panel: an independent replication. J Clin Oncol. 2010;28(15):2493–8.
58. Braun K, Sjoberg DD, Vickers AJ, Lilja H, Bjartell AS. A four-kallikrein panel predicts high-grade cancer on biopsy: independent validation in a community cohort. Eur Urol. 2016;69(3):505–11.

59. Bryant RJ, Sjoberg DD, Vickers AJ, Robinson MC, Kumar R, Marsden L, et al. Predicting high-grade cancer at ten-core prostate biopsy using four kallikrein markers measured in blood in the ProtecT study. J Natl Cancer Inst. 2015;107(7):djv095.

60. Russo GI, Regis F, Castelli T, Favilla V, Privitera S, Giardina R, et al. A systematic review and meta-analysis of the diagnostic accuracy of prostate health index and 4-Kallikrein panel score in predicting overall and high-grade prostate cancer. Clin Genitourin Cancer. 2017;15(4):429–39 e1.

61. Vickers A, Vertosick EA, Sjoberg DD, Roobol MJ, Hamdy F, Neal D, et al. Properties of the 4-Kallikrein panel outside the diagnostic gray zone: meta-analysis of patients with positive digital rectal examination or prostate specific antigen 10 ng/ml and above. J Urol. 2017;197(3 Pt 1):607–13.

62. Punnen S, Nahar B, Prakash NS, Sjoberg DD, Zappala SM, Parekh DJ. The 4Kscore predicts the grade and stage of prostate cancer in the radical prostatectomy specimen: results from a multi-institutional prospective trial. Eur Urol Focus. 2017;3(1):94–9.

63. Carlsson S, Maschino A, Schroder F, Bangma C, Steyerberg EW, van der Kwast T, et al. Predictive value of four kallikrein markers for pathologically insignificant compared with aggressive prostate cancer in radical prostatectomy specimens: results from the European Randomized Study of Screening for Prostate Cancer section Rotterdam. Eur Urol. 2013;64(5):693–9.

64. Bussemakers MJ, van Bokhoven A, Verhaegh GW, Smit FP, Karthaus HF, Schalken JA, et al. DD3: a new prostate-specific gene, highly overexpressed in prostate cancer. Cancer Res. 1999;59(23):5975–9.

65. Hessels D, Klein Gunnewiek JM, van Oort I, Karthaus HF, van Leenders GJ, van Balken B, et al. DD3(PCA3)-based molecular urine analysis for the diagnosis of prostate cancer. Eur Urol. 2003;44(1):8–15; discussion -6.

66. Carroll PR, Parsons JK, Andriole G, Bahnson RR, Castle EP, Catalona WJ, et al. NCCN guidelines insights: prostate cancer early detection, version 2.2016. J Natl Compr Cancer Netw. 2016;14(5):509–19.

67. Marks LS, Fradet Y, Deras IL, Blase A, Mathis J, Aubin SM, et al. PCA3 molecular urine assay for prostate cancer in men undergoing repeat biopsy. Urology. 2007;69(3):532–5.

68. Haese A, de la Taille A, van Poppel H, Marberger M, Stenzl A, Mulders PF, et al. Clinical utility of the PCA3 urine assay in European men scheduled for repeat biopsy. Eur Urol. 2008;54(5):1081–8.

69. Wei JT, Feng Z, Partin AW, Brown E, Thompson I, Sokoll L, et al. Can urinary PCA3 supplement PSA in the early detection of prostate cancer? J Clin Oncol. 2014;32(36):4066–72.

70. Tomlins SA, Day JR, Lonigro RJ, Hovelson DH, Siddiqui J, Kunju LP, et al. Urine TMPRSS2:ERG Plus PCA3 for individualized prostate cancer risk assessment. Eur Urol. 2016;70(1):45–53.

71. Leyten GH, Hessels D, Smit FP, Jannink SA, de Jong H, Melchers WJ, et al. Identification of a candidate gene panel for the early diagnosis of prostate cancer. Clin Cancer Res. 2015;21(13):3061–70.

72. Van Neste L, Hendriks RJ, Dijkstra S, Trooskens G, Cornel EB, Jannink SA, et al. Detection of high-grade prostate cancer using a urinary molecular biomarker-based risk score. Eur Urol. 2016;70(5):740–8.

73. Dijkstra S, Govers TM, Hendriks RJ, Schalken JA, Van Criekinge W, Van Neste L, et al. Cost-effectiveness of a new urinary biomarker-based risk score compared to standard of care in prostate cancer diagnostics – a decision analytical model. BJU Int. 2017;120(5):659–65.

74. Bjurlin MA, Meng X, Le Nobin J, Wysock JS, Lepor H, Rosenkrantz AB, et al. Optimization of prostate biopsy: the role of magnetic resonance imaging targeted biopsy in detection, localization and risk assessment. J Urol. 2014;192(3):648–58.

75. Meng X, Rosenkrantz AB, Mendhiratta N, Fenstermaker M, Huang R, Wysock JS, et al. Relationship between Prebiopsy multiparametric magnetic resonance imaging (MRI),

biopsy indication, and MRI-ultrasound fusion-targeted prostate biopsy outcomes. Eur Urol. 2016;69(3):512–7.

76. Liddell H, Jyoti R, Haxhimolla HZ. Mp-MRI prostate characterised PIRADS 3 lesions are associated with a low risk of clinically significant prostate cancer – a retrospective review of 92 biopsied PIRADS 3 lesions. Curr Urol. 2015;8(2):96–100.

77. Kuru TH, Roethke MC, Rieker P, Roth W, Fenchel M, Hohenfellner M, et al. Histology core-specific evaluation of the European Society of Urogenital Radiology (ESUR) standardised scoring system of multiparametric magnetic resonance imaging (mpMRI) of the prostate. BJU Int. 2013;112(8):1080–7.

78. NiMhurchu E, O'Kelly F, Murphy IG, Lavelle LP, Collins CD, Lennon G, et al. Predictive value of PI-RADS classification in MRI-directed transrectal ultrasound guided prostate biopsy. Clin Radiol. 2016;71(4):375–80.

79. Park SY, Jung DC, Oh YT, Cho NH, Choi YD, Rha KH, et al. Prostate cancer: PI-RADS version 2 helps preoperatively predict clinically significant cancers. Radiology. 2016;280(1):108–16.

80. Martorana E, Pirola GM, Scialpi M, Micali S, Iseppi A, Bonetti LR, et al. Lesion volume predicts prostate cancer risk and aggressiveness: validation of its value alone and matched with prostate imaging reporting and data system score. BJU Int. 2017;120(1):92–103.

81. Min JH, Park BK, Park JJ, Park SY, Kim CK. Preoperative assessment of prostate cancer using prebiopsy MRI. AJR Am J Roentgenol. 2014;203(2):341–6.

82. Bjurlin MA, Taneja SS. Prediagnostic risk assessment with prostate MRI and MRI-targeted biopsy. Urol Clin North Am. 2017;44(4):535–46.

83. Mertan FV, Greer MD, Shih JH, George AK, Kongnyuy M, Muthigi A, et al. Prospective evaluation of the prostate imaging reporting and data system version 2 for prostate cancer detection. J Urol. 2016;196:690–6.

84. Borofsky MS, Rosenkrantz AB, Abraham N, Jain R, Taneja SS. Does suspicion of prostate cancer on integrated T2 and diffusion-weighted MRI predict more adverse pathology on radical prostatectomy? Urology. 2013;81(6):1279–83.

85. de Rooij M, Hamoen EH, Futterer JJ, Barentsz JO, Rovers MM. Accuracy of multi-parametric MRI for prostate cancer detection: a meta-analysis. AJR Am J Roentgenol. 2014;202(2):343–51.

86. Giles SL, Morgan VA, Riches SF, Thomas K, Parker C, deSouza NM. Apparent diffusion coefficient as a predictive biomarker of prostate cancer progression: value of fast and slow diffusion components. AJR Am J Roentgenol. 2011;196(3):586–91.

87. van As NJ, de Souza NM, Riches SF, Morgan VA, Sohaib SA, Dearnaley DP, et al. A study of diffusion-weighted magnetic resonance imaging in men with untreated localised prostate cancer on active surveillance. Eur Urol. 2009;56(6):981–7.

88. Henderson DR, de Souza NM, Thomas K, Riches SF, Morgan VA, Sohaib SA, et al. Nine-year follow-up for a study of diffusion-weighted magnetic resonance imaging in a prospective prostate cancer active surveillance cohort. Eur Urol. 2016;69(6):1028–33.

89. Tamada T, Dani H, Taneja SS, Rosenkrantz AB. The role of whole-lesion apparent diffusion coefficient analysis for predicting outcomes of prostate cancer patients on active surveillance. Abdom Radiol (NY). 2017;42:2340–5.

90. De Cobelli F, Ravelli S, Esposito A, Giganti F, Gallina A, Montorsi F, et al. Apparent diffusion coefficient value and ratio as noninvasive potential biomarkers to predict prostate cancer grading: comparison with prostate biopsy and radical prostatectomy specimen. AJR Am J Roentgenol. 2015;204(3):550–7.

91. Lee H, Kim CK, Park BK, Sung HH, Han DH, Jeon HG, et al. Accuracy of preoperative multiparametric magnetic resonance imaging for prediction of unfavorable pathology in patients with localized prostate cancer undergoing radical prostatectomy. World J Urol. 2016;35:929–34.

92. Park JJ, Kim CK, Park SY, Park BK, Lee HM, Cho SW. Prostate cancer: role of pretreatment multiparametric 3-T MRI in predicting biochemical recurrence after radical prostatectomy. AJR Am J Roentgenol. 2014;202(5):W459–65.

93. Yoon MY, Park J, Cho JY, Jeong CW, Ku JH, Kim HH, et al. Predicting biochemical recurrence in patients with high-risk prostate cancer using the apparent diffusion coefficient of magnetic resonance imaging. Investig Clin Urol. 2017;58(1):12–9.
94. Kim TH, Kim CK, Park BK, Jeon HG, Jeong BC, Seo SI, et al. Relationship between Gleason score and apparent diffusion coefficients of diffusion-weighted magnetic resonance imaging in prostate cancer patients. Can Urol Assoc J. 2016;10(11–12):E377–E82.
95. Niu XK, He WF, Zhang Y, Das SK, Li J, Xiong Y, et al. Developing a new PI-RADS v2-based nomogram for forecasting high-grade prostate cancer. Clin Radiol. 2017;72:458–64.
96. Fang D, Zhao C, Ren D, Yu W, Wang R, Wang H, et al. Could magnetic resonance imaging help to identify the presence of prostate cancer before initial biopsy? The development of Nomogram predicting the outcomes of prostate biopsy in the Chinese population. Ann Surg Oncol. 2016;23(13):4284–92.
97. Bjurlin MA, Sarkar S, Venkataraman R, Mendhiratta N, Meng X, Rosenkrantz AB, Huang WC, Lepor H, Taneja SS. Prediction of prostate cancer risk among men undergoing combined MRI-targeted and systematic biopsy using novel pre-biopsy nomograms that incorporate MRI findings. Urology. 2018;112:112–20.
98. Bjurlin MA, Renson A, Rais-Bahrami S, Truong M, Rosenkrantz AB, Huang R, et al. Predicting benign prostate pathology on magnetic resonance imaging/ultrasound fusion biopsy in men with a prior negative 12-core systematic biopsy: external validation of a prognostic nomogram. Eur Urol Focus. 2018:pii: S2405–4569(18)30122–6. https://doi.org/10.1016/j.euf.2018.05.005.
99. NCCN Guidelines Version 3.2016.
100. Ficarra V, Novara G, Ahlering TE, Costello A, Eastham JA, Graefen M, et al. Systematic review and meta-analysis of studies reporting potency rates after robot-assisted radical prostatectomy. Eur Urol. 2012;62(3):418–30.
101. Ficarra V, Novara G, Rosen RC, Artibani W, Carroll PR, Costello A, et al. Systematic review and meta-analysis of studies reporting urinary continence recovery after robot-assisted radical prostatectomy. Eur Urol. 2012;62(3):405–17.
102. Frey A, Pedersen C, Lindberg H, Bisbjerg R, Sonksen J, Fode M. Prevalence and predicting factors for commonly neglected sexual side effects to external-beam radiation therapy for prostate cancer. J Sex Med. 2017;14(4):558–65.
103. Frey AU, Sønksen J, Fode M. Neglected side effects after radical prostatectomy: a systematic review. J Sex Med. 2014;11(2):374–85.
104. Galvin DJ, Eastham JA. Critical appraisal of outcomes following open radical prostatectomy. Curr Opin Urol. 2009;19(3):297–302.
105. Resnick MJ, Koyama T, Fan KH, Albertsen PC, Goodman M, Hamilton AS, et al. Long-term functional outcomes after treatment for localized prostate cancer. N Engl J Med. 2013;368(5):436–45.
106. Zhu Z, Zhang J, Liu Y, Chen M, Guo P, Li K. Efficacy and toxicity of external-beam radiation therapy for localised prostate cancer: a network meta-analysis. Br J Cancer. 2014;110(10):2396–404.
107. Hamdy FC, Donovan JL, Lane JA, Mason M, Metcalfe C, Holding P, et al. 10-year outcomes after monitoring, surgery, or radiotherapy for localized prostate cancer. N Engl J Med. 2016;375(15):1415–24.
108. Wilt TJ, Brawer MK, Jones KM, Barry MJ, Aronson WJ, Fox S, et al. Radical prostatectomy versus observation for localized prostate cancer. N Engl J Med. 2012;367(3):203–13.
109. Wilt TJ, Jones KM, Barry MJ, Andriole GL, Culkin D, Wheeler T, et al. Follow-up of prostatectomy versus observation for early prostate cancer. N Engl J Med. 2017;377(2):132–42.
110. Cooperberg MR, Carroll PR. Trends in management for patients with localized prostate cancer, 1990-2013. JAMA. 2015;314(1):80–2.
111. Womble PR, Montie JE, Ye Z, Linsell SM, Lane BR, Miller DC. Contemporary use of initial active surveillance among men in Michigan with low-risk prostate cancer. Eur Urol. 2015;67(1):44–50.

112. Chen RC, Rumble RB, Loblaw DA, Finelli A, Ehdaie B, Cooperberg MR, et al. Active surveillance for the management of localized prostate cancer (Cancer Care Ontario Guideline): American Society of Clinical Oncology Clinical Practice Guideline Endorsement. J Clin Oncol. 2016;34(18):2182–90.

113. D'Amico AV, Whittington R, Malkowicz S, et al. Biochemical outcome after radical prostatectomy, external beam radiation therapy, or interstitial radiation therapy for clinically localized prostate cancer. JAMA. 1998;280(11):969–74.

114. Sanda MG, Cadeddu JA, Kirkby E, Chen RC, Crispino T, Fontanarosa J, et al. Clinically localized prostate cancer: AUA/ASTRO/SUO guideline. Part I: risk stratification, shared decision making, and care options. J Urol. 2018;199(3):683–90.

115. Godtman RA, Holmberg E, Khatami A, Stranne J, Hugosson J. Outcome following active surveillance of men with screen-detected prostate cancer. Results from the Göteborg randomised population-based prostate cancer screening trial. Eur Urol. 2013;63(1):101–7.

116. Klotz L, Vesprini D, Sethukavalan P, Jethava V, Zhang L, Jain S, et al. Long-term follow-up of a large active surveillance cohort of patients with prostate cancer. J Clin Oncol. 2015;33(3):272–7.

117. Selvadurai ED, Singhera M, Thomas K, Mohammed K, Woode-Amissah R, Horwich A, et al. Medium-term outcomes of active surveillance for localised prostate cancer. Eur Urol. 2013;64(6):981–7.

118. Tosoian JJ, Trock BJ, Landis P, Feng Z, Epstein JI, Partin AW, et al. Active surveillance program for prostate cancer: an update of the Johns Hopkins experience. J Clin Oncol. 2011;29(16):2185–90.

119. Welty CJ, Cowan JE, Nguyen H, Shinohara K, Perez N, Greene KL, et al. Extended followup and risk factors for disease reclassification in a large active surveillance cohort for localized prostate cancer. J Urol. 2015;193(3):807–11.

120. Ahmed HU. The index lesion and the origin of prostate cancer. N Engl J Med. 2009;361(17):1704–6.

121. Liu W, Laitinen S, Khan S, Vihinen M, Kowalski J, Yu G, et al. Copy number analysis indicates monoclonal origin of lethal metastatic prostate cancer. Nat Med. 2009;15(5):559–65.

122. Ahmed HU, Freeman A, Kirkham A, Sahu M, Scott R, Allen C, et al. Focal therapy for localized prostate cancer: a phase I/II trial. J Urol. 2011;185(4):1246–55.

123. Valerio M, Ahmed HU, Emberton M, Lawrentschuk N, Lazzeri M, Montironi R, et al. The role of focal therapy in the management of localised prostate cancer: a systematic review. Eur Urol. 2014;66(4):732–51.

124. Onik G, Narayan P, Vaughan D, Dineen M, Brunelle R. Focal "nerve-sparing" cryosurgery for treatment of primary prostate cancer: a new approach to preserving potency. Urology. 2002;60(1):109–14.

125. Ellis DS, Manny TB Jr, Rewcastle JC. Focal cryosurgery followed by penile rehabilitation as primary treatment for localized prostate cancer: initial results. Urology. 2007;70(6 Suppl):9–15.

126. Lambert EH, Bolte K, Masson P, Katz AE. Focal cryosurgery: encouraging health outcomes for unifocal prostate cancer. Urology. 2007;69(6):1117–20.

127. Mouraviev V, Johansen TE, Polascik TJ. Contemporary results of focal therapy for prostate cancer using cryoablation. J Endourol. 2010;24(5):827–34.

128. Ward JF, Jones JS. Focal cryotherapy for localized prostate cancer: a report from the national Cryo On-Line Database (COLD) Registry. BJU Int. 2012;109(11):1648–54.

129. Tay KJ, Polascik TJ, Elshafei A, Cher ML, Given RW, Mouraviev V, et al. Primary cryotherapy for high-grade clinically localized prostate cancer: oncologic and functional outcomes from the COLD registry. J Endourol. 2016;30(1):43–8.

130. Ahmed HU, Freeman A, Kirkham A, Sahu M, Scott R, Allen C, et al. Focal therapy for localized prostate cancer: a phase I/II trial. J Urol. 2011;185(4):1246–54.

131. El Fegoun AB, Barret E, Prapotnich D, Soon S, Cathelineau X, Rozet F, et al. Focal therapy with high-intensity focused ultrasound for prostate cancer in the elderly. A feasibility study with 10 years follow-up. Int Braz J Urol. 2011;37(2):213–9; discussion 20–2.

132. Muto S, Yoshii T, Saito K, Kamiyama Y, Ide H, Horie S. Focal therapy with high-intensity-focused ultrasound in the treatment of localized prostate cancer. Jpn J Clin Oncol. 2008;38(3):192–9.

133. Guillaumier S, Peters M, Arya M, Afzal N, Charman S, Dudderidge T, et al. A multicentre study of 5-year outcomes following focal therapy in treating clinically significant nonmetastatic prostate cancer. Eur Urol. 2018;74(4):422–29.

134. Lindner U, Weersink RA, Haider MA, Gertner MR, Davidson SR, Atri M, et al. Image guided photothermal focal therapy for localized prostate cancer: phase I trial. J Urol. 2009;182(4):1371–7.

135. Chen YY, Hossack T, Woo H. Long-term results of bipolar radiofrequency needle ablation of the prostate for lower urinary tract symptoms. J Endourol. 2011;25(5):837–40.

136. Hu B, Hu B, Chen L, Li J, Huang J. Contrast-enhanced ultrasonography evaluation of radiofrequency ablation of the prostate: a canine model. J Endourol. 2010;24(1):89–93.

137. Richstone L, Ziegelbaum M, Okeke Z, Faure A, Kaye JD, Sette MJ, et al. Ablation of bull prostate using novel bipolar radiofrequency ablation probe. J Endourol. 2009;23(1):11–6.

Chapter 10
Gastroenterology in the Aging Male

Alina Wong, Rebecca Kosowicz, and Cynthia W. Ko

Introduction

Gastrointestinal disorders in aging men are frequent with substantial impacts upon patients' quality of life. Diagnostic and management approaches must consider the unique pathophysiology, differential diagnosis, and potential for benefit in aging men. Gastroesophageal reflux disease, constipation, diarrhea, and iron deficiency anemia from occult gastrointestinal bleeding are all frequent problems that need to be addressed in this population. Providers caring for aging men must also consider screening for gastrointestinal cancers, most prominently colorectal cancer, whose incidence increases with age. Decisions about initiating or continuing colorectal cancer screening in this population should balance the likelihood of benefit against the potential for harms from screening. This chapter will review the pathophysiology, differential diagnosis, and management considerations for common gastrointestinal conditions in older men, including gastroesophageal reflux, diarrhea, constipation, occult gastrointestinal bleeding, and iron deficiency anemia. It will also outline considerations and approaches for colorectal cancer screening in this population.

Gastroesophageal Reflux Disease

Gastroesophageal reflux disease (GERD) affects around 40% of adults in the United States and increases in prevalence with age. Of the population with GERD, 10–20% have symptoms at least once weekly [1]. Per American College of Gastroenterology

A. Wong · R. Kosowicz · C. W. Ko (✉)
Department of Medicine, Division of Gastroenterology, University of Washington, Seattle, WA, USA
e-mail: cwko@u.washington.edu

© Springer Nature Switzerland AG 2021
J. P. Alukal et al. (eds.), *Design and Implementation of the Modern Men's Health Center*, https://doi.org/10.1007/978-3-030-54482-9_10

(ACG) guidelines, GERD is defined as "symptoms or complications resulting from the reflux of gastric contents into the esophagus or beyond, into the oral cavity or lung" [2]. Quality of life, especially with nocturnal symptoms, is significantly affected with increased time off work and decreased productivity. Complications of GERD include erosive esophagitis, esophageal strictures, Barrett's esophagus, and esophageal adenocarcinoma. While symptoms of acid reflux decrease with age, complications such as erosive esophagitis and Barrett's esophagus increase in frequency after age 50, especially in Caucasian men.

Pathophysiology

Gastroesophageal reflux disease can result from a multitude of factors including motility disorders (gastroparesis, esophageal dysmotility), damaging factors (increased gastric acid production), decreased protective factors (reduced saliva and bicarbonate production), and mechanical factors (hiatal hernia, obesity, and obstructive sleep apnea). While disorders such as Zollinger-Ellison syndrome can cause increased gastric production, acid overproduction is a rare cause of GERD in general.

GERD most often occurs due to transient LES relaxations (tLESR), which allow for acid reflux into the esophagus [3]. The lower esophageal sphincter (LES) acts as a barrier to the reflux of stomach contents. LES incompetence increases in frequency with age and contributes to the higher prevalence of GERD in the elderly [4]. Other considerations in the elderly include reduced gastric emptying, decreased esophageal mucosal resistance, impaired esophageal acid clearance due to dysmotility, increased reflux of bile salts, difficulty maintaining upright position, and medication side effects [5, 6]. Medications used to treat patients' other comorbid conditions such as nonsteroidal anti-inflammatory drugs (NSAIDS), potassium or iron supplements, and bisphosphonates can directly injure the esophageal mucosa. Decreased pain perception results in fewer symptoms and subsequently increases the rate of GERD complications in the elderly [7, 8].

Evaluation

Typical symptoms of GERD include heartburn and acid regurgitation and are usually sufficient for diagnosis. GERD can also manifest atypically with symptoms including chest pain, cough, wheezing, hoarseness, sore throat, and globus sensation. The frequency of severe heartburn symptoms declines with age secondary to a decrease in esophageal pain perception; however, extra-intestinal symptoms such as atypical chest pain, laryngitis, chronic cough, and aspiration increase with age.

Typical symptoms of heartburn and acid reflux warrant a trial of acid suppressive therapy such as proton pump inhibitors (PPIs) or histamine receptor-2 (H2) antagonists. Resolution of symptoms with treatment and relapse of symptoms with discontinuation of symptoms is diagnostic of GERD. In contrast, patients with atypical symptoms should be evaluated first for other more concerning etiologies such as cardiac chest pain prior to a trial of acid suppressive therapy.

Further evaluation with upper endoscopy or esophageal pH studies is unnecessary in most patients with GERD in the absence of warning signs such as weight loss, dysphagia, anemia, or gastrointestinal bleeding. However, due to the higher incidence of complications in the elderly, prompt evaluation should be performed for atypical symptoms, symptoms unresponsive to standard acid suppressive therapy, patients with warning signs such as dysphagia or weight loss, and patients with risk factors for Barrett's esophagus such as Caucasian ethnicity, older age, obesity, family history of esophageal cancer, and history of smoking. Ambulatory esophageal manometry and pH monitoring can be considered for patients with atypical symptoms, refractory symptoms in well-established GERD, and for preoperative confirmation of GERD in order to better characterize the underlying pathophysiology.

Treatment

The goals of treatment are resolution of symptoms as well as management and prevention of complications. The cornerstone of treatment is lifestyle modifications along with acid suppressive therapy. Lifestyle modifications focus on weight loss; tobacco cessation; restriction of coffee, spicy, and acidic foods; head of bed elevation; and avoidance of oral intake at least 3 h prior to lying down. Medications that can exacerbate symptoms or potentiate the effects of GERD in the elderly such as NSAIDS, potassium tablets, bisphosphonates, beta-blockers, and calcium blockers are avoided as medically feasible.

Acid suppression can be accomplished with H2 antagonists and PPIs. H2 antagonists work by blocking histamine stimulation of parietal cells. On the other hand, PPIs irreversibly block the hydrogen-potassium-ATPase pump, which acts in the final step of acid production. Multiple studies have shown that PPIs are more effective than H2 antagonists in controlling acid symptoms and healing erosive esophagitis. PPIs are highly effective, and 80% of patients demonstrate healing of erosive reflux disease after 8 weeks of therapy [9]. Maintenance PPI therapy is continued for patients who relapse with discontinuation of medication or have complications of reflux disease such as erosive esophagitis or Barrett's esophagus. Although PPIs are the most effective therapy for acid suppression, they have garnered much press for possible adverse effects with long-term use. Reported complications include dementia, osteoporosis, infections, and kidney injury, among many others [10]. While most associated severe adverse effects of PPIs lack sufficient evidence and these associations remain controversial, physicians must use PPIs judiciously with specific consideration of appropriate indications, dosing, duration of therapy, and consideration of step-down therapy to H2 receptor antagonists.

Complications

Complications of GERD include Barrett's esophagus and esophageal adenocarcinoma. Esophageal adenocarcinoma is increasing in incidence and is the sixth leading cause of cancer death in the world [11, 12]. The strongest risk factor for esophageal adenocarcinoma is Barrett's esophagus, which increases risk of this malignancy 30- to 50-fold [13, 14]. Barrett's esophagus is defined as the replacement of squamous esophageal epithelium by intestinal epithelium. Diagnosis requires endoscopic evidence of columnar mucosa in the esophagus with histologic confirmation of intestinal metaplasia with goblet cells. Risk factors for Barrett's esophagus include age over 50, male sex, chronic reflux disease, Caucasian race, smoking, and obesity, particularly central obesity [15, 16].

Despite retrospective studies showing that adenocarcinomas diagnosed in screening programs tend to be earlier stage, screening and surveillance for Barrett's esophagus remain controversial. The main questions revolve around whom to screen, as symptomatic GERD remains a poor predictor of Barrett's esophagus on endoscopy and the overall incidence of adenocarcinoma in Barrett's esophagus is low [17]. Subsequently, gastrointestinal society guidelines recommend only screening the highest-risk populations. For example, the ACG recommends screening for Barrett's esophagus in men with chronic (>5 years) and/or frequent (weekly or more) symptoms of gastroesophageal reflux and two or more risk factors for Barrett's esophagus including age over 50 years, Caucasian race, presence of central obesity, history of smoking, or a family history of Barrett's esophagus or esophageal adenocarcinoma [18].

Conventional upper endoscopy remains the gold standard for screening and surveillance of Barrett's esophagus. The goal of screening and surveillance programs is to detect and treat early dysplasia to help decrease the incidence of esophageal adenocarcinoma. Surveillance in patients with established Barrett's esophagus involves periodic endoscopy with collection of biopsy specimens to evaluate for dysplasia. Given the costs and specialist expertise required for upper endoscopy, investigators are studying other techniques for Barrett's detection. These include transnasal endoscopy, cytosponge, biomarkers, and most recently breath testing [19–23]. However, more studies are needed, especially randomized controlled trials, to address accuracy and long-term follow-up of these new techniques.

PPIs remain the mainstay of medical treatment for Barrett's esophagus even in patients without reflux symptoms. Patients found to have low- or high-grade dysplasia on surveillance can often be managed endoscopically with ablative therapy and close follow-up surveillance [18].

Summary

GERD is common among the elderly who tend to have fewer or more atypical symptoms but are more prone to complications. It is important to recognize and adequately treat the symptoms of GERD to prevent erosive esophagitis, peptic strictures, gastrointestinal bleeding, Barrett's esophagus, and esophageal adenocarcinoma. Treatment is similar to that of younger patients, but special attention needs to be paid to patient comorbidities and potential side effects of medical therapy.

Diarrhea

Diarrhea can be considered acute or chronic depending on the duration of symptoms. Acute diarrhea is defined as the passage of three or more loose or liquid stools above one's baseline in a 24-h period, with duration less than 14 days [24]. Diarrhea is considered chronic when symptoms persist for more than 4 weeks. Because of varying patient perceptions of stool frequency and consistency, fecal weight over 200 g per day is often used as an objective definition of diarrhea.

Chronic diarrhea affects 3–7% of the population per year. In community dwelling residents aged 65–93 years, 14.2% reported chronic diarrhea [25]. Fecal incontinence more than once a week was reported in 3.7 per 100 of the elderly population. However, only 23% of subjects had seen a physician for these symptoms within the prior year. With aging, the prevalence of risk factors for diarrhea including comorbidities such as diabetes, poor nutritional status, use of predisposing medications, and prior gastrointestinal surgeries increases. Residence in a group home or nursing facility may incur increased risk for diarrhea, specifically with *Clostridium difficile* infection.

Pathophysiology

Physiologic changes which can predispose to diarrhea with aging include loss of enteric neurons, changes in gut microbiota, and lactose intolerance. Chronic diarrhea can be classified as watery, inflammatory, or fatty in etiology. Watery diarrhea can be further classified as secretory or osmotic in etiology and may arise from multiple etiologies. Inflammatory etiologies include inflammatory bowel disease or microscopic colitis. Steatorrhea may arise from pancreatic insufficiency or other malabsorptive disorders. Although unlikely to be of new onset in the elderly man, irritable bowel syndrome can be diarrhea predominant. The diagnosis of diarrhea-predominant irritable bowel syndrome can be made using the criteria from the Rome Foundation, which include abdominal pain occurring at least 1 day per week in the last 3 months associated with change in stool form or frequency or associated with defecation. These symptoms should have been present for at least 6 months prior to diagnosis [26].

Medications such as antibiotics, laxatives, metformin, and magnesium-containing supplements are common culprits for diarrhea and should be considered in both acute and chronic diarrhea. Short bowel syndrome is a malabsorptive condition causing diarrhea and can be seen from surgical resection after treatment of malignancy, Crohn's disease, trauma, radiation, or vascular insufficiency. After surgeries such as gastrectomy or cholecystectomy, diarrhea can occur due to dumping syndrome or bile salt malabsorption. Radiation enteritis or proctitis is important to consider as people age and risk of malignancy increases. Small intestinal bacterial overgrowth can be seen with disordered gut motility in diabetes or scleroderma. Less commonly, thyrotoxicosis and lymphoma can present with diarrhea.

Chronic diarrhea can also be due to structural causes. In the elderly, a large fecal burden in the colon can paradoxically present as post-obstructive overflow diarrhea. Fecal incontinence is often reported as diarrhea; one etiology may be decreased rectal compliance which can be seen with age. Overflow diarrhea and incontinence can often be differentiated from true diarrhea with a careful history and physical examination.

Evaluation

A thorough patient history can distinguish causes of diarrhea, starting determining whether diarrhea is acute or chronic. Patients with acute diarrhea should be evaluated for viral or bacterial infectious causes. Testing for *Clostridium difficile* should also be performed. Exposure to less hygienic environments with poorly cooked foods and unclean water increases one's risks for bacterial, mycobacterial, and parasitic infections. Comorbidities resulting in immunocompromise or use of immunosuppressive therapy also increase risk of chronic bacterial and viral infections.

It is important to assess for alarm features of weight loss, rectal bleeding or anemia, nocturnal diarrhea, and progressive abdominal pain which suggest need for more urgent and intensive evaluation. Understanding medication usage, diet, medical, psychological, and surgical history is a cornerstone of a complete evaluation. The physical exam should assess orthostatic changes, hydration, and nutrition to identify those in need for more urgent intervention.

Additional laboratory evaluation can include measurement of electrolytes and renal function, complete blood counts, thyroid-stimulating hormone, and C-reactive protein or sedimentation rate to look for evidence of inflammatory disease. Stool analysis for fecal fat and elastase can be used to evaluate for steatorrhea. Fecal sodium and potassium levels allow calculation of a stool osmolar gap. An osmolar gap less than 50 mOsm/kg indicates secretory diarrhea, and an osmotic gap greater than 125 mOsm/kg indicates osmotic diarrhea.

In situations where the individual patient is at high risk of spreading disease burden to others, or during known or suspected outbreaks, diagnostic evaluation for infection should be performed (2). Stool samples can be evaluated for bacterial, viral, and parasitic causes. *Clostridium difficile* infection can be evaluated by assays for *C. difficile* toxins. For more chronic diarrhea or with an appropriate exposure history, ova and parasites are tested in stool. Celiac disease testing with tissue transglutaminase antibody and serum IgA levels should be considered in the appropriate host. Hydrogen breath testing can be used to evaluate for small intestinal bacterial overgrowth or carbohydrate malabsorption.

Evaluation with endoscopy and colonoscopy may be needed for evaluation of structural causes like masses or strictures or to take biopsy samples to rule out celiac disease, microscopic colitis, or inflammatory bowel disease. Imaging studies such as CT scans are useful if there is steatorrhea to rule out pancreatic abnormalities, if there is suspicion of inflammatory bowel disease, or to look for structural abnormalities [27].

Treatment

The cornerstone of supporting elderly patients with diarrhea is ensuring adequate hydration to meet volume output demands. In patients without documented positive findings on stool testing, the use of antibiotics in acute community-acquired diarrhea is discouraged as most of this diarrhea is viral in origin [24]. After ensuring adequate hydration and nutrition, management requires identifying and addressing the underlying cause, often elucidated on the history and physical exam. For diarrhea without an identified etiology after appropriate evaluation, therapeutic trials are reasonable [27]. Commonly, separate trials of lactose, fructose, and gluten avoidance provide diagnoses or relief of symptoms. Fiber can be used for stool bulking, or bile acid-binding resins such as cholestyramine can provide symptom relief. Antidiarrheal medications such as loperamide or diphenoxylate-atropine work to slow gut transit by evoking a segmenting motor pattern that promotes increased fluid absorption.

Summary

Diarrhea is common as men age, but many do not seek medical care for this symptom [25]. With aging, physiologic changes, increasing comorbidities, more frequent medication use, and environmental exposures can predispose to diarrhea. Long-term care facilities pose increased risk for acquisition and spread of infections. As mobility decreases and food security becomes challenging, elderly patients with diarrhea are susceptible to malnutrition and fluid imbalance. Physicians are encouraged to identify acute or chronic diarrhea and identify underlying etiologies with a history and physical exam. Additional testing may be necessary, but therapeutic trials are successful in many.

Constipation

Constipation affects around 30% of the general population and increases in prevalence with age. It is more common in females than males, affecting 34% of women and 26% of men age 85 years and over [28]. Constipation also affects up to 80% of residents in long-term care facilities [29]. It has been associated with anxiety and poor health perception and can lead to complications such as fecal impaction, overflow incontinence, sigmoid volvulus, colonic pseudo-obstruction, rectal prolapse, and urinary retention and infection. It also exerts high economic costs on the healthcare system. In the United States, around 820 million dollars are spent on laxatives per year [30].

Constipation describes symptoms of infrequent stools or difficult stool passage. It can be primary or secondary in etiology. Primary etiologies include functional or slow transit constipation, pelvic floor defecatory disorders, or constipation-predominant irritable bowel syndrome. Secondary constipation may be secondary to structural abnormalities (colorectal cancer, stricture, rectocele), endocrine disorders (diabetes mellitus, hyperthyroidism), infiltrative diseases (scleroderma, amyloidosis), neurologic diseases (central nervous system lesions, spinal cord disease), or medications.

Pathophysiology

Constipation occurs due to changes in colonic motility and physiology. Intrinsic changes in the elderly predispose them to constipation. Constipation can be classified into three categories: anorectal disorders, slow transit constipation, or normal transit constipation. Pelvic floor function changes predisposing to constipation include diminished resting and maximal anal sphincter pressure, decreased maximal squeeze pressure and loss of rectal wall elasticity, and fibro-fatty degeneration and increased thickness of the internal anal sphincter with aging [31, 32]. Anorectal disorders can result from lack of coordination between abdominal muscle contraction and pelvic floor relaxation, anal stenosis, anal fissures, rectocele, hemorrhoids, or due to urogynecologic diseases.

Constipation due to impaired colonic transit has been associated with myenteric nervous system dysfunction, increased collagen deposition in the left colon resulting in impaired colon and rectal compliance and dysmotility, impaired segmental motor coordination, and increased binding of plasma endorphins to intestinal receptors [33, 34]. Slow transit constipation can be associated with endocrine and metabolic disorders such as hypothyroidism, hypercalcemia, diabetes, or infiltrative and neurologic diseases. On the other hand, normal transit constipation can be classified as irritable bowel syndrome (IBS) or functional constipation. Criteria from the Rome Foundation define functional constipation as two or more of the following: straining, hard or lumpy stools, sensation of incomplete evacuation, sensation of anorectal obstruction or blockage, or manual maneuvers to assist defecation in at least 25% of evacuations and/or fewer than three defecations per week [35]. These criteria need to be fulfilled for the last 3 months with symptom onset at least 6 months prior to diagnosis. In functional constipation, the patient may have abdominal pain, but it is not associated with bowel movements.

Other contributing factors in the elderly include increased comorbidities, polypharmacy, and decreased mobility. Common offending medications include those with anticholinergic effects, opioids, calcium channel blockers, iron supplements, and NSAIDs [36, 37]. Lifestyle factors such as diminished fluid intake, low-fiber diets, and decreased mobility increase the risk of constipation in the elderly. Other contributing factors include neurocognitive disorders, myopathic diseases, endocrine abnormalities, spinal cord injury, and mood disorders.

Evaluation

Initial evaluation includes a thorough history and physical examination focusing on differentiating between primary and secondary causes of constipation. The Bristol stool score is a visual aid that can be used to help patients characterize stool quality and pattern. Rome Foundation criteria may be used to diagnose functional constipation or constipation-predominant irritable bowel syndrome [35]. During the primary evaluation, it is important to determine if the patient has any alarm signs such as weight loss, hematochezia, iron deficiency anemia, family history of colorectal cancer or inflammatory bowel disease, or positive fecal immunochemical testing. It is also important to distinguish between new-onset constipation and chronic constipation as a change in bowel habits could represent a colorectal malignancy. If any alarm features are present, patients should be evaluated further with colonoscopy unless this is not consistent with their goals of care. Physical exam needs to include a digital rectal exam to evaluate for fecal impaction and anorectal disorders.

In the absence of alarm features, the clinician should evaluate for secondary causes of constipation, inadequate dietary intake of calories and fiber, history of emotional or physical abuse, and symptoms suggestive of abnormal defecation such as prolonged straining, sensation of anorectal blockage, difficulty in evacuating soft stools, and digital maneuvers to help evacuate stool. It is important to obtain a careful medication and diet history and to evaluate for any underlying systemic illnesses. Initial laboratory workup for secondary causes of constipation includes thyroid-stimulating hormone, hemoglobin A1c, hemoglobin, mean corpuscular volume, and calcium to exclude secondary causes of constipation and assess for alarm features.

Once secondary causes of constipation are ruled out, a therapeutic trial of fiber supplementation or osmotic laxatives such as polyethylene glycol is undertaken. If constipation continues, then more specialized testing is pursued. Anorectal manometry can be performed to diagnose pelvic floor dyssynergia, and treatment usually consists of pelvic floor physical therapy and biofeedback training. Colonic transit time can be assessed with a radiopaque marker tests or a wireless motility capsule. Radiopaque markers can be ingested and an abdominal x-ray used to count the remaining markers on days three and five. Delayed colonic transit is defined as eight or more markers seen on day three or five or more markers seen on day five. The wireless motility capsule gives a more complete assessment of gastrointestinal tract transit time, measuring gastric emptying, as well as small bowel and colonic transit time. Of note, if anorectal manometry is abnormal, there is no need to perform colonic transit testing as 50% of patients with a defecatory disorder will have delayed transit [38].

Treatment

Initial management of constipation includes reassurance and education. It is important to counsel patients about diet, exercise, and regular toileting. Increasing dietary fiber with either diet or supplements increases stool weight and accelerates colonic transit. Patients can increase dietary fiber intake by including more fruits, vegetables, nuts, and bran in their diet. As most Americans consume less than half the recommended daily intake of fiber [39], fiber supplementation should also be begun. Fiber supplementation is started at a low dose and slowly increased to a goal of 12–15 g per day as it can cause bloating, distention, and flatulence. A response is usually seen over several weeks. In normal transit constipation, 80% of patients will have a response to fiber supplementation [40]. While there has been an interest recently in probiotics and meta-analyses have shown possible effectiveness of *Bifidobacterium lactis, Lactobacillus casei,* and *Escherichia coli* Nissle, these agents have not been validated for the treatment of functional constipation [41–43].

In addition to fiber supplementation and lifestyle modifications, initial management of constipation includes a therapeutic laxative trial. Osmotic laxatives (such as polyethylene glycol, lactulose, or magnesium) are composed of poorly absorbed ions that create an osmotic gradient within the intestinal lumen causing increased stool water content. According to a recent meta-analysis, the number needed to treat was 3 to improve constipation with osmotic laxatives [44]. There is insufficient data to support stool softeners and while effective, stimulant laxatives are associated with abdominal cramping and electrolyte abnormalities and are thus not considered first-line therapy.

Despite the wide range of available laxatives, approximately half of constipated patients do not achieve adequate alleviation of symptoms with the aforementioned laxatives. New agents have subsequently been developed. One new class of drugs is the secretagogues. Lubiprostone acts by activating type 2 chloride channels in the intestine, thus increasing chloride, water, and sodium secretion into the intestinal lumen. Lubiprostone has been effective in increasing number of spontaneous bowel movements in randomized controlled trials compared to placebo. While the percentage of elderly patients included in the trials varied, in one of these studies as many as 10% of participants were elderly [45]. Lubiprostone does not cause electrolyte abnormalities, but side effects include nausea and headache. Linaclotide and plecanatide are guanylate cyclase-C agonists which increase the secretion of chloride, bicarbonate, and water into the intestinal lumen. The most common side effect is diarrhea, but in randomized controlled trials, <5% of patients discontinued linaclotide secondary to adverse events [46].

Summary

Constipation affects a large proportion of elderly patients and is especially common in long-term care facilities. It is associated with anxiety and poor health perception and can result in serious complications such as fecal impaction, colonic pseudo-obstruction, and urinary retention and infection. Evaluation focuses on differentiating between primary and secondary causes of constipation and assessing for alarm features that would warrant early endoscopic evaluation. If secondary causes of constipation are ruled out and a therapeutic trial of fiber supplementation or osmotic laxatives is unsuccessful, further assessment with anorectal manometry and colonic transit testing can be pursued to distinguish between pelvic floor disorders, slow transit constipation, and normal transit constipation. Treatment consists of lifestyle modifications and a therapeutic laxative trial, but special attention needs to be paid to potential side effects such as dehydration, electrolyte imbalance, and hepatotoxicity.

Iron Deficiency Anemia and Occult Gastrointestinal Bleeding

Gastrointestinal bleeding can be from an upper or lower source in the gastrointestinal (GI) tract. The bleeding may be visible to the eye, such as in melena (black, tarry stool), hematochezia (bright red blood per rectum), and coffee-colored emesis or hematemesis. Visible GI bleeding typically requires a more urgent workup and will not be discussed in this chapter. Instead, we will focus on chronic or occult GI bleeding, which presents most often as a clinically stable patient with iron deficiency anemia without visible GI blood loss. The prevalence of iron deficiency anemia in the United States is estimated at 5% in postmenopausal women and 2% of adult men [47]. The prevalence of occult GI bleeding is 1 in 20 in all adults. Often, fecal occult blood testing will be the initial indicator of GI pathology. Iron deficiency anemia can result from occult GI blood loss or iron malabsorption. Patients with iron deficiency anemia have a 31-times greater risk of GI malignancy compared to those with normal hemoglobin and iron saturation levels [48]. The prevalence of anemia increases with age and is as high as 26% in men over 85 years old. Anemia in the elderly has been associated with decreased physical performance, increased number of falls, frailty, decreased cognition, dementia, hospitalization, and increased mortality [49]. Therefore, anemia requires particular attention and evaluation in elderly men [50].

Pathophysiology

The differential diagnosis of presumed GI bleeding and iron deficiency anemia is divided into inflammatory, vascular, or neoplastic etiologies. Occult GI bleeding with iron deficiency anemia can be seen with lesions of the GI tract such as neoplasms, angiodysplasia, or mucosal ulcers. In the elderly especially, ulcers can appear in the rectum and can be constipation-induced or a complication of rectal prolapse. Peptic ulcer disease can be seen from *Helicobacter pylori* infection, NSAID use, or malignancy. NSAID use can induce small bowel or colonic ulcers or generalized colopathy in addition to gastric or duodenal ulcers. Gastrointestinal neoplasms commonly present as occult blood loss and can be in the stomach, small bowel, or colon.

In the absence of a structural GI lesion, another potential etiology for iron deficiency anemia is malabsorption from gastric or small intestinal disorders. Causes include celiac disease, *Helicobacter pylori* infection, gastric hypochlorhydria, inflammatory bowel disease, and surgical resections which impair iron absorption such as gastric bypass surgery.

Evaluation

Anemia is diagnosed with a hemoglobin concentration below the fifth percentile. Therefore, older white men are considered anemic with hemoglobin level less than 13.2 g/dL and older black men with a hemoglobin level less than 12.7 g/dL [49]. Iron deficiency is diagnosed using ferritin less than 50 mcg/L and transferrin saturation of less than 15%, along with a mean corpuscular volume of red blood cells less than 80 fL. As these indices can be altered by acute infection or inflammation, malnutrition, hemolysis, thalassemia, and anemia of chronic disease, other causes of anemia should be considered. Tissue transglutaminase antibodies and serum IgA levels can be used to evaluate for celiac disease.

Evaluation of iron deficiency anemia or occult GI bleeding is done initially with upper and lower endoscopy. However, prior to the endoscopic evaluation, diagnoses may be suspected from the history, physical exam, and laboratory assessment. Symptoms of abdominal pain, diarrhea, weight loss, and anorexia can narrow the differential diagnosis. Medication usage, especially the use of NSAIDs which cause gastrointestinal ulcers or anticoagulants/antiplatelet agents which can precipitate bleeding from an undiagnosed source, should be assessed. Physical exam may suggest specific causes of iron deficiency anemia or occult bleeding; for instance, skin changes may represent extra-intestinal signs of celiac disease or inflammatory bowel disease, or stigmata of chronic liver disease which point to portal hypertensive gastropathy or colopathy may be present.

The appropriateness for endoscopy should be assessed on an individual basis. In the elderly, consideration should be made to comorbidities that increase risk of peri-procedural harm from colonoscopy preparation or sedation or from specific procedure-related complications such as gastrointestinal perforations or post-polypectomy hemorrhage. Dehydration and falls should be considered especially with decreased mobility in the setting of colon lavage. In asymptomatic patients with positive fecal occult blood testing who are not iron deficient, a colonoscopy is performed first. If this is negative, additional testing is not necessarily indicated. An upper endoscopy should be performed if the patient is symptomatic or has iron deficiency anemia. Biopsies of the stomach for *Helicobacter pylori* or gastric atrophy and of the duodenum for celiac disease are often done at this time. If the upper and lower endoscopy do not identify a source of blood loss, the small bowel can be evaluated using a wireless capsule endoscopy [51]. Deep enteroscopy through push or double balloon technique may be used in patients not eligible for video capsule endoscopy or if a lesion is found on small bowel capsule endoscopy. Other evaluation of the small bowel may include an upper gastrointestinal series with small bowel follow-through or a CT or MR enterography. However, if an asymptomatic patient has positive fecal occult blood testing but is not anemic, small bowel investigation is not necessary.

Treatment

Treatment of chronic occult GI bleeding depends on the etiology found. In general, however, iron deficiency anemia should also be addressed with oral iron replacement using ferrous sulfate or ferrous gluconate. Some patients require intravenous iron replacement if iron deficiency is severe, oral iron is poorly tolerated, or they are unable to absorb oral iron due to prior gastrointestinal surgeries.

Vascular ectasias, if found in an area accessible with endoscopy, can be treated with endoscopic techniques such as argon plasma coagulation. Bleeding from malignancy is unlikely to be controlled endoscopically and management should address the underlying malignancy. Inflammatory bowel disease is managed by a gastroenterologist to control the underlying disease, and ischemic colitis is most often managed conservatively with optimization of vascular perfusion.

Summary

As men age, occult GI bleeding comes with distinct considerations. For example, comorbidities are more common and may increases risks associated with endoscopic evaluation. As the use of anticoagulant and antiplatelet agents is more common, management decisions become more complex and should balance risks and benefits of these therapies. Special care in colonoscopy preparation is advised in the elderly, given the increased susceptibility to dehydration and risk of falls. Primary care clinicians should take care to assess the appropriateness of fecal occult blood testing in this population and use shared decision-making to determine the appropriate extent of workup.

Colorectal Cancer Screening and Surveillance

Colorectal cancer (CRC) is the third most commonly diagnosed cancer in men and the second leading cause of cancer death in the United States [52]. CRC incidence increases with age and is consistently higher in men than in women in all age groups.

In US men of ages 50–54 years, the annual incidence of CRC is 66.7 per 100,000 and the annual mortality is 16.4 per 100,000. In men of ages 75–79 years, the annual incidence of CRC increases to 232.4 per 100,000 and mortality to 98.5 per 100,000 [52]. Because of the high incidence and mortality from CRC, as well as the effectiveness of screening, the US Preventive Services Task Force and other leading organizations recommend screening in average-risk individuals beginning at age 45 or 50 years and routinely continuing until age 75 years [53–55]. These guidelines also recommend individualized decision-making regarding screening for individuals of ages 76–85 years depending on patient preferences and against routine screening for individuals over the age of 85 years. Recent declines in the incidence of and mortality from CRC in older age groups have been attributed to more widespread adoption of screening [56, 57].

Patients with a genetic cancer syndrome such as familial adenomatous polyposis or Lynch syndrome, a family history of CRC, or a personal history of inflammatory bowel disease are considered at higher risk for CRC and require more intensive colonoscopy-based screening at intervals determined by the underlying condition. Patients who have a personal history of CRC, colorectal adenomas, or sessile serrated polyps should enter a surveillance program, undergoing colonoscopy at intervals determined by the number, size, and histology of prior polyps [58].

CRC is believed to begin as a precursor lesion – the adenomatous or sessile serrated polyp. Screening has the potential to identify and remove these precursor lesions, preventing malignant transformation and decreasing cancer incidence. In addition, screening can provide early detection of asymptomatic cancers, allowing earlier stage at diagnosis and potentially decreasing cancer mortality. In the United States, screening most commonly occurs by testing for fecal occult blood by either guaiac-based or immunochemical assays (FOBT or FIT, respectively) or by colonoscopy. Flexible sigmoidoscopy is also a recommended option but is relatively uncommon. FOBT and flexible sigmoidoscopy screening are supported by randomized clinical trials, while evidence for colonoscopy has been extrapolated from the sigmoidoscopy trials and supported primarily by observational data. Randomized trials of FOBT have demonstrated a 9–22% reduction in CRC mortality with biennial screening and 32% reduction with annual screening [59–65]. Patients with positive results on FOBT/FIT should undergo follow-up colonoscopy to detect and remove polyps and repeating the FOBT/FIT is generally not appropriate. Ideally, FOBT/FIT should be performed annually rather than biennially due to greater effectiveness in decreasing CRC mortality [62].

Colonoscopy in patients at average risk for colorectal cancer is recommended every 10 years [53, 54]. In the United States, it is the most widely utilized screening test as it has the greatest potential for detection and removal of colorectal polyps. Colonoscopy also has a higher risk of harm than FOBT/FIT or flexible sigmoidoscopy, with potentially severe complications such as gastrointestinal bleeding, cardiovascular events, colon perforation, and death [66–69]. The risks of these serious complications increase with age [66, 70, 71].

Prior RCTs of screening FOBT and flexible sigmoidoscopy have enrolled subjects up to the age 65–75 years [59, 61, 64, 65, 72–74]. Only one randomized trial of FOBT randomized subjects up to 80 years of age [62]. Therefore, the effectiveness of screening in older individuals is much less certain than in individuals under the age of 65–75 years. Although CRC incidence increases with age, the competing risks for mortality from other comorbid conditions make CRC screening less likely to be beneficial in this population. Decreases in CRC incidence and mortality are generally not seen for at least 5–10 years after screening initiation [63, 65, 75, 76]. Therefore, screening patients with a life expectancy of less than 5–10 years is unlikely to be beneficial.

The risks associated with screening itself and complications after screening or surveillance colonoscopy increase with age [66, 70, 71, 77]. In addition to a patient's chronological age, physiologic age should be considered. Modeling studies suggest that physiologic age may be more influential than chronologic age in influencing the benefit-to-harm ratio in cancer screening in general [78–80]. Relatively younger individuals with high levels of comorbidity may be less likely to benefit from screening than healthy older individuals. Comorbid conditions also increase the risk of adverse events after colonoscopy, including serious cardiopulmonary and gastrointestinal complications [66, 70, 71, 77]. Use of antiplatelet or anticoagulant medications for cardiovascular or cerebrovascular comorbidities increases the risk of bleeding complications after colonoscopy [69]. Thus, with comorbidity, the likelihood of screening benefit decreases because of competing mortality risks, while the risk of screening-related adverse events increases. Online tools are available for estimating physiologic age, life expectancy, and screening-related benefits and harms [81, 82]. Use of these tools may be helpful in shared decision-making with patients about the desirability of pursuing or continuing cancer screening [83, 84]. Patients are amenable to discussions about cessation of cancer screening if the discussion is properly framed around age and health status rather than life expectancy [83].

Overall, the benefits of screening in individuals over the age of 75 years are uncertain because of lack of evidence from rigorous randomized trials. The potential benefits must be balanced against the competing risks for mortality and the higher risk of colonoscopy-related complications. Therefore, the decision to initiate or continue screening in older men must be individualized in context of the likelihood of benefit, the risk of colonoscopy-related complications, and the individual's projected life expectancy [84]. Modeling studies support individualized decision-making incorporating likelihood of benefit and harm based on prior screening history, age, and comorbid conditions [78, 79]. Given the competing risks of mortality and increased risk of screening-related complications, individualized decision-making about the harms and benefits of screening is recommended in older men.

Conclusions

Gastrointestinal conditions in aging men are common with potential impacts on quality of life and functional status, as well as high medical costs. The unique pathophysiologic factors in an older population require different approaches to diagnosis and management. In particular, changes in gastrointestinal function such as altered gut transit must be considered, and contributions of comorbidities or concomitant medications may affect diagnosis and management. This chapter has outlined the pathophysiology and management options for common gastrointestinal conditions in light of the unique considerations in this patient population.

References

1. Singh S, Garg SK, Singh PP, Iyer PG, El-Serag HB. Acid-suppressive medications and risk of oesophageal adenocarcinoma in patients with Barrett's oesophagus: a systematic review and meta-analysis. Gut. 2014;63(8):1229–37.
2. Katz PO, Gerson LB, Vela MF. Guidelines for the diagnosis and management of gastroesophageal reflux disease. Am J Gastroenterol. 2013;108(3):308–28; quiz 29.
3. Hershcovici T, Mashimo H, Fass R. The lower esophageal sphincter. Neurogastroenterol Motil. 2011;23(9):819–30.
4. Huang X, Zhu HM, Deng CZ, Porro GB, Sangaletti O, Pace F. Gastroesophageal reflux: the features in elderly patients. World J Gastroenterol. 1999;5(5):421–3.
5. Lee J, Anggiansah A, Anggiansah R, Young A, Wong T, Fox M. Effects of age on the gastroesophageal junction, esophageal motility, and reflux disease. Clin Gastroenterol Hepatol. 2007;5(12):1392–8.
6. Chait MM. Gastroesophageal reflux disease: important considerations for the older patients. World J Gastrointest Endosc. 2010;2(12):388–96.
7. Johnson DA, Fennerty MB. Heartburn severity underestimates erosive esophagitis severity in elderly patients with gastroesophageal reflux disease. Gastroenterology. 2004;126(3):660–4.
8. Fass R, Pulliam G, Johnson C, Garewal HS, Sampliner RE. Symptom severity and oesophageal chemosensitivity to acid in older and young patients with gastro-oesophageal reflux. Age Ageing. 2000;29(2):125–30.
9. Chiba N, De Gara CJ, Wilkinson JM, Hunt RH. Speed of healing and symptom relief in grade II to IV gastroesophageal reflux disease: a meta-analysis. Gastroenterology. 1997;112(6):1798–810.
10. Malfertheiner P, Kandulski A, Venerito M. Proton-pump inhibitors: understanding the complications and risks. Nat Rev Gastroenterol Hepatol. 2017;14(12):697–710.
11. Pennathur A, Gibson MK, Jobe BA, Luketich JD. Oesophageal carcinoma. Lancet. 2013;381(9864):400–12.
12. Torre LA, Bray F, Siegel RL, Ferlay J, Lortet-Tieulent J, Jemal A. Global cancer statistics, 2012. CA Cancer J Clin. 2015;65(2):87–108.
13. Bhat S, Coleman HG, Yousef F, Johnston BT, McManus DT, Gavin AT, et al. Risk of malignant progression in Barrett's esophagus patients: results from a large population-based study. J Natl Cancer Inst. 2011;103(13):1049–57.
14. Lagergren J. Adenocarcinoma of oesophagus: what exactly is the size of the problem and who is at risk? Gut. 2005;54 Suppl 1:i1–5.
15. Rubenstein JH, Mattek N, Eisen G. Age- and sex-specific yield of Barrett's esophagus by endoscopy indication. Gastrointest Endosc. 2010;71(1):21–7.
16. Rubenstein JH, Morgenstern H, Appelman H, Scheiman J, Schoenfeld P, McMahon LF, et al. Prediction of Barrett's esophagus among men. Am J Gastroenterol. 2013;108(3):353–62.
17. El-Serag HB, Sweet S, Winchester CC, Dent J. Update on the epidemiology of gastro-oesophageal reflux disease: a systematic review. Gut. 2014;63(6):871–80.
18. Shaheen NJ, Falk GW, Iyer PG, Gerson LB. Gastroenterology ACo. ACG clinical guideline: diagnosis and management of Barrett's Esophagus. Am J Gastroenterol. 2016;111(1):30–50; quiz 1.

19. Shariff MK, Bird-Lieberman EL, O'Donovan M, Abdullahi Z, Liu X, Blazeby J, et al. Randomized crossover study comparing efficacy of transnasal endoscopy with that of standard endoscopy to detect Barrett's esophagus. Gastrointest Endosc. 2012;75(5):954–61.
20. Kadri SR, Lao-Sirieix P, O'Donovan M, Debiram I, Das M, Blazeby JM, et al. Acceptability and accuracy of a non-endoscopic screening test for Barrett's oesophagus in primary care: cohort study. BMJ. 2010;341:c4372.
21. Benaglia T, Sharples LD, Fitzgerald RC, Lyratzopoulos G. Health benefits and cost effectiveness of endoscopic and nonendoscopic cytosponge screening for Barrett's esophagus. Gastroenterology. 2013;144(1):62–73.e6.
22. Ross-Innes CS, Chettouh H, Achilleos A, Galeano-Dalmau N, Debiram-Beecham I, MacRae S, et al. Risk stratification of Barrett's oesophagus using a non-endoscopic sampling method coupled with a biomarker panel: a cohort study. Lancet Gastroenterol Hepatol. 2017;2(1):23–31.
23. Chan DK, Zakko L, Visrodia KH, Leggett CL, Lutzke LS, Clemens MA, et al. Breath testing for Barrett's Esophagus using exhaled volatile organic compound profiling with an electronic nose device. Gastroenterology. 2017;152(1):24–6.
24. Riddle MS, DuPont HL, Connor BA. ACG clinical guideline: diagnosis, treatment, and prevention of acute diarrheal infections in adults. Am J Gastroenterol. 2016;111(5):602–22.
25. Talley NJ, O'Keefe EA, Zinsmeister AR, Melton LJ 3rd. Prevalence of gastrointestinal symptoms in the elderly: a population-based study. Gastroenterology. 1992;102(3):895–901.
26. Lacy BE, Patel NK. Rome criteria and a diagnostic approach to irritable bowel syndrome. J Clin Med. 2017;6(11):99.
27. Schiller LR, Pardi DS, Sellin JH. Chronic diarrhea: diagnosis and management. Clin Gastroenterol Hepatol. 2017;15(2):182–93 e3.
28. Harris LA. Prevalence and ramifications of chronic constipation. Manag Care Interface. 2005;18(8):23–30.
29. Kinnunen O. Study of constipation in a geriatric hospital, day hospital, old people's home and at home. Aging (Milano). 1991;3(2):161–70.
30. Dennison C, Prasad M, Lloyd A, Bhattacharyya SK, Dhawan R, Coyne K. The health-related quality of life and economic burden of constipation. PharmacoEconomics. 2005;23(5):461–76.
31. Fox JC, Fletcher JG, Zinsmeister AR, Seide B, Riederer SJ, Bharucha AE. Effect of aging on anorectal and pelvic floor functions in females. Dis Colon Rectum. 2006;49(11):1726–35.
32. Roach M, Christie JA. Fecal incontinence in the elderly. Geriatrics. 2008;63(2):13–22.
33. Camilleri M, Lee JS, Viramontes B, Bharucha AE, Tangalos EG. Insights into the pathophysiology and mechanisms of constipation, irritable bowel syndrome, and diverticulosis in older people. J Am Geriatr Soc. 2000;48(9):1142–50.
34. Varma JS, Bradnock J, Smith RG, Smith AN. Constipation in the elderly. A physiologic study. Dis Colon Rectum. 1988;31(2):111–5.
35. Drossman DA. The functional gastrointestinal disorders and the Rome III process. Gastroenterology. 2006;130(5):1377–90.
36. Traube M, McCallum RW. Calcium-channel blockers and the gastrointestinal tract. American College of Gastroenterology's committee on FDA related matters. Am J Gastroenterol. 1984;79(11):892–6.
37. Ness J, Hoth A, Barnett MJ, Shorr RI, Kaboli PJ. Anticholinergic medications in community-dwelling older veterans: prevalence of anticholinergic symptoms, symptom burden, and adverse drug events. Am J Geriatr Pharmacother. 2006;4(1):42–51.
38. Bharucha AE, Pemberton JH, Locke GR. American Gastroenterological Association technical review on constipation. Gastroenterology. 2013;144(1):218–38.
39. Cash BD, Chang L, Sabesin SM, Vitat P. Update on the management of adults with chronic idiopathic constipation. J Fam Pract. 2007;56(6 Suppl Update):S13–9; quiz S20.
40. Suares NC, Ford AC. Systematic review: the effects of fibre in the management of chronic idiopathic constipation. Aliment Pharmacol Ther. 2011;33(8):895–901.
41. Yang YX, He M, Hu G, Wei J, Pages P, Yang XH, et al. Effect of a fermented milk containing Bifidobacterium lactis DN-173010 on Chinese constipated women. World J Gastroenterol. 2008;14(40):6237–43.

42. Koebnick C, Wagner I, Leitzmann P, Stern U, Zunft HJ. Probiotic beverage containing lactoba-cillus casei Shirota improves gastrointestinal symptoms in patients with chronic constipation. Can J Gastroenterol. 2003;17(11):655–9.
43. Möllenbrink M, Bruckschen E. Treatment of chronic constipation with physiologic Escherichia coli bacteria. Results of a clinical study of the effectiveness and tolerance of microbiological therapy with the E. coli Nissle 1917 strain (Mutaflor). Med Klin (Munich). 1994;89(11):587–93.
44. Ford AC, Suares NC. Effect of laxatives and pharmacological therapies in chronic idiopathic constipation: systematic review and meta-analysis. Gut. 2011;60(2):209–18.
45. Johanson JF, Morton D, Geenen J, Ueno R. Multicenter, 4-week, double-blind, randomized, placebo-controlled trial of lubiprostone, a locally-acting type-2 chloride channel activator, in patients with chronic constipation. Am J Gastroenterol. 2008;103(1):170–7.
46. Baffy N, Foxx-Orenstein AE, Harris LA, Sterler S. Intractable constipation in the elderly. Curr Treat Options Gastroenterol. 2017;15(3):363–81.
47. Looker AC, Dallman PR, Carroll MD, Gunter EW, Johnson CL. Prevalence of iron deficiency in the United States. JAMA. 1997;277(12):973–6.
48. Ioannou GN, Rockey DC, Bryson CL, Weiss NS. Iron deficiency and gastrointestinal malig-nancy: a population-based cohort study. Am J Med. 2002;113(4):276–80.
49. Goodnough LT, Schrier SL. Evaluation and management of anemia in the elderly. Am J Hematol. 2014;89(1):88–96.
50. Guralnik JM, Eisenstaedt RS, Ferrucci L, Klein HG, Woodman RC. Prevalence of anemia in persons 65 years and older in the United States: evidence for a high rate of unexplained ane-mia. Blood. 2004;104(8):2263–8.
51. Gerson LB, Fidler JL, Cave DR, Leighton JA. ACG clinical guideline: diagnosis and manage-ment of small bowel bleeding. Am J Gastroenterol. 2015;110(9):1265–87; quiz 88.
52. Noone AM, Howlander N, Krapcho M, Miller D, Brest A, Yu M, et al. SEER cancer statistics review, 1975–2015. Bethesda: National Cancer Institute; 2018.
53. Bibbins-Domingo K, Grossman DC, Curry SJ, Davidson KW, Epling JW Jr, Garcia FA, et al. Screening for colorectal cancer: US Preventive Services Task Force recommendation state-ment. JAMA. 2016;315(23):2564–75.
54. Rex DK, Boland CR, Dominitz JA, Giardiello FM, Johnson DA, Kaltenbach T, et al. Colorectal cancer screening: recommendations for physicians and patients from the U.S. Multi-Society Task Force on Colorectal Cancer. Am J Gastroenterol. 2017;112(7):1016–30.
55. Wolf AMD, Fontham ETH, Church TR, Flowers CR, Guerra CE, LaMonte SJ, et al. Colorectal cancer screening for average-risk adults: 2018 guideline update from the American Cancer Society. CA Cancer J Clin. 2018;68:250–81.
56. Yang DX, Gross CP, Soulos PR, Yu JB. Estimating the magnitude of colorectal cancers pre-vented during the era of screening: 1976 to 2009. Cancer. 2014;120(18):2893–901.
57. Doubeni CA. The impact of colorectal cancer screening on the US population: is it time to celebrate? Cancer. 2014;120(18):2810–3.
58. Lieberman DA, Rex DK, Winawer SJ, Giardiello FM, Johnson DA, Levin TR. Guidelines for colonoscopy surveillance after screening and polypectomy: a consensus update by the US Multi-Society Task Force on Colorectal Cancer. Gastroenterology. 2012;143(3):844–57.
59. Kronborg O, Fenger C, Olsen J, Jorgensen OD, Sondergaard O. Randomised study of screen-ing for colorectal cancer with faecal-occult-blood test. Lancet. 1996;348:1467–71.
60. Scholefield JH, Moss S, Sufi F, Mangham CM, Hardcastle JD. Effect of faecal occult blood screening on mortality from colorectal cancer: results from a randomised controlled trial. Gut. 2002;50(6):840–4.
61. Hardcastle JD, Chamberlain JO, Robinson MHE, Moss SM, Amar SS, Balfour TW, et al. Randomised controlled trial of faecal-occult-blood screening for colorectal cancer. Lancet. 1996;348:1472–7.

62. Mandel JS, Bond JH, Church TR, Snover DC, Bradley GM, Schuman LM, et al. Reducing mortality from colorectal cancer by screening for fecal occult blood. N Engl J Med. 1993;328:1365–71.
63. Mandel JS, Church TR, Bond JH, Ederer F, Geisser MS, Mongin SJ, et al. The effect of fecal occult-blood screening on the incidence of colorectal cancer. N Engl J Med. 2000;343(22):1603–7.
64. Faivre J, Dancourt V, Lejeune C, Tazi MA, Lamour J, Gerard D, et al. Reduction in colorectal cancer mortality by fecal occult blood screening in a French controlled study. Gastroenterology. 2004;126(7):1674–80.
65. Holme O, Loberg M, Kalager M, Bretthauer M, Hernan MA, Aas E, et al. Effect of flexible sigmoidoscopy screening on colorectal cancer incidence and mortality: a randomized clinical trial. JAMA. 2014;312(6):606–15.
66. Warren JL, Klabunde CN, Mariotto AB, Meekins A, Topor M, Brown ML, et al. Adverse events after outpatient colonoscopy in the Medicare population. Ann Intern Med. 2009;150(12):849–57.
67. Levin TR, Conell C, Shapiro JA, Chazan SG, Nadel MR, Selby JV. Complications of screening flexible sigmoidoscopy. Gastroenterology. 2002;123(6):1786–92.
68. Levin TR, Zhao W, Conell C, Seeff LC, Manninen DL, Shapiro JA, et al. Complications of colonoscopy in an integrated health care delivery system. Ann Intern Med. 2006;145(12):880–6.
69. Ko CW, Riffle S, Michaels L, Morris C, Holub J, Shapiro JA, et al. Serious complications within 30 days of screening and surveillance colonoscopy are uncommon. Clin Gastroenterol Hepatol. 2009;8(2):166–73.
70. Wang L, Mannalithara A, Singh G, Ladabaum U. Low rates of gastrointestinal and non-gastrointestinal complications for screening or surveillance colonoscopies in a population-based study. Gastroenterology. 2018;154(3):540–55 e8.
71. Rabeneck L, Paszat LF, Hilsden RJ, Saskin R, Leddin D, Grunfeld E, et al. Bleeding and perforation after outpatient colonoscopy and their risk factors in usual clinical practice. Gastroenterology. 2008;135(6):1899–906, 906 e1.
72. Atkin WS, Edwards R, Kralj-Hans I, Wooldrage K, Hart AR, Northover JM, et al. Once-only flexible sigmoidoscopy screening in prevention of colorectal cancer: a multicentre randomised controlled trial. Lancet. 2010;375(9726):1624–33.
73. Schoen RE, Pinsky PF, Weissfeld JL, Yokochi LA, Church T, Laiyemo AO, et al. Colorectal-cancer incidence and mortality with screening flexible sigmoidoscopy. N Engl J Med. 2012;366(25):2345–57.
74. Segnan N, Armaroli P, Bonelli L, Risio M, Sciallero S, Zappa M, et al. Once-only sigmoidoscopy in colorectal cancer screening: follow-up findings of the Italian Randomized Controlled Trial--SCORE. J Natl Cancer Inst. 2011;103:1310–22.
75. Atkin W, Wooldrage K, Parkin DM, Kralj-Hans I, MacRae E, Shah U, et al. Long term effects of once-only flexible sigmoidoscopy screening after 17 years of follow-up: the UK Flexible Sigmoidoscopy Screening randomised controlled trial. Lancet. 2017;389(10076):1299–311.
76. Lee SJ, Boscardin WJ, Stijacic-Cenzer I, Conell-Price J, O'Brien S, Walter LC. Time lag to benefit after screening for breast and colorectal cancer: meta-analysis of survival data from the United States, Sweden, United Kingdom, and Denmark. BMJ. 2013;346:e8441.
77. Tran AH, Man Ngor EW, Wu BU. Surveillance colonoscopy in elderly patients: a retrospective cohort study. JAMA Intern Med. 2014;174(10):1675–82.
78. Lansdorp-Vogelaar I, Gulati R, Mariotto AB, Schechter CB, de Carvalho TM, Knudsen AB, et al. Personalizing age of cancer screening cessation based on comorbid conditions: model estimates of harms and benefits. Ann Intern Med. 2014;161(2):104–12.
79. van Hees F, Habbema JD, Meester RG, Lansdorp-Vogelaar I, van Ballegooijen M, Zauber AG. Should colorectal cancer screening be considered in elderly persons without previous screening? A cost-effectiveness analysis. Ann Intern Med. 2014;160(11):750–9.

80. Ko CW, Sonnenberg A. Comparing risks and benefits of colorectal cancer screening in elderly patients. Gastroenterology. 2005;129(4):1163–70.
81. Lee S, Smith A, Widera E, Yourman L, Schonberg M, Ahalt C. ePrognosis [cited 2018 June 18]. Available from: https://eprognosis.ucsf.edu.
82. Cruz M, Covinsky K, Widera EW, Stijacic-Cenzer I, Lee SJ. Predicting 10-year mortality for older adults. JAMA. 2013;309(9):874–6.
83. Schoenborn NL, Lee K, Pollack CE, Armacost K, Dy SM, Bridges JFP, et al. Older adults' views and communication preferences about cancer screening cessation. JAMA Intern Med. 2017;177(8):1121–8.
84. Walter LC, Covinsky KE. Cancer screening in elderly patients: a framework for individualized decision making. JAMA. 2001;285(21):2750–6.

Chapter 11
Dermatology in the Aging Man

Vanessa L. Pascoe, Maryam Safaee, and Michi Shinohara

Introduction

Dermatologic care is a key component for optimal men's health, particularly for aging men. In the United States, about 27% of the population is seen annually by a physician for a skin condition [1]. The burden of skin disease increases with age, with those over 65 years old having double the number of skin problems per visit compared to younger patients [1]. Detecting a serious skin problem, such as skin cancer, is common during routine dermatologic exam. In a single institution study, skin cancer was diagnosed in 7% of patients presenting for "routine dermatologic care," especially in older men (mean age 70) [2]. Even seemingly benign skin conditions like rosacea [3] and psoriasis [4] can have significant impact on quality of life.

Aging Skin

Age-related skin changes are inevitable. Men are more highly impacted by aging in the skin; furthermore, men are perceived to appear older than their chronologic age relative to women [5]. Expected changes with aging include dry skin (xerosis),

---

Vanessa L. Pascoe and Maryam Safaee have equally contributed.

V. L. Pascoe
Department of Dermatology, Beth Israel Deaconess Medical Center, Boston, MA, USA
e-mail: vpascoe@bidmc.harvard.edu

M. Safaee
Tibor Rubin Veteran's Administration Medical Center, Long Beach, CA, USA
e-mail: maryam.safaee@va.gov

M. Shinohara (✉)
University of Washington, Division of Dermatology, Seattle, WA, USA
e-mail: mshinoha@uw.edu

© Springer Nature Switzerland AG 2021
J. P. Alukal et al. (eds.), *Design and Implementation of the Modern Men's Health Center*, https://doi.org/10.1007/978-3-030-54482-9_11

wrinkling, fragility, and skin growths, among others. Some changes in the skin, such as laxity and wrinkling, are predictable ("intrinsic" or chronologic aging), while others are caused or exacerbated by external causes (smoking and UV exposure) [6]. All layers of the skin are affected by aging, and there are accompanying functional and disease-related implications.

Wound Healing

A major feature of aging skin is diminished capacity to regenerate or heal after injury. The epidermis thins by as much as 50% by age 80, which, along with degradation in elastin fibers, leads to increased fragility, decreased tensile strength, and slower wound healing [7, 8].

Vitamin D Production

The epidermis is also a major contributor to vitamin D3 synthesis. Age-induced epidermal thinning leads to decreased vitamin D3 production, resulting in age-related vitamin D deficiency [9].

Dry Skin and Itching

The stratum corneum is a lipid rich layer that serves as a hydrophobic barrier, keeping the environment out and water in. Aged skin develops alterations in several key lipids, predisposing to age-related xerosis [10]. Filaggrin in particular is markedly diminished in the legs, which may explain a particular propensity toward dry skin on the lower legs with age [11].

Immunosenescence

The skin is an immune organ and has a robust presence by both the innate and adaptive immune systems. As such, the skin is also subject to normal age-related immune dysregulation, or immunosenescence [12]. Immunosenescence decreases the effectiveness of skin-delivered vaccines in the elderly and increases the risk of skin infections [12]. Decreased immune surveillance also predisposes toward skin cancer [13]. This general state of dysregulation of the skin immune system also predisposes toward pruritus and dermatitis in the aged [14].

Photoaging

Age-related changes in the skin are worsened by ultraviolet (UV) light exposure [13]. Men are more susceptible to photoaging compared to women. Men have a higher prevalence of sunburn and are less likely to use sunscreen, with only 21.7% of men reporting that they are "very likely" to use sunscreen (compared with 41% of women) [15].

Wrinkling is exacerbated by UV-induced decrease in collagen production and increase in matrix metalloproteinases and other enzymes that degrade existing collagen and elastins [6, 16]. Aged skin has a reduced capacity to compensate for reactive oxygen species (ROS)-induced inflammation. Exposure to other ROS inducers, such as smoking or UV exposure, leads to further downstream inflammation and activation of skin-aging pathways [16].

Hallmarks of photoaged skin include wrinkling, dyspigmentation, and telangiectasia, collectively referred to as dermatoheliosis (Fig. 11.1). Erythema in sun-damaged areas may be prominent and fixed, particularly on the neck of fair-skinned individuals, termed chronic heliodermatitis [17]. "Solar elastosis" refers to the UV-induced degradation of dermal elastin networks and leads to a variety of clinical manifestations. These include a beaded, "chicken-skin" like appearance particularly apparent on the neck (Fig. 11.2); thickened skin with geometric, linear indentations (cutis rhomboidalis nuchae; Fig. 11.3); and a papulonodular presentation on the face with cysts and comedones (Favre-Racouchot syndrome; Fig. 11.4) [18]. Photodamage also affects the skin vasculature, resulting in telangiectasia and actinic purpura independent of coagulopathy (Fig. 11.5) [18, 19], the latter of which is often of substantial concern to patients in the authors' experience.

The optimal approach to photoaging is prevention. Daily use of sunscreen (see section below for recommendations) has been shown in several large trials to slow or prevent the signs of photoaging [20]. Once photoaging occurs, the most extensive evidence exists for treatment with retinoids [19]. The use of retinoids causes epidermal thickening, increases collagen I production, and reduces UV induction of collagen-degrading enzymes [19].

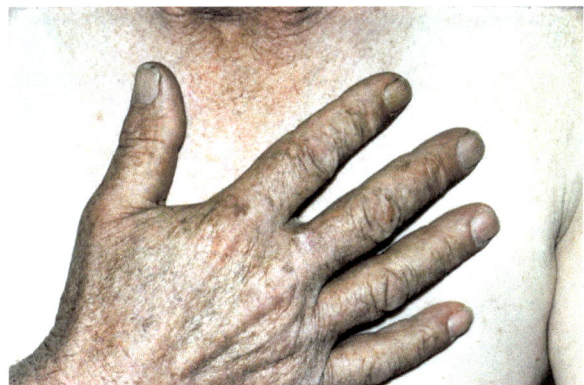

Fig. 11.1 Dermatoheliosis: severe photodamage, with wrinkling, dyspigmentation, and telangiectasia on sun-exposed skin

Fig. 11.2 Solar elastosis, demonstrating a beaded, "chicken skin" appearance on the neck

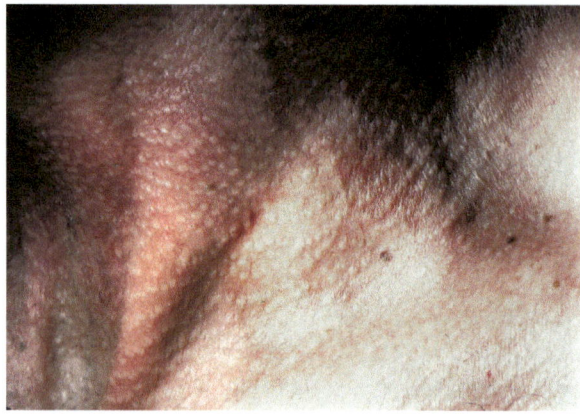

Fig. 11.3 Cutis rhomboidalis nuchae

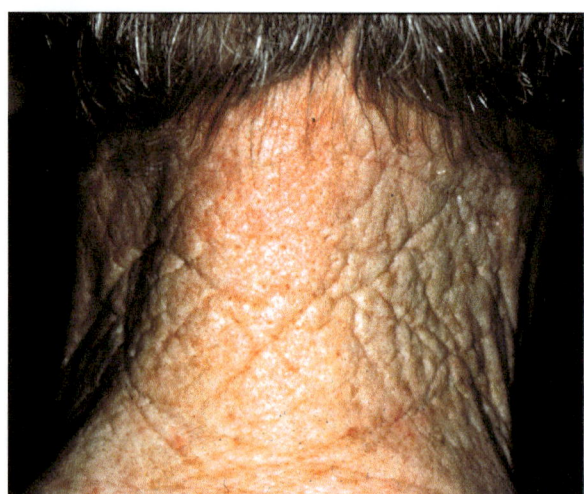

Skin Neoplasia

It is inevitable that as we age, new growths occur on the skin, most of which are benign. The incidence of skin cancer, however, also increases with age, particularly in conjunction with other exposures such as sun exposure. This section describes the spectrum of select benign and malignant cutaneous growths that can occur in the aging male, with an emphasis on the common, and the serious.

Fig. 11.4 Favre-
Racouchot syndrome, with
comedones and cysts from
photodamage

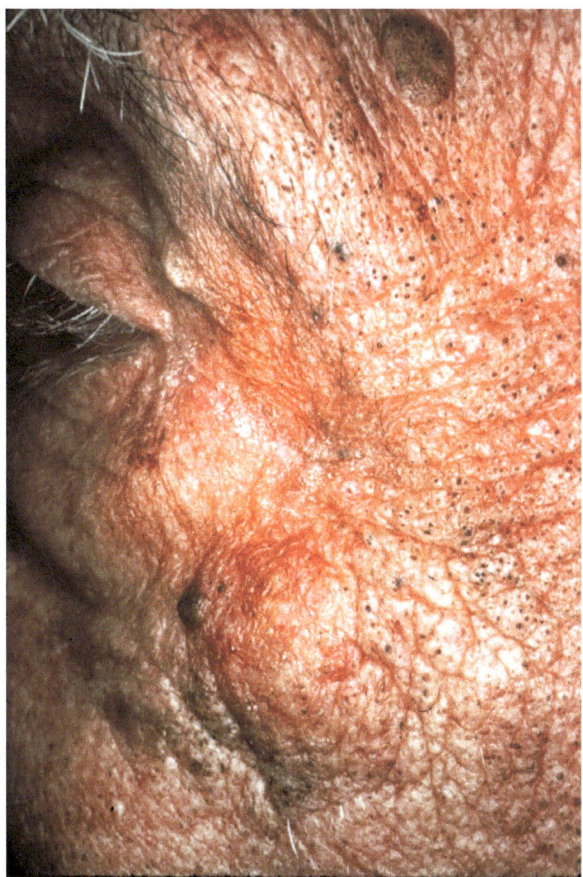

Fig. 11.5 Actinic purpura

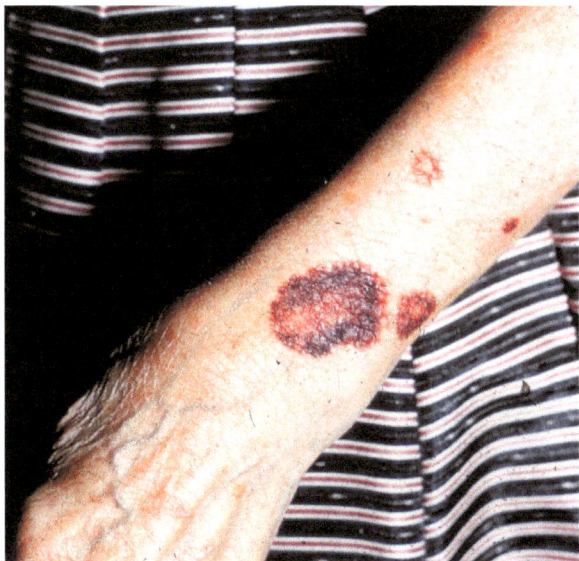

Benign Growths

Acrochordons (skin tags) are outgrowths of normal skin and are present in up to 50% of adults, often appearing as skin-colored pedunculated papules on thin stalks. The incidence of acrochordons increases with age [21] and in those with obesity and/or diabetes [22]. They often occur at sites of friction, such as the neck, axillae, or groin, and are asymptomatic unless there is rubbing on jewelry or clothing or if blood supply gets cut off and infarction occurs. Treatment of acrochordons consists of liquid nitrogen cryotherapy, electrodessication, or removal with forceps and fine-tipped scissors.

Seborrheic keratoses (SK) are one of the most common benign skin lesions, typically developing after the fourth decade. SKs are proliferations of immature keratinocytes that can develop on any hair-bearing surface, but have a predilection for the trunk, head, and neck. Their pathogenesis is not well understood, but sun exposure is thought to play a role [23]. SKs can have a varied appearance, but the classic description is of a well-demarcated, round, or oval brown papule with a verrucous surface and a waxy, stuck-on appearance [24] (Fig. 11.6). SKs are benign and treatment is not required. Patients may find SKs cosmetically bothersome, and lesions can become pruritic or irritated/inflamed. Treatments for symptomatic lesions include liquid nitrogen cryotherapy, curettage/excision, electrodessication, and a novel topical agent containing 40% hydrogen peroxide [25].

Skin Cancer

Skin cancer is the most common cancer in the United States, with more than 2 million cases annually [26]. The number of skin cancers diagnosed in the United States every year exceeds all other cancers combined [27]. The incidence of skin cancer has been increasing over the past couple of decades [28], likely in part due to

Fig. 11.6 Numerous seborrheic keratoses

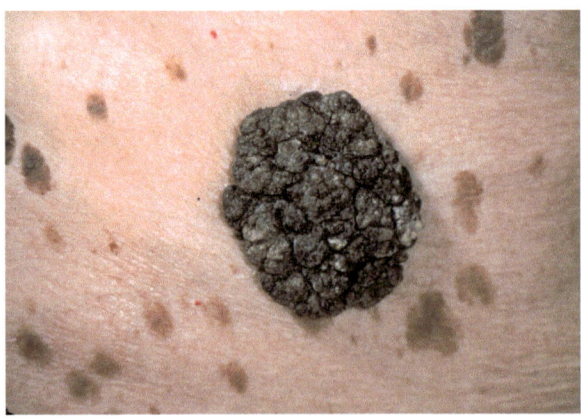

Fig. 11.7 Basal cell carcinoma, with characteristic peripheral translucent or "pearly" rim and central erosion

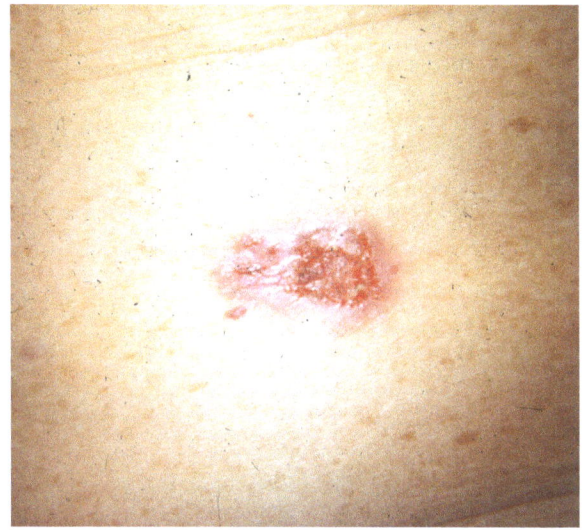

improved detection [29], but also due to an aging population. Factors that increase risk for skin cancer include a history of significant sun exposure – in particular blistering sunburns, fair skin, Northern European descent, indoor tanning bed use, as well as long-term immunosuppressive therapy [30]. Skin cancers are divided into non-melanoma skin cancers (NMSC, including basal cell carcinoma and squamous cell carcinoma) and melanoma.

Basal cell carcinoma (BCC) is the most common skin cancer in the United States [31]. Incidence of BCC increases with age and is 30% higher in men than in women [32]. BCCs classically present in sun-exposed skin as pearly papules with telangiectasias and tend to ulcerate and bleed (Fig. 11.7). Superficial BCCs may present as pink, scaly, thin papules that may mimic dermatitis [33] (Fig. 11.8). Skin biopsy is required to make the diagnosis. Therapies for BCC include surgical excision, Mohs surgery, electrodessication and curettage, and topical agents [34], with selection of therapy dependent on both tumor and patient factors. BCCs very rarely metastasize or become life-threatening, but they can be locally invasive and destructive [35] (Fig. 11.9) and a cause of significant morbidity.

Cutaneous squamous cell carcinoma (SCC) is the second most common skin cancer, accounting for 20% of non-melanoma skin cancers [36]. Men are twice as likely to develop SCC compared with women [37], and incidence of SCC increases with age. SCCs typically present as pink papules or plaques with hyperkeratosis and scaling and sometimes ulceration (Fig. 11.10). SCCs can develop anywhere, but favor sun-exposed areas such as the head and neck [38]. Skin biopsy is required to make the diagnosis. Unlike BCCs, 2–5% of SCCs metastasize [39], necessitating prompt recognition and treatment. Treatments for SCC include surgical excision, Mohs surgery, electrosurgery, topical treatments, and radiation therapy.

Melanoma, though less common than BCC or SCC, is the leading cause of skin cancer death [40]. Melanoma can develop from normal-appearing skin or from

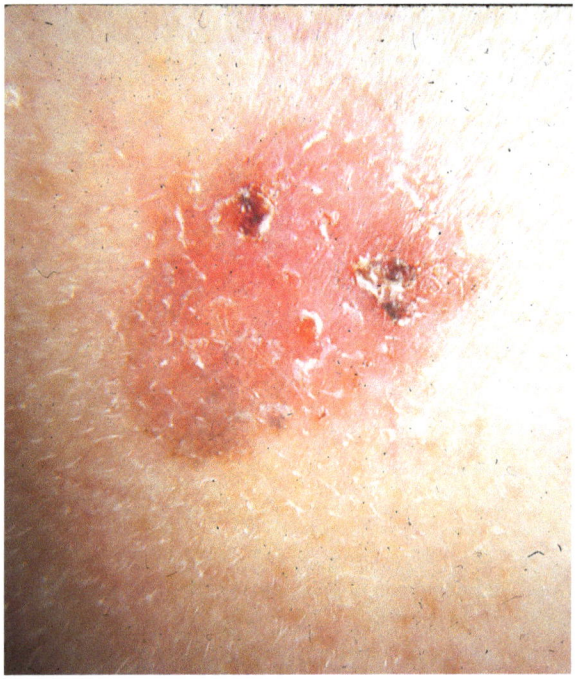

Fig. 11.8 Superficial/ multifocal basal cell carcinoma often mimics dermatitis, but often has small erosions that can provide a clue to the diagnosis

pre-existing nevi that undergo malignant transformation. Worrisome clinical features of pigmented lesions that might indicate melanoma are described by the "ABCDE" rule: Asymmetry (one half differs from the other), Borders (uneven, jagged), Color (multiple colors), Diameter (larger than a pencil eraser), and Evolution (changing in size, color, shape over time) [41] (Fig. 11.11). Melanomas can occur anywhere on the skin and can also be found in non-sun-exposed areas. In men, the most common locations for melanoma are the chest and back [42]. In those with darker skin, melanomas are more common on the palms of the hands, soles of the feet, and under the nails.

Risk factors for melanoma include UV exposure (including severe blistering sunburns, tanning bed use), fair skin/light hair/freckling, greater than 50 nevi, atypical nevi, first-degree relative with melanoma, and immunosuppression [43]. The prognosis for melanoma is primarily dependent on tumor characteristics, with 10-year survival rates for stage IA and IV melanomas of 95% and 10–15%, respectively. Although melanoma is less common in men compared to women, men have worse outcomes, and it's unclear whether this is because of protective factors in women or melanoma stimulating factors in men [44]. Most melanomas are detected by patients or family members, but when melanomas are detected by physicians, they are detected in earlier stages, emphasizing the benefits of complete skin exam [45].

Merkel cell carcinoma (MCC) is a rare but aggressive skin cancer. MCC is thought to arise from skin Merkel cells, which are neuroendocrine cells that are

Fig. 11.9 Locally destructive basal cell carcinoma

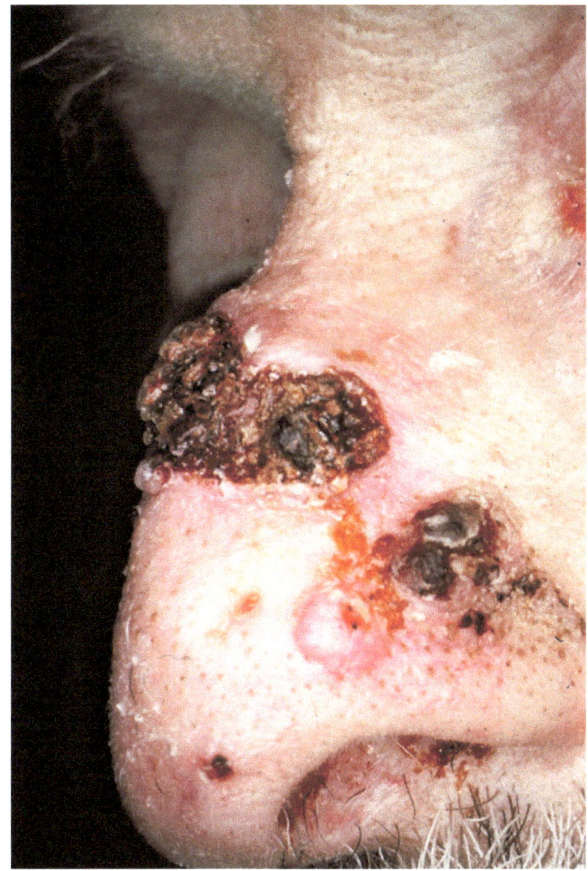

Fig. 11.10 Squamous cell carcinoma, with an eroded and verrucous or warty appearance

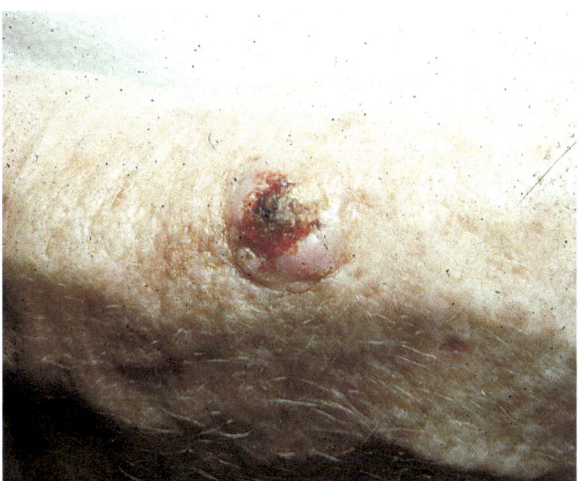

Fig. 11.11 Malignant melanoma demonstrating variable pigmentation, irregular border, and large size

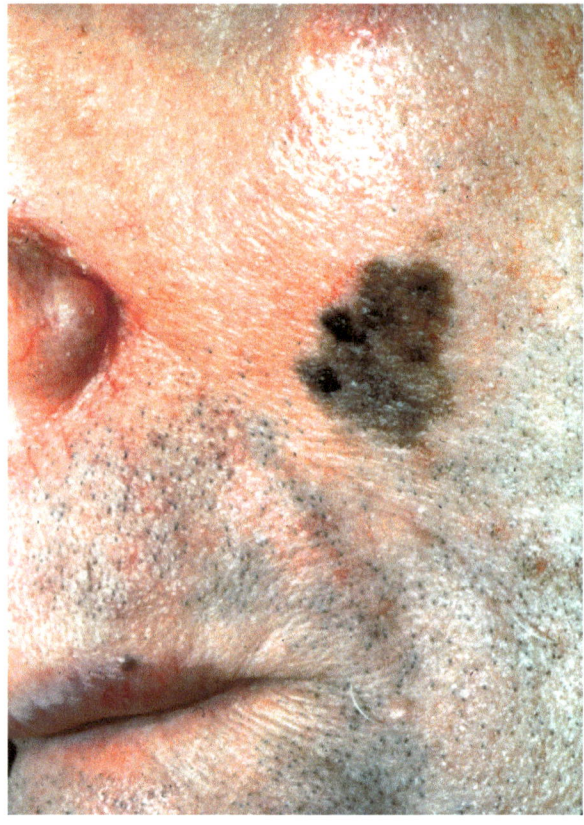

postulated to serve as "touch cells." MCC predominantly affects older adults (average age 75) and is more common in men compared to women [46, 47]. Risk factors for MCC include UV exposure and immunosuppression [48]. A major discovery in recent years was the finding that the majority of cases of MCC are associated with an oncogenic virus, the Merkel cell polyomavirus [49]. The Merkel cell polyomavirus is ubiquitous and can be detected in as many as 60–80% of the general population. In addition to the Merkel cell polyomavirus, development of MCC requires multiple factors, most notably UV exposure [50].

MCC presents most frequently in sun-exposed areas as a rapidly growing, painless, firm, shiny, skin-colored or bluish red, and subcutaneous nodule [51] (Fig. 11.12). It is diagnosed by skin biopsy. Patients with MCC should undergo complete staging including imaging; current guidelines for staging and treatment are available from the National Comprehensive Cancer Network (NCCN.org). The overall survival of patients with MCC at 5 years is approximately 51% for local disease and drops to 14% for metastatic disease [50]. Given the aggressive potential of MCC, patients are best cared for by multidisciplinary teams of dermatology, oncology, surgical oncology, and radiation oncology with experience treating those with MCC.

Fig. 11.12 Merkel cell
carcinoma. The appearance
can be somewhat
nondescript

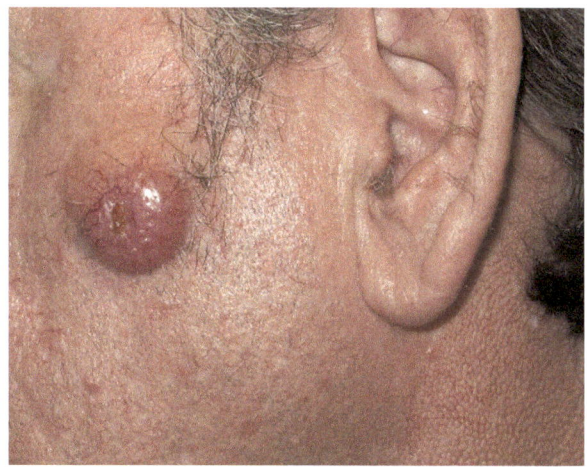

Preventative Care and Recommendations for Photoprotection

Photoprotection can prevent skin cancers as well as photoaging [52]. When most people think of sun protection, they usually think of sunscreen, but photoprotection also includes sun protective clothing and sun protective behavior.

Sunscreen is effective at preventing photoaging. Daily users of broad-spectrum sunscreen are 24% less likely to show increased aging [53]. Today's sunscreen comes in a range of sun protective factor (SPF), active sunscreen ingredients (chemical sunscreen vs physical blocker), and vehicles for application.

Chemical sunscreens are widely included in sunscreens because of ease of application. They work by absorbing UV radiation [54]. Examples of chemical sunscreens include avobenzone and octinoxate. Most chemical blockers are used in combination, as some are more effective against UVA and others UVB. Disadvantages to chemical blockers include photo-instability, necessitating frequent reapplication, and a higher rate of cutaneous reactions, ranging from irritant and allergic contact dermatitis to phototoxic and photoallergic reactions [55]. Oxybenzone is the most frequent cause of sunscreen-induced contact dermatitis, though the rate is still quite low, at less than 0.1% [56].

Physical blockers include mineral compounds such as zinc oxide and titanium dioxide, which work by reflecting and scattering UV light. In the past, physical blocker sunscreens appeared as a white film on the skin, rendering them unpopular. The development of nanoparticles has resulted in improved transparency and usability, but at a higher cost.

In general, daily use of a sunscreen that is broad-spectrum (UVA and UVB protection), SPF 30 or higher, applied liberally 15–30 min before sun exposure, and reapplied at least every 2 h while outdoors and hourly if swimming or sweating is recommended. Most adults do not apply adequate amounts of sunscreen [57]. The amount necessary to cover an average-sized adult is roughly equivalent to six teaspoons or a shot glass [58].

There are additional non-sunscreen methods to prevent sun exposure, including sun protective clothing, including broadbrimmed hats, long sleeves, tightly woven and/or dark fabrics, or fabrics with an official UPF rating of 30 and above [59]. Sun protective fashion has come a long way – stylish options exist. Broadbrimmed hats protect the particularly vulnerable scalp and ears in aging men.

Finally, we recommend sun avoidance (seeking shade or staying indoors), particularly between the hours of 10 am and 4 pm when UV radiation is strongest [60]. It is also important to mention that the concept of a "base tan" is a myth; tanning beds and sun tans do not provide adequate protection against future UV exposure [61], and there is no such thing as a safe tan.

Common Dermatoses in the Aging Man

Xerosis and Asteatotic Dermatitis

Xerosis (dry skin) is the most common dermatologic condition in the elderly, affecting more than 50% of adults aged 65 or older [62]. Xerosis causes rough, dry skin, often with fine scaling, and most commonly affects the shins. Pruritus is common [63]. Severely xerotic skin may have redness, cracking, and/or adherent platelike scale with pruritus. This is known as eczema craquelé or asteatotic dermatitis (Fig. 11.13). With age, the skin's natural barrier function becomes impaired, decreasing water retention capability [64] due to a combination of decreased surface acidity [65] and decreased production of lipid barrier precursors [66]. In addition, medications such as diuretics, cholesterol-lowering agents, antiandrogens, and cimetidine can contribute to xerosis [67]. Xerosis can lead to significant pruritus and render elderly males at increased risk of contact dermatitis [68].

Treatment of xerosis involves restoring the damaged stratum corneum and maintaining moisture content through a combination of bathing habits, emollients, and if possible avoidance of cold, dry environments [69]. One should limit bathing frequency (at most once daily), duration (less than 10 min), and use of warm (not hot) water. A gentle, non-scented soap should be used and restricted to only the axillae and groin unless required in other areas. Immediately after bathing, a thick emollient cream or ointment should be applied to the skin [70]. A humidifier may be beneficial during dry winter months [69]. If the xerosis is pruritic or has progressed to eczema craquelé or asteatotic dermatitis, topical corticosteroids may also be required.

Drug Eruptions

In the United States, between the ages of 65 and 74, 75% of the population has two or greater chronic medical conditions, and between the ages of 75 and 84, this number rises to 81% [71]. With this comes increasing medication exposure. Drug

Fig. 11.13 Severe xerosis or "eczema craquelé"

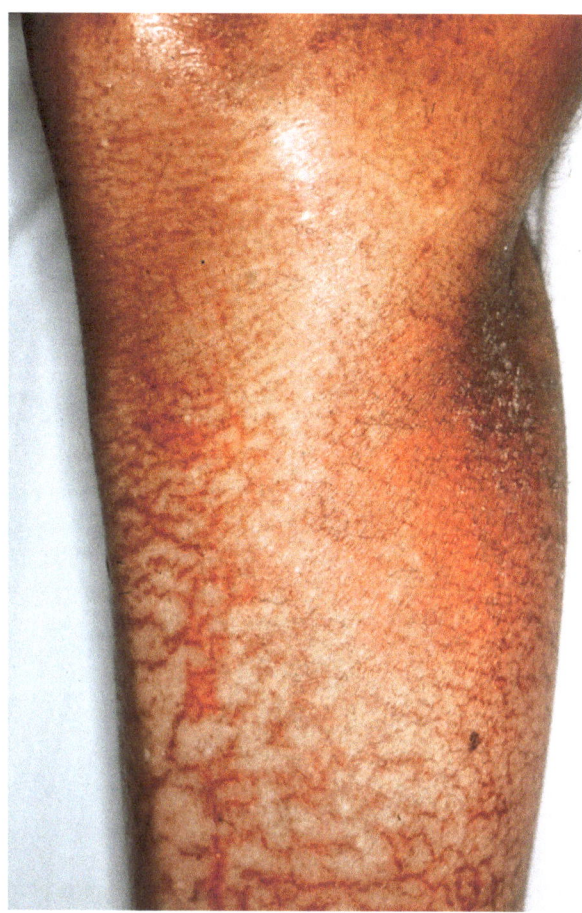

eruptions are estimated to occur in 2% of individuals exposed to medications [72]. The most common culprits are penicillins, cephalosporins, sulfonamide antibiotics, allopurinol, and aromatic anti-seizure medications [73].

Uncomplicated morbilliform eruptions account for 95% of cutaneous drug reactions [73]. Morbilliform eruptions typically occur 1–2 weeks after initial exposure to a medication, though can appear sooner with re-exposure [74]. Exam shows morbilliform ("measles-like") symmetric erythematous macules and papules initially on the trunk and then spreading peripherally to involve the extremities [75] (Fig. 11.14). They are usually pruritic, not painful, and generally spare the mucosae. Low-grade fever is common [74]. The differential includes a viral exanthem. If there is mucosal involvement, blistering, cutaneous pain, a high fever, or facial edema/erythema, more complicated drug eruptions such as drug reaction with eosinophilia and systemic symptoms (DRESS) or Stevens-Johnson syndrome (SJS)/ toxic epidermal necrolysis (TEN) should be considered [74]. Treatment of a morbilliform drug exanthem is discontinuation of the offending drug and supportive care

Fig. 11.14 Morbilliform drug eruption most commonly starts in the intertriginous areas and spreads to the trunk and extremities

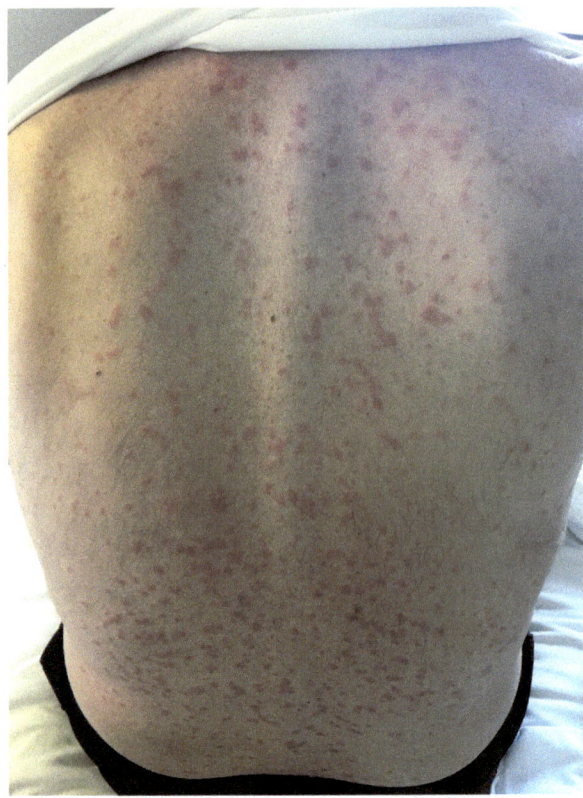

with mid-potency topical corticosteroids and antihistamines can help ease pruritus while waiting for the eruption to resolve [75]. If left alone, the rash typically spontaneously resolves in 1–2 weeks.

Not all drug eruptions are acute. Common chronic drug eruptions seen in the outpatient setting include an eczematous dermatitis to calcium channel blockers [76] and hydrochlorothiazide-induced photosensitivity and lichenoid drug eruption [77].

Eruption of Senescence

Pruritus is common in patients over 65 years of age [78]. This can be multifactorial; however, some older adults with generalized pruritus may also present with a non-specific eczematous dermatitis with pink pruritic papules and occasional plaques. Often the pruritus is out of proportion to the cutaneous findings. This has been termed "eruption of senescence" and is thought to be due to a decrease in Th1 cell-mediated immunity and shift to a Th2 predominant state [14, 79].

Psoriasis

Psoriasis is a common chronic inflammatory skin condition, affecting 2% of the American and European population [80]. Although psoriasis is equally prevalent in men and women, men, on average, have more severe disease than women [81]. Psoriasis may progressively worsen with age or wax and wane in severity [82]. Psoriasis is a clinical diagnosis, made by a comprehensive history and physical examination with an emphasis on a full skin exam, paying particular attention to body sites with a predilection for psoriatic plaques.

Plaque psoriasis, also known as psoriasis vulgaris, is the most common presentation of psoriasis and accounts for 90% of cases [80, 82]. Lesions typically present as well-demarcated erythematous plaques covered by silvery scale (Fig. 11.15). Plaques can be limited or extensive. The most frequent body areas of involvement include the extensor surfaces of the forearms, shins, gluteal cleft, periumbilical, retro-auricular, and scalp. Other variants of psoriasis include guttate psoriasis, characterized by numerous teardrop-shaped erythematous scaly spots; inverse psoriasis (also known as flexural) involving in skin folds such as the axillae or groin; pustular psoriasis; and erythrodermic psoriasis, which, although rare, can be life-threatening [80].

Nail involvement occurs in up to 55% of those with psoriasis [83] and usually occurs after the onset of cutaneous disease but occasionally may be the first manifestation of psoriasis [84]. It is important to also inquire about joint involvement in psoriasis, as up to 30% of patients will develop psoriatic arthritis (PsA) [85]. PsA is an inflammatory, asymmetric, polyarthritis which commonly presents with warmth, redness, swelling, and pain of affected joints. Patients with PsA describe stiffness after prolonged periods of inactivity which improves with activity. The peripheral and/or axial joints can be affected [86]. Radiographs and MRI are recommended if PsA is suspected [87]. In addition to articular disease, other features of PsA include

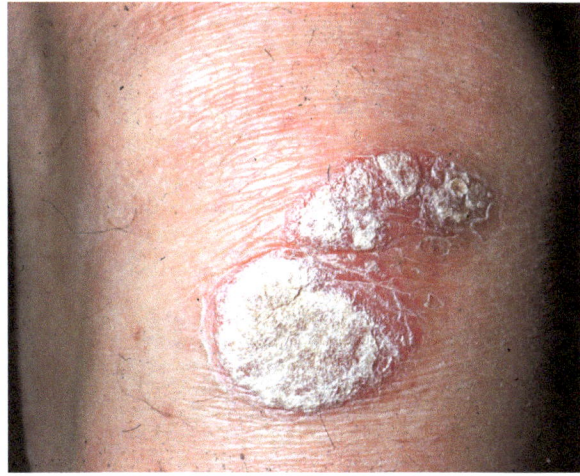

Fig. 11.15 Psoriasis vulgaris. Note well-demarcated plaque with silvery scale on an extensor surface

enthesitis (inflammation at the site of the insertion of tendons or ligaments), tenosynovitis, and dactylitis (diffuse swelling of an entire finger or toe).

In recent years there has been a considerable influx of treatment options for patients with psoriasis. The mainstay of therapy for patients with mild or localized disease includes topical steroids, topical calcineurin inhibitors, and phototherapy. For moderate to severe disease, systemic therapies are utilized. The role of anti-TNF and newer-generation biologic therapies has dramatically changed the management of severe psoriasis and allowed patients to achieve almost complete remission in what was once a chronic and difficult to treat condition [88].

Recent evidence suggests patients with psoriasis may have an increased association with cardiovascular disease, including increased risk for myocardial infarction, coronary artery disease, stroke, and diabetes [89]. Patients with severe psoriasis have, on average, a 4-year decrease in their life expectancy likely due in part to the increased prevalence of coronary artery disease [90]. Based on these findings, guidelines have been proposed for the screening and counseling of patients with psoriasis. These include informing patients with moderate to severe psoriasis of the increased risk of CAD associated with their psoriasis; screening for family history of heart disease and/or risk factors for diabetes mellitus, hypertension, or dyslipidemia; and at least annual measurements of blood pressure, lipid profile, and blood glucose levels [90].

Bullous Pemphigoid

Bullous pemphigoid (BP) is an autoimmune blistering skin disorder that most frequently affects the elderly. Age is one of the most important risk factors for BP, with an almost 300-fold higher relative risk for patients >90 years of age when compared to patients ≤60 years [91]. Men have a higher overall incidence of developing BP in their lifetime [92].

Patients with BP present with tense, often widespread, bullae on the skin and describe intense pruritus. The bullae can range anywhere from 1 to 4 cm, contain clear fluid, and leave behind erosions and crusted lesions (Fig. 11.16). BP lesions predominate on the trunk and the flexural aspects of the limbs. The oral cavity is involved in approximately 10–30% of patients [91]. During the early stages of BP, there may be nonspecific pruritus, either alone or in combination with an eczematous, papular, or urticarial eruption. This "pre-bullous" phase of BP can persist for several weeks to months before bullae develop [93].

The diagnosis of BP is based on clinical features combined with skin biopsy. Direct immunofluorescence (DIF) on a specimen of perilesional (unaffected) skin is performed to look for autoantibody deposition in the skin. The diagnosis of BP can also be established with serologic tests such as ELISA against the target antigens, BP180 and BP230, which are proteins located at the dermal-epidermal junction that are important for epidermal basement membrane adhesion [91].

Fig. 11.16 Bullous pemphigoid, with tense blisters admixed with ruptured blisters and erosion

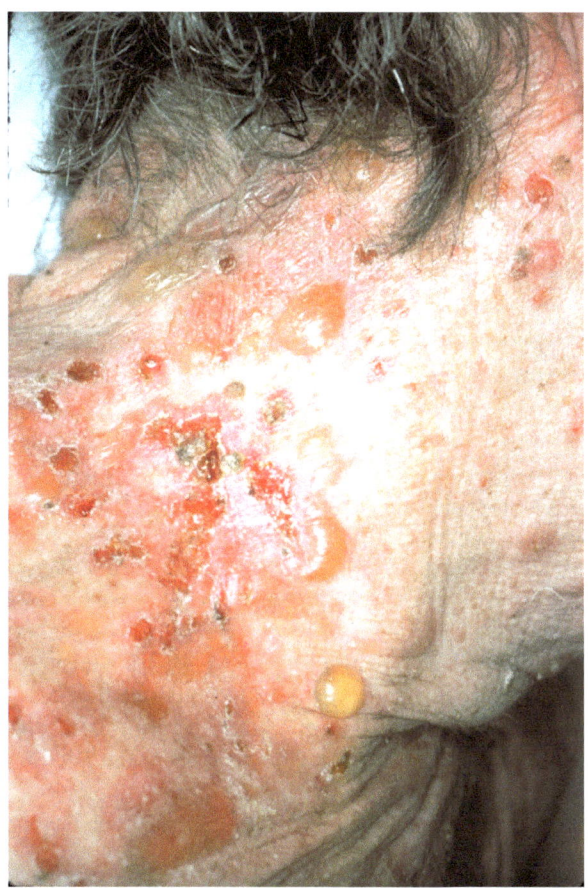

Treatment for BP depends on the degree of cutaneous involvement and severity of symptoms. If the disease is mild and localized, superpotent topical steroids can be utilized. In more severe or extensive disease, systemic steroids or immunomodulators are often necessary, and consultation with a dermatologist is warranted [91].

Disorders of Skin Appendages in the Aging Male: Nails and Hair

Nails

As men age, they may note changes in their finger- and toenails. The growth rate and morphology of the nail plate change with age, resulting in thicker nails with alterations in contour, surface texture, and color [94]. The mechanism for this is unclear, but may be due to a combination of factors including poor blood circulation in the distal extremities and recurrent trauma through life [95].

In addition to physiologic changes, there are nail disorders that are more likely to appear in the aging male. These include brittle nails, onychocryptosis (ingrown toenails), and onychomycosis.

Onychomycosis

Onychomycosis, one of the most common nail conditions, is a fungal infection of the nail unit. The incidence of onychomycosis increases with advancing age, and males are more commonly affected than females [96, 97]. Besides age and male gender, other risk factors for onychomycosis include peripheral vascular disease and diabetes [98].

Dermatophytes from the *Trichophyton, Epidermophyton*, and *Microsporum* families can all cause onychomycosis; however, *Trichophyton* genus is most commonly implicated [99]. Onychomycosis due to dermatophytes is more specifically called tinea unguium. Distal/lateral subungual onychomycosis is the most common clinical presentation of dermatophyte onychomycosis, characterized by nailplate thickening, onycholysis (lifting of the nail from the nail bed), and the presence of subungual debris (Fig. 11.17). Although a diagnosis of onychomycosis is often assumed based on clinical findings, confirming the diagnosis with laboratory studies before treatment can be cost-effective and is recommended to avoid incorrect diagnosis and treatment failures [100].

There are several ways to obtain an adequate sample for evaluation of onychomycosis. The diseased nail should be clipped back as far as possible. Subungual debris overlying the nail bed can then be obtained with a curette. Specimens can be analyzed using direct microscopy using potassium hydroxide (KOH), a rapid and inexpensive method to confirm the presence of fungal hyphae. Periodic acid-Schiff (PAS) staining of the nail plate is less rapid and more expensive, but has greater sensitivity and specificity [96, 101]. Both KOH and PAS can be used in combination with culture of the subungual debris to guide therapy.

Fig. 11.17 Onychomycosis. The great toenails are often first affected

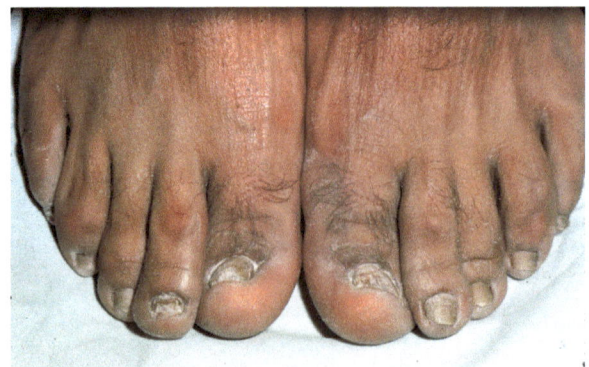

Treatment of onychomycosis is not mandatory, but there are certain circumstances where treatment is recommended. This includes patients experiencing discomfort or pain with infected nails, immunosuppressed patients, or those with a history of lower leg cellulitis or diabetes mellitus [96]. Oral antifungal therapies provide the best cure rates for onychomycosis. Oral terbinafine is considered a first-line agent, given at a dose of 250 mg daily for 6 weeks for fingernails and 16 weeks for toenails [102].

Aging Hair

Hair graying is one of the most recognizable signs of aging, with the age of onset and rate of progression in large part influenced by one's genetics [103]. Hair pigment is derived from follicular melanocytes that transfer pigment to the hair shaft, and there is a gradual loss of follicular melanocytes over time [104].

Alopecia

Hair loss with age is universal and can be considered a marker of generalized senescence. This age-related hair thinning or "alopecia of senescence" typically occurs after the age of 50 and presents with a gradual diffuse reduction in hair density and diameter [105]. Androgenetic (patterned) alopecia (AA), also known as male pattern baldness, is common, occurring in almost 50% of men by the age of 50, with the highest prevalence in white men [103]. In AA, large caliber hairs progressively become finer and thinner in a process known as miniaturization, ultimately leading to overall decreased coverage of the scalp. These changes are most readily observed along the frontal hairline and vertex or crown of the scalp.

There is a genetic predisposition to AA, and the role of androgens is well documented. In AA, there is a substantial increase of testosterone conversion to dihydrotestosterone (DHT) by the enzyme 5-alpha-reductase. DHT's affinity for the androgen receptor is five times that of testosterone. Its binding induces miniaturization of androgen-sensitive hair follicles [106].

First-line therapy for AA includes topical minoxidil and oral finasteride, both of which have been extensively studied and have been shown to induce some degree of hair regrowth and reversal of miniaturization [107]. Neither agent can completely reverse AA, however, and men should be counseled that halting progression of hair loss is a more realistic goal than hair regrowth [108].

The exact mechanism of action of topical minoxidil on hair regrowth is unknown. It may promote hair growth by increasing the duration of the anagen (growing) phase while decreasing the telogen (resting) phase, leading to enlargement of miniaturized hairs [109]. The recommended administration of topical minoxidil for AA is two times daily to the scalp, continued for at least 4 months to assess efficacy. Of note, men should be counseled that topical minoxidil can initially induce a telogen effluvium [110] resulting in transient hair loss. Optimally, topical minoxidil is used indefinitely, as discontinuation will reverse its effects [111].

Finasteride works by competitively inhibiting 5-alpha-reductase and inhibits conversion of testosterone to DHT. The recommended dose of finasteride for AA is 1 mg by mouth per day, with treatment continuation for least 12 months to assess full efficacy [112]. Patients may experience sexual dysfunction, including erectile dysfunction, decreased libido, and ejaculatory dysfunction. These sexual side effects may increase with age [113].

Hair transplantation surgery has undergone significant improvements, both in technique and outcomes. This modality of hair restoration involves harvesting hair follicles from the occiput and surgically transferring them to the affected frontal or vertex scalp. As hair follicles on the occipital scalp are androgen independent, transplanted hair follicles are unaffected by further androgen influence in their new location [103]. This method of hair harvesting is dependent on adequate supply of donor hair and can be costly. Many hair transplantation experts recommend that patients undergoing the procedure also continue medical therapy with minoxidil and/or finasteride [114]. Patients seeking hair transplantation surgery should be counseled to invest in consultation with a knowledgeable and experienced surgeon.

Cosmetic Treatments and Procedures in the Aging Man

Men are increasing their utilization of cosmetic treatments. In 2017, men received 9% of all nonsurgical cosmetic procedures, a 30% increase over the previous 5 years [115]. Understanding the relevant differences in facial anatomy between men and women is important to ensure patient satisfaction and prevent complications. Men, in general, have thicker skin and increased facial muscle mass compared to women [116]. Characteristically male faces are square, with flatter eyebrows, prominent zygomatic arches, larger jaws, and more prominent chins compared to women [116, 117].

Botulinum Toxin

Botulinum toxin injection is the most common cosmetic procedure performed in men [115, 118]. Over 160,000 men yearly undergo botulinum toxin injection for cosmetic purposes [115]. A survey study of men found that "facial wrinkles" are one of the highest priorities for men when asked about facial aesthetics. The periorbital area (crow's feet, tear troughs) and forehead lines were of particular concern. Men have more facial musculature compared to women that, in conjunction with the normal age-related loss of subcutaneous tissue, results in more prominent wrinkling (rhytids) [119]. In contrast to women, the appearance of the lips and perioral wrinkling are of lower concern to men [120].

Due to increased muscle mass as compared to women, men may not respond to "usual" doses of botulinum toxin, leading some experts to advocate increasing doses of botulinum toxin for men [118]. Aging men in particular are more susceptible to brow ptosis, which may be exacerbated or unmasked by botulinum toxin treatment of the frontalis muscle [118].

Soft Tissue Fillers

The injection of soft tissue fillers, including hyaluronic acid, calcium hydroxylapatite, poly-L-lactic acid, and polymethyl methacrylate, is the second most common cosmetic procedure pursued by men [115]. Fillers are utilized for soft tissue augmentation, to enhance features (such as the chin), or to compensate for age-related loss of volume in the face [116]. Careful attention to the volume of filler used is required in men. Men generally prefer to have fewer, more effective treatments rather than a series of treatments; however, this approach can risk overtreatment and result in a feminized appearance [121].

Retinoids

Topical retinoids are first-line therapy for photoaging. Retinoids exert their effects on the skin by increasing collagen production, inducing epidermal hyperplasia, and decreasing keratinocyte and melanocyte atypia [122]. It is important to inform patients of the potential for local skin irritation with the use of topical retinoids, particularly when starting use. Common side effects include dryness, redness, scaling, and stinging. Counseling patients of these expected reactions may decrease nonadherence [123].

Currently available retinoids include tretinoin, tazarotene, and adapalene. Tretinoin comes in several concentrations, allowing for easy dose titration. Adapalene has the advantage of being available without a prescription and is generally less irritating than the other retinoids.

References

1. Lim HW, Collins SAB, Resneck JS Jr, et al. The burden of skin disease in the United States. J Am Acad Dermatol. 2017;76(5):958–72.e2.
2. Enamandram M, Duncan LM, Kimball AB. Delivering value in dermatology: insights from skin cancer detection in routine clinical visits. J Am Acad Dermatol. 2015;72(2):310–3.
3. Moustafa F, Lewallen RS, Feldman SR. The psychological impact of rosacea and the influence of current management options. J Am Acad Dermatol. 2014;71(5):973–80.
4. de Korte J, Sprangers MA, Mombers FM, Bos JD. Quality of life in patients with psoriasis: a systematic literature review. J Investig Dermatol Symp Proc. 2004;9(2):140–7.

5. Bulpitt CJ, Markowe HL, Shipley MJ. Why do some people look older than they should? Postgrad Med J. 2001;77(911):578–81.
6. Gilchrest BA. Photoaging. J Invest Dermatol. 2013;133(E1):E2–6.
7. Wulf HC, Sandby-Moller J, Kobayasi T, Gniadecki R. Skin aging and natural photoprotection. Micron (Oxford, England: 1993). 2004;35(3):185–91.
8. Rittie L, Fisher GJ. Natural and sun-induced aging of human skin. Cold Spring Harb Perspect Med. 2015;5(1):a015370.
9. MacLaughlin J, Holick MF. Aging decreases the capacity of human skin to produce vitamin D3. J Clin Invest. 1985;76(4):1536–8.
10. Starr NJ, Johnson DJ, Wibawa J, et al. Age-related changes to human stratum corneum lipids detected using time-of-flight secondary ion mass spectrometry following in vivo sampling. Anal Chem. 2016;88(8):4400–8.
11. Tezuka T, Qing J, Saheki M, Kusuda S, Takahashi M. Terminal differentiation of facial epidermis of the aged: immunohistochemical studies. Dermatology (Basel, Switzerland). 1994;188(1):21–4.
12. Mahbub S, Brubaker AL, Kovacs EJ. Aging of the innate immune system: an update. Curr Immunol Rev. 2011;7(1):104–15.
13. Gilchrest BA. Skin aging and photoaging: an overview. J Am Acad Dermatol. 1989;21(3 Pt 2):610–3.
14. Berger TG, Steinhoff M. Pruritus in elderly patients--eruptions of senescence. Semin Cutan Med Surg. 2011;30(2):113–7.
15. Buller DB, Cokkinides V, Hall HI, et al. Prevalence of sunburn, sun protection, and indoor tanning behaviors among Americans: review from national surveys and case studies of 3 states. J Am Acad Dermatol. 2011;65(5 Suppl 1):S114–23.
16. Pillai S, Oresajo C, Hayward J. Ultraviolet radiation and skin aging: roles of reactive oxygen species, inflammation and protease activation, and strategies for prevention of inflammation-induced matrix degradation – a review. Int J Cosmet Sci. 2005;27(1):17–34.
17. Lavker RM, Kligman AM. Chronic heliodermatitis: a morphologic evaluation of chronic actinic dermal damage with emphasis on the role of mast cells. J Invest Dermatol. 1988;90(3):325–30.
18. Goldberg LH, Altman A. Benign skin changes associated with chronic sunlight exposure. Cutis. 1984;34(1):33–8, 40.
19. Gilchrest BA. A review of skin ageing and its medical therapy. Br J Dermatol. 1996;135(6):867–75.
20. Iannacone MR, Hughes MC, Green AC. Effects of sunscreen on skin cancer and photoaging. Photodermatol Photoimmunol Photomed. 2014;30(2–3):55–61.
21. Banik R, Lubach D. Skin tags: localization and frequencies according to sex and age. Dermatologica. 1987;174(4):180–3.
22. Kahana M, Grossman E, Feinstein A, Ronnen M, Cohen M, Millet MS. Skin tags: a cutaneous marker for diabetes mellitus. Acta Derm Venereol. 1987;67(2):175–7.
23. Yeatman JM, Kilkenny M, Marks R. The prevalence of seborrhoeic keratoses in an Australian population: does exposure to sunlight play a part in their frequency? Br J Dermatol. 1997;137(3):411–4.
24. Hafner C, Vogt T. Seborrheic keratosis. J Dtsch Dermatol Ges. 2008;6(8):664–77.
25. Baumann LS, Blauvelt A, Draelos ZD, et al. Safety and efficacy of hydrogen peroxide topical solution, 40% (w/w) in patients with seborrheic keratoses: results from two identical, randomized, double-blind, placebo-controlled, phase 3 studies (A-101-SEBK-301/302). J Am Acad Dermatol. 2018;79:869–77.
26. Kim RH, Armstrong AW. Nonmelanoma skin cancer. Dermatol Clin. 2012;30(30):125–39, ix.
27. American Cancer Society. https://www.cancer.org/cancer/skin-cancer/prevention-and-early-detection.html.
28. Rogers HW, Weinstock MA, Harris AR, et al. Incidence estimate of nonmelanoma skin cancer in the United States, 2006. Arch Dermatol. 2010;146(3):283–7.

29. Hacker SM, Flowers FP. Squamous cell carcinoma of the skin. Will heightened awareness of risk factors slow its increase? Postgrad Med. 1993;93(8):115–21, 25–6.
30. Zanetti R, Rosso S, Martinez C, et al. Comparison of risk patterns in carcinoma and melanoma of the skin in men: a multi-Centre case-case-control study. Br J Cancer. 2006;94(5):743–51.
31. Telfer NR, Colver GB, Morton CA, British Association of D. Guidelines for the management of basal cell carcinoma. Br J Dermatol. 2008;159(1):35–48.
32. Hannuksela-Svahn A, Pukkala E, Karvonen J. Basal cell skin carcinoma and other nonmelanoma skin cancers in Finland from 1956 through 1995. Arch Dermatol. 1999;135(7):781–6.
33. Marzuka AG, Book SE. Basal cell carcinoma: pathogenesis, epidemiology, clinical features, diagnosis, histopathology, and management. Yale J Biol Med. 2015;88(2):167–79.
34. Clark CM, Furniss M, Mackay-Wiggan JM. Basal cell carcinoma: an evidence-based treatment update. Am J Clin Dermatol. 2014;15(3):197–216.
35. von Domarus H, Stevens PJ. Metastatic basal cell carcinoma. Report of five cases and review of 170 cases in the literature. J Am Acad Dermatol. 1984;10(13):1043–60.
36. Alam M, Ratner D. Cutaneous squamous-cell carcinoma. N Engl J Med. 2001;344(13):975–83.
37. Peterson K, Baseman JB, Alderete JF. Molecular cloning of Treponema pallidum outer envelope fibronectin binding proteins, P1 and P2. Genitourin Med. 1987;63(6):355–60.
38. English DR, Armstrong BK, Kricker A, Winter MG, Heenan PJ, Randell PL. Demographic characteristics, pigmentary and cutaneous risk factors for squamous cell carcinoma of the skin: a case-control study. Int J Cancer. 1998;76(5):628–34.
39. Brougham ND, Dennett ER, Cameron R, Tan ST. The incidence of metastasis from cutaneous squamous cell carcinoma and the impact of its risk factors. J Surg Oncol. 2012;106(7):811–5.
40. Morales AV, Advani R, Horwitz SM, et al. Indolent primary cutaneous B-cell lymphoma: experience using systemic rituximab. J Am Acad Dermatol. 2008;59(6):953–7.
41. Goodson AG, Grossman D. Strategies for early melanoma detection: approaches to the patient with nevi. J Am Acad Dermatol. 2009;60(5):719–35; quiz 36–8.
42. Chevalier V, Barbe C, Le Clainche A, et al. Comparison of anatomical locations of cutaneous melanoma in men and women: a population-based study in France. Br J Dermatol. 2014;171(3):595–601.
43. Tucker MA. Melanoma epidemiology. Hematol Oncol Clin North Am. 2009;23(3):383–95, vii.
44. Swetter SM, Johnson TM, Miller DR, Layton CJ, Brooks KR, Geller AC. Melanoma in middle-aged and older men: a multi-institutional survey study of factors related to tumor thickness. Arch Dermatol. 2009;145(4):397–404.
45. Swetter SM, Pollitt RA, Johnson TM, Brooks DR, Geller AC. Behavioral determinants of successful early melanoma detection: role of self and physician skin examination. Cancer. 2012;118(15):3725–34.
46. Albores-Saavedra J, Batich K, Chable-Montero F, Sagy N, Schwartz AM, Henson DE. Merkel cell carcinoma demographics, morphology, and survival based on 3870 cases: a population based study. J Cutan Pathol. 2010;37(1):20–7.
47. Tothill R, Estall V, Rischin D. Merkel cell carcinoma: emerging biology, current approaches, and future directions. Am Soc Clin Oncol Educ Book. 2015;35:e519–26.
48. Church CD, Nghiem P. How does the Merkel polyomavirus lead to a lethal cancer? Many answers, many questions, and a new mouse model. J Invest Dermatol. 2015;135(5):1221–4.
49. Feng H, Shuda M, Chang Y, Moore PS. Clonal integration of a polyomavirus in human Merkel cell carcinoma. Science. 2008;319(5866):1096–100.
50. Coggshall K, Tello TL, North JP, Yu SS. Merkel cell carcinoma: an update and review: pathogenesis, diagnosis, and staging. J Am Acad Dermatol. 2018;78(3):433–42.
51. Heath M, Jaimes N, Lemos B, et al. Clinical characteristics of Merkel cell carcinoma at diagnosis in 195 patients: the AEIOU features. J Am Acad Dermatol. 2008;58(3):375–81.
52. Green A, Battistutta D, Hart V, et al. The Nambour Skin Cancer and Actinic Eye Disease Prevention Trial: design and baseline characteristics of participants. Control Clin Trials. 1994;15(6):512–22.

53. Hughes MC, Williams GM, Baker P, Green AC. Sunscreen and prevention of skin aging: a randomized trial. Ann Intern Med. 2013;158(11):781–90.
54. Sambandan DR, Ratner D. Sunscreens: an overview and update. J Am Acad Dermatol. 2011;64(4):748–58.
55. Heurung AR, Raju SI, Warshaw EM. Adverse reactions to sunscreen agents: epidemiology, responsible irritants and allergens, clinical characteristics, and management. Dermatitis. 2014;25(6):289–326.
56. Studer HP. The economist's point of view: cascades of money for health. Krankenpfl Soins Infirm. 1996;89(7):78–82.
57. Heerfordt IM. Sunscreen use at Danish beaches and how to improve coverage. Dan Med J. 2018;155(4):88–90.
58. Isedeh P, Osterwalder U, Lim HW. Teaspoon rule revisited: proper amount of sunscreen application. Photodermatol Photoimmunol Photomed. 2013;29(1):55–6.
59. Gies P. Photoprotection by clothing. Photodermatol Photoimmunol Photomed. 2007;23(6):264–74.
60. Wang SQ, Balagula Y, Osterwalder U. Photoprotection: a review of the current and future technologies. Dermatol Ther. 2010;23(1):31–47.
61. Miyamura Y, Coelho SG, Schlenz K, et al. The deceptive nature of UVA tanning versus the modest protective effects of UVB tanning on human skin. Pigment Cell Melanoma Res. 2011;24(1):136–47.
62. Paul C, Maumus-Robert S, Mazereeuw-Hautier J, Guyen CN, Saudez X, Schmitt AM. Prevalence and risk factors for xerosis in the elderly: a cross-sectional epidemiological study in primary care. Dermatology. 2011;223(3):260–5.
63. Bolognia J, Schaffer J, Cerroni L. Dermatology. 4th ed. Amsterdam, Netherlands: Elsevier; 2018.
64. Ghadially R, Brown BE, Sequeira-Martin SM, Feingold KR, Elias PM. The aged epidermal permeability barrier. Structural, functional, and lipid biochemical abnormalities in humans and a senescent murine model. J Clin Invest. 1995;95(5):2281–90.
65. Choi EH, Man MQ, Xu P, et al. Stratum corneum acidification is impaired in moderately aged human and murine skin. J Invest Dermatol. 2007;127(12):2847–56.
66. Jensen JM, Forl M, Winoto-Morbach S, et al. Acid and neutral sphingomyelinase, ceramide synthase, and acid ceramidase activities in cutaneous aging. Exp Dermatol. 2005;14(8):609–18.
67. Elias PM, Ghadially R. The aged epidermal permeability barrier: basis for functional abnormalities. Clin Geriatr Med. 2002;18(1):103–20, vii.
68. Prakash AV, Davis MD. Contact dermatitis in older adults: a review of the literature. Am J Clin Dermatol. 2010;11(6):373–81.
69. White-Chu EF, Reddy M. Dry skin in the elderly: complexities of a common problem. Clin Dermatol. 2011;29(1):37–42.
70. Berger TG, Shive M, Harper GM. Pruritus in the older patient: a clinical review. JAMA. 2013;310(22):2443–50.
71. Ornstein SM, Nietert PJ, Jenkins RG, Litvin CB. The prevalence of chronic diseases and multimorbidity in primary care practice: a PPRNet report. J Am Board Fam Med. 2013;26(5):518–24.
72. Bigby M, Jick S, Jick H, Arndt K. Drug-induced cutaneous reactions. A report from the Boston Collaborative Drug Surveillance Program on 15,438 consecutive inpatients, 1975 to 1982. JAMA. 1986;256(24):3358–63.
73. Bigby M. Rates of cutaneous reactions to drugs. Arch Dermatol. 2001;137(6):765–70.
74. Stern RS. Clinical practice. Exanthematous drug eruptions. N Engl J Med. 2012;366(26):2492–501.
75. Biesbroeck LK, Shinohara MM. Inpatient consultative dermatology. Med Clin North Am. 2015;99(6):1349–64.

76. Joly P, Benoit-Corven C, Baricault S, et al. Chronic eczematous eruptions of the elderly are associated with chronic exposure to calcium channel blockers: results from a case-control study. J Invest Dermatol. 2007;127(12):2766–71.
77. Pascoe VL, Fenves AZ, Wofford J, Jackson JM, Menter A, Kimball AB. The spectrum of nephrocutaneous diseases and associations: inflammatory and medication-related nephrocutaneous associations. J Am Acad Dermatol. 2016;74(2):247–70; quiz 71-2.
78. Valdes-Rodriguez R, Mollanazar NK, Gonzalez-Muro J, et al. Itch prevalence and characteristics in a Hispanic geriatric population: a comprehensive study using a standardized itch questionnaire. Acta Derm Venereol. 2015;95(4):417–21.
79. Xu AZ, Tripathi SV, Kau AL, Schaffer A, Kim BS. Immune dysregulation underlies a subset of patients with chronic idiopathic pruritus. J Am Acad Dermatol. 2016;74(5):1017–20.
80. Boehncke WH, Schon MP. Psoriasis. Lancet (London, England). 2015;386(9997):983–94.
81. Hagg D, Eriksson M, Sundstrom A, Schmitt-Egenolf M. The higher proportion of men with psoriasis treated with biologics may be explained by more severe disease in men. PLoS One. 2013;8(5):e63619.
82. Lebwohl M. Psoriasis. Lancet (London, England). 2003;361(9364):1197–204.
83. Oram Y, Akkaya AD. Treatment of nail psoriasis: common concepts and new trends. Dermatol Res Pract. 2013;2013:180496.
84. Klaassen KM, van de Kerkhof PC, Pasch MC. Nail psoriasis: a questionnaire-based survey. Br J Dermatol. 2013;169(2):314–9.
85. Henes JC, Ziupa E, Eisfelder M, et al. High prevalence of psoriatic arthritis in dermatological patients with psoriasis: a cross-sectional study. Rheumatol Int. 2014;34(2):227–34.
86. Moll JM, Wright V. Psoriatic arthritis. Semin Arthritis Rheum. 1973;3(1):55–78.
87. Offidani A, Cellini A, Valeri G, Giovagnoni A. Subclinical joint involvement in psoriasis: magnetic resonance imaging and X-ray findings. Acta Derm Venereol. 1998;78(6):463–5.
88. Armstrong AW, Siegel MP, Bagel J, et al. From the Medical Board of the National Psoriasis Foundation: treatment targets for plaque psoriasis. J Am Acad Dermatol. 2017;76(2):290–8.
89. Mehta NN, Azfar RS, Shin DB, Neimann AL, Troxel AB, Gelfand JM. Patients with severe psoriasis are at increased risk of cardiovascular mortality: cohort study using the General Practice Research Database. Eur Heart J. 2010;31(8):1000–6.
90. Friedewald VE, Cather JC, Gelfand JM, et al. AJC editor's consensus: psoriasis and coronary artery disease. Am J Cardiol. 2008;102(12):1631–43.
91. Bernard P, Antonicelli F. Bullous pemphigoid: a review of its diagnosis, associations and treatment. Am J Clin Dermatol. 2017;18(4):513–28.
92. Jung M, Kippes W, Messer G, Zillikens D, Rzany B. Increased risk of bullous pemphigoid in male and very old patients: a population-based study on incidence. J Am Acad Dermatol. 1999;41(2 Pt 1):266–8.
93. Di Zenzo G, Marazza G, Borradori L. Bullous pemphigoid: physiopathology, clinical features and management. Adv Dermatol. 2007;23:257–88.
94. Abdullah L, Abbas O. Common nail changes and disorders in older people: diagnosis and management. Can Fam Physician. 2011;57(2):173–81.
95. Singh G, Haneef NS, Uday A. Nail changes and disorders among the elderly. Indian J Dermatol Venereol Leprol. 2005;71(6):386–92.
96. Elewski BE. The effect of toenail onychomycosis on patient quality of life. Int J Dermatol. 1997;36(10):754–6.
97. Sigurgeirsson B, Baran R. The prevalence of onychomycosis in the global population: a literature study. J Eur Acad Dermatol Venereol. 2014;28(11):1480–91.
98. Gupta AK, Daigle D, Foley KA. The prevalence of culture-confirmed toenail onychomycosis in at-risk patient populations. J Eur Acad Dermatol Venereol. 2015;29(6):1039–44.
99. Ameen M, Lear JT, Madan V, Mohd Mustapa MF, Richardson M, Hughes JR, et al. British Association of Dermatologists' guidelines for the management of onychomycosis 2014. Br J Dermatol. 2014;171(5):937–58.

100. Lipner SR, Scher RK. Part I: Onychomycosis: clinical overview and diagnosis. J Am Acad Dermatol. 2018;80:835–51.
101. Biesbroeck LK, Fleckman P. Nail disease for the primary care provider. Med Clin North Am. 2015;99(6):1213–26.
102. Warshaw EM, Fett DD, Bloomfield HE, et al. Pulse versus continuous terbinafine for onychomycosis: a randomized, double-blind, controlled trial. J Am Acad Dermatol. 2005;53(4):578–84.
103. Mirmirani P. Age-related hair changes in men: mechanisms and management of alopecia and graying. Maturitas. 2015;80(1):58–62.
104. Commo S, Gaillard O, Bernard BA. Human hair greying is linked to a specific depletion of hair follicle melanocytes affecting both the bulb and the outer root sheath. Br J Dermatol. 2004;150(3):435–43.
105. Hordinsky M, Sawaya M, Roberts JL. Hair loss and hirsutism in the elderly. Clin Geriatr Med. 2002;18(1):121–33, vii.
106. Ellis JA, Sinclair R, Harrap SB. Androgenetic alopecia: pathogenesis and potential for therapy. Expert Rev Mol Med. 2002;4(22):1–11.
107. Varothai S, Bergfeld WF. Androgenetic alopecia: an evidence-based treatment update. Am J Clin Dermatol. 2014;15(3):217–30.
108. Saraswat A, Kumar B. Minoxidil vs finasteride in the treatment of men with androgenetic alopecia. Arch Dermatol. 2003;139(9):1219–21.
109. Messenger AG, Rundegren J. Minoxidil: mechanisms of action on hair growth. Br J Dermatol. 2004;150(2):186–94.
110. Bardelli A, Rebora A. Telogen effluvium and minoxidil. J Am Acad Dermatol. 1989;21(3 Pt 1):572–3.
111. Olsen EA, Weiner MS. Topical minoxidil in male pattern baldness: effects of discontinuation of treatment. J Am Acad Dermatol. 1987;17(1):97–101.
112. Mella JM, Perret MC, Manzotti M, Catalano HN, Guyatt G. Efficacy and safety of finasteride therapy for androgenetic alopecia: a systematic review. Arch Dermatol. 2010;146(10):1141–50.
113. Olsen EA, Whiting DA, Savin R, et al. Global photographic assessment of men aged 18 to 60 years with male pattern hair loss receiving finasteride 1 mg or placebo. J Am Acad Dermatol. 2012;67(3):379–86.
114. Avram M, Rogers N. Contemporary hair transplantation. Dermatol Surg. 2009;35(11):1705–19.
115. Surgery ASfAP. https://surgery.org/sites/default/files/ASAPS-Stats2017.pdf.
116. Rossi AM, Fitzgerald R, Humphrey S. Facial soft tissue augmentation in males: an anatomical and practical approach. Dermatol Surg. 2017;43 Suppl 2:S131–s9.
117. Farhadian JA, Bloom BS, Brauer JA. Male aesthetics: a review of facial anatomy and pertinent clinical implications. J Drugs Dermatol. 2015;14(9):1029–34.
118. Green JB, Keaney TC. Aesthetic treatment with botulinum toxin: approaches specific to men. Dermatol Surg. 2017;43 Suppl 2:S153–s6.
119. Sadick NS. The pathophysiology of the male aging face and body. Dermatol Clin. 2018;36(1):1–4.
120. Jagdeo J, Keaney T, Narurkar V, Kolodziejczyk J, Gallagher CJ. Facial treatment preferences among aesthetically oriented men. Dermatol Surg. 2016;42(10):1155–63.
121. Sadick NS. Volumetric structural rejuvenation for the male face. Dermatol Clin. 2018;36(1):43–8.
122. Cho S, Lowe L, Hamilton TA, Fisher GJ, Voorhees JJ, Kang S. Long-term treatment of photoaged human skin with topical retinoic acid improves epidermal cell atypia and thickens the collagen band in papillary dermis. J Am Acad Dermatol. 2005;53(5):769–74.
123. Samuel M, Brooke RC, Hollis S, Griffiths CE. Interventions for photodamaged skin. Cochrane Database Syst Rev. 2005;(1):Cd001782.

Chapter 12
Men's Health and Psychiatry

Molly M. Shores

This chapter will provide a broad overview of differences in prevalent mental health disorders between men and women. These differences may be related to testosterone effects on brain structure and function, which will be briefly reviewed. The remainder of the chapter will focus on the association of endogenous testosterone with mood disorders and the use of exogenous testosterone in the treatment of mood disorders.

Mental Health Disorders in Men

The need to consider men's distinct mental health-care needs is indicated by the large differences in prevalent mental health conditions between men and women. Women have twice the rate of major depression, anxiety, and PTSD as men, while men have twice the rate of substance use disorders and three to four times the rates of autism and ADHD as women [1–4]. The potential biologic basis for the greater prevalence of autism and ADHD in males is beyond the scope of this article and has been reviewed elsewhere [5, 6]. However, studies have suggested that both autism and ADHD are associated with higher levels of prenatal testosterone and that autism may be an extreme variant of male characteristics [7–9]. The etiology of these disorders is complex, and in addition to potential effects of fetal testosterone levels, other potential causes include genetic, epigenetic, immune, and environmental factors [5, 6].

M. M. Shores (✉)
VA Puget Sound Health Care System, University of Washington, Department of Psychiatry and Behavioral Sciences, Seattle, WA, USA
e-mail: mxs@uw.edu

© Springer Nature Switzerland AG 2021   231
J. P. Alukal et al. (eds.), *Design and Implementation of the Modern Men's Health Center*, https://doi.org/10.1007/978-3-030-54482-9_12

Substance Use Disorders

Men have higher rates of all substance use disorders than women, which is likely related to both cultural factors and to biologic differences, such as differences in drug metabolism, neuroendocrine factors, and brain structure and function. However, although men have a greater prevalence for substance use disorders than women, they have similar treatment outcomes [10]. The most common substance use disorders in men are alcohol, cannabis, cocaine, hallucinogens, and opiates [4]. In men, substance use disorders increase during periods of transition such as college, marriage, parenthood, and retirement. Substance use disorders also increase with social stressors, such as bereavement, divorce, work stress, and unemployment [4].

Opiate Use Disorder

Over the past decade opiate use disorders and mortality from opioid overdose have reached an "epidemic" level in the United States [11–16]. The full assessment and management of opioid use disorder are beyond the scope of this article and have been reviewed elsewhere [17]. However, in addition to providing treatment with psychosocial interventions, opiate substitution is recommended for treatment consideration as it has been shown to be highly effective in decreasing opioid relapse, morbidity, and mortality. Buprenorphine and methadone have similar effects in decreasing risk for relapse, but buprenorphine is associated with less adverse effects and a lower risk for overdose [18–20]. Chronic opiate use in men is associated with testosterone deficiency, and it is estimated that approximately 5 million men in the United States have opioid-induced androgen deficiency [21, 22]. Opiate-induced androgen deficiency is associated with increased irritability, fatigue, and decreased libido and sexual function. A recent study found that testosterone replacement in men with opioid-induced androgen deficiency improved libido and quality of life and decreased pain in men on chronic opiates [23]. The Endocrine Society Clinical Guidelines recommend that men with chronic opiate treatment be screened for testosterone deficiency and evaluated for testosterone replacement therapy [24].

Depressive Disorders

Depressive disorders are a common condition in men with a prevalence of approximately 5–6% for major depression and a similar prevalence for subthreshold depressive disorders. Although men have a lower prevalence of depressive illness than women, they have a markedly higher rate of suicide. Risk factors for suicide in men include increasing age, Caucasian race, veteran status, history of mental illness, psychosocial stressors, and having access to lethal means. However, since suicide is a rare event, risk factors alone cannot adequately predict suicide. Interventions that have been shown to decrease the suicide rate are limiting access to lethal means such as guns, educating primary care providers about depression treatment, and integrating mental health care into primary care settings [25–29]. The management and assessment of suicide risk have been reviewed in more detail elsewhere [30, 31].

Depressive illness increases in men with aging and has a significant impact on well-being as it is associated with decreased quality of life, increased mortality, and increased morbidity from multiple conditions, including diabetes, COPD, and coronary artery disease [32–36]. The type of depressive disorders common in medically ill, primary-care patients are less severe, subthreshold depressive disorders [37–39]. These less severe mood disorders are also characteristic of the depressive illnesses associated with androgen deficiency [40, 41]. However, although subthreshold depressive disorders are not as severe as major depression, they are also associated with decreased quality of life, impaired function, and morbidity and mortality [42–45]. Treatment for subthreshold disorders with antidepressants or therapy has shown minimal benefits, while mental health care that is integrated into primary care clinics has shown better results [46].

Finally, the lower prevalence of depression in men could also be related to detection bias as men are less likely than women to engage in preventative health care or to seek either medical or mental health care, despite the fact that men have greater overall mortality and a much higher suicide rate than women [47–49]. Men also may be more concerned about stigma of having a mental health disorder and more reluctant than women to discuss emotions [4, 48–50]. Since men may have difficulties in seeking mental health care, providers could help to facilitate engagement in care by using a medical model for mental illness and reviewing that untreated mental illness may increase medical morbidity and mortality.

Testosterone and the Male Brain

The lower prevalence of depression and anxiety disorders in men, which has also been observed in a large multinational study [51], suggests that testosterone may have protective effects to decrease the risk for depressive and anxiety disorders. Androgen receptors in the brain are densely located in the hippocampus, amygdala, and dorsolateral prefrontal cortex, which are crucial in regulating mood, arousal, stress, and memory [52]. During the prenatal period and the first year of life, androgens masculinize the male brain via organizational and activational effects. Organizational effects occur at critical times in development and result in permanent changes in brain structure, synapses, and circuits [53]. Examples of organizational effects of testosterone are that males generally have a larger amygdala, sexually dimorphic nucleus, and greater left-right asymmetry than females [52–55]. Activational effects of testosterone are effects that are acute and transient and occur throughout the life cycle and include regulation of nerve growth factors, neuropeptides, neurotransmitters, and neurogenesis. In animal models, testosterone regulates neuronal plasticity and increases neurogenesis in the hippocampus in conjunction with antidepressant treatment [56–59]. Testosterone stimulates mitogen-activated protein kinase (MAPK), which appears to play a role in mood regulation as both lithium and valproic acid increase the expression of MAPK [54]. In male rats, metabolites of testosterone modulate GABA-A receptors in the cortex and hippocampus, which may contribute to anxiolytic effects of testosterone [60]. In animal models, testosterone increases the firing of serotonergic neurons, increases serotonin release, and increases serotonin $5HT_{2a}$ receptor density in the forebrain [61, 62]. In female to male transgendered individuals, testosterone increases serotonin binding in the amygdala, caudate, putamen, and median raphe and increases hypothalamic neuroplasticity [63–65]. In hypogonadal men, testosterone increases cerebral flow and increases cerebral glucose metabolism [66, 67]. In healthy young men, testosterone increases amygdala activation in response to images of fear or anger [68]. Low testosterone levels are associated with increased hypothalamic-pituitary-adrenal (HPA) axis hyperactivity, which may occur with depression or stress [69]. In conclusion, the potential association between testosterone and depression is complex as androgen receptors are densely located in areas of the brain that regulate mood, stress, and arousal, and testosterone has multiple effects on brain structure and function. Finally testosterone may impact brain function not only due to direct effects of testosterone but also due to effects of the metabolites of testosterone, dihydrotestosterone (DHT) and estrogen.

Testosterone, Aging, and Depressive Disorders

Aging. Testosterone levels begin to decline in middle age, and low testosterone levels are present in approximately 20% of men in primary care settings [70]. However, the prevalence of hypogonadism, e.g., repeated low morning testosterone levels plus signs or symptoms of hypogonadism, occurs at a lower rate in approximately 3–6% of older men [71–73]. In addition to the age-related decrease in testosterone levels, testosterone also decreases with stress, medications, obesity, diabetes, inactivity, and acute or chronic illness [74, 75], and age-associated low testosterone levels may be related more to medical morbidity than to age [76]. Age-related decreases in testosterone levels are not necessarily a permanent condition as more than 50% of men with low testosterone had normal testosterone levels at follow-up, with normalization being more likely in younger, leaner men [77].

Testosterone and Depression

Aging is associated with a decrease in testosterone levels and an increase in depressive illness, particularly subthreshold depressive disorders [33, 45]. Given the many effects that testosterone has on the brain, it is feasible that declining levels of testosterone may be linked to depressive illness in men. Furthermore some symptoms of hypogonadism, such as decreased libido, irritability, anorexia, decreased concentration, and fatigue, overlap with symptoms of major depression. However, the potential relationship between testosterone and depression is complex because many conditions are independently associated with depression and testosterone deficiency and prior studies have produced conflicting results on the association between testosterone and mood disorders [64].

Low Serum Testosterone Levels and Prevalent Depressive Illness

Multiple epidemiologic studies have examined the association of testosterone levels and prevalent depressive symptoms and found that low free testosterone [78–80], bioavailable testosterone [81, 82], and total testosterone levels were associated with increased depressive symptoms [78, 79, 83, 84]. Although most cross-sectional studies found that low testosterone levels were associated with depressive illness, some studies did not [41, 85] detect an association with depressive symptoms but did note that low testosterone was associated with increased anxiety [85].

Low Serum Testosterone Levels and Incident Depressive Illness

Several prospective studies examined whether men with low testosterone had an increased risk for incident depressive illness compared to men with normal testosterone levels. In a study of veterans, men with repeatedly low total testosterone had an increased risk for incident depression with the greatest risk in men aged 50–65 years, with an adjusted hazard ratio (aHR) of 3.2, 95% confidence interval (95% CI) (1.7–5.9). In contrast, veterans with low testosterone levels who were older than 65 did not have an increased risk for depression with aHR of 1.4, 95% CI (0.7–2.6) [86, 87]. In a study of elderly men, low free testosterone was associated with an increased risk for incident depressive symptoms with aHR of 1.99, 95% CI (1.17–3.37) [80]. In a large study of elderly Australian community-dwelling elderly men, those with very low total testosterone levels (<6.4 nmol/L (184 ng/dL)) had an increased risk for incident depression with aHR of 1.86, 95% CI (1.05–3.31). Strengths of this study were that it was a large prospective study of over 3000 men that used a well-validated clinical database and had stringent criteria to exclude prevalent or past depression. Weaknesses were that there was a low rate of incident depression of only 4% and a high dropout rate of 30%, which suggests the possibility of survivorship bias [88]. In a study of men followed in primary care, baseline testosterone levels were not associated with incident depression, but longitudinal increases in testosterone over a 1-year period were associated with decreased risk for depression with aHR of 0.84, 95%CI (0.72–0.98) [89]. Finally, one prospective study found an association between low testosterone and incident depression in unadjusted analyses, but this did not persist in adjusted analyses [90].

Threshold Level for Low Testosterone and Depressive Symptoms

Several studies noted an inverse association between testosterone levels and mood, with depressive illness increasing with lower testosterone levels [86–88], but once testosterone was in the physiologic range, there were no correlations between testosterone levels and mood [91–94]. The threshold at which depressive symptoms increase significantly in relation to low testosterone has been reported to range from 230 to 288 ng/dL of total testosterone; at levels below this, the risk for prevalent depressive illness increases significantly [79, 87, 95].

Testosterone Levels, Androgen Receptor Polymorphisms, and Depression

Other studies examined whether serum testosterone and androgen receptor polymorphisms are associated with depressive symptoms. An increased number of androgen receptor cytosine, adenine, and guanine (CAG) repeats has been associated with androgen receptor insensitivity. This polymorphism of increased CAGs could result in a man with normal testosterone levels having hypogonadal symptoms due to androgen receptor insensitivity [96]. In studies of older men, those with increased CAGs had increased depressive symptoms despite having normal testosterone levels [97, 98]. In younger men, the presence of increased CAGs and low testosterone were associated with depressive symptoms [99]. However, some studies found no association with an increased number of CAGs and depressive symptoms [100–102].

Testosterone in Men with Diagnosed Depressive Illness

While these prior studies examined the association between low testosterone levels and mood symptoms, other studies examined if men with diagnosed depressive illness had decreased testosterone levels. In a cross-sectional study, men with major depression had lower TT and BAT levels and a greater prevalence of biochemical hypogonadism (34% vs 6% by BAT) than nondepressed men [103]. In depressed men, testosterone levels were lower during the depressive episode, but normalized following remission of the depression [104–106]. In contrast, men with major depression and an intact HPA axis did not have lower testosterone levels. However, if HPA hyperactivity with hyper-cortisolemia was present, then testosterone levels were lower in depressed [106, 107] and also in nondepressed men [107]. In men with major depression, those with low total testosterone or free testosterone had more persistent depressive illness over a 3-year follow-up period than men with normal testosterone levels [79]. In a study of men with different depressive disorders, men with dysthymia had significantly lower testosterone levels compared to controls and men with major depression [40].

In conclusion, most studies reported an association between lower testosterone levels and increased depressive symptoms with a testosterone threshold level for depressive illness ranging from 230 to 288 ng/dl of total testosterone. Men with diagnosed depression had variable testosterone levels, with some studies reporting no difference between depressed men and controls, [40, 108, 109], while others found that testosterone levels were lower in men with dysthymia or with major depression with a hyperactive HPA axis with elevated cortisol [40, 107].

High Serum Testosterone and Mood Disorders

A limited number of research studies have been conducted to examine the effect of high testosterone levels on mood in men. In one study, high-dose testosterone cypionate (up to 600 mg/week) for 6 weeks in eugonadal men was associated with increased manic and aggressive symptoms. The mood responses were variable though, with most men (84%) having few mood symptoms while some men (4%) had marked mood symptoms [110]. Men who have high testosterone levels from anabolic-androgenic steroid (AAS) abuse have been reported to have depression, hypomania, mania, irritability, and aggressive behavior. A recent review reported that short-term AAS use was associated with hypomanic symptoms, while long-term use and discontinuation were both associated with depression [111]. After stopping AAS, it may take months-years for the hypothalamic-pituitary-gonadal (HPG) axis to normalize and some men have persistent symptoms [111, 112]. Finally, an observational study reported that higher testosterone levels were associated with aggressive behavior in a study of male patients with dementia in analyses that controlled for underlying psychosis and agitation [113].

Although these studies reported increased aggression and adverse mood effects with high serum testosterone levels, other studies reported no significant changes in mood with high testosterone levels. In a randomized controlled trial of eugonadal men treated with 200 mg of intramuscular (IM) testosterone, treatment wasn't associated with adverse mood effects or aggressive behavior, and the only factor associated with aggressiveness was baseline impulsivity [114]. In a study of eugonadal men treated with testosterone undecanoate 1000 mg, placebo, or washout in a randomized crossover design, testosterone treatment was associated with increased anger, irritability, and decreased fatigue. However, the changes in anger and irritability were mild, and there was no change in aggressive behavior [115]. In conclusion, most studies that treated men with high doses of testosterone did not detect a significant change in mood or aggression. However, the mood effects of high testosterone levels were variable, with some men reporting marked changes in mood. The factors associated with an increased risk for mood changes with high levels of testosterone are unclear. In addition, acute AAS has been associated with hypomania, while chronic AAS abuse and AAS withdrawal have been associated with depression.

Testosterone Treatment and Mood Disorders

Despite the cross-sectional and prospective studies that reported an association between low testosterone levels and depressive illness, treatment trials have reported conflicting results on the effectiveness of testosterone treatment for mood disorders. This section will briefly review some selected studies of testosterone treatment in mood disorders and then summarize several recent meta-analyses.

Testosterone Treatment in HIV+ Men

In a randomized, double-blind, placebo-controlled trial in men with hypogonadism and AIDS wasting syndrome, testosterone was associated with a significant decrease in depressive symptoms, with the decrease in depressive symptoms correlated with an increase in weight [116]. In a double-blind, placebo-controlled 6-week trial of IM T (200–400 mg) in HIV+ men with borderline low total testosterone levels, testosterone was associated with decreased fatigue, decreased depressive symptoms, and increased libido. Treatment was also associated with a significant increase in muscle mass that was greater in men with AIDS wasting syndrome [117]. In a placebo-controlled study, the effects of testosterone (up to 400 mg IM every 2 weeks.), fluoxetine, or placebo were examined on depression and fatigue in HIV+ men. Although testosterone-treated men had an improvement in mood and energy, there was a high placebo response rate and no significant difference between treatment groups. However, testosterone was significantly more effective in decreasing fatigue [118].

Testosterone Treatment in Men with Hypogonadism or Depression

In one of the largest trials of testosterone treatment and depression, 170 men with hypogonadism, metabolic syndrome, and depression were treated with testosterone undecanoate for 30 weeks. Testosterone decreased depressive symptoms, with the greatest response in men with total testosterone levels <7.7 nmol/L (222 ng/dL) [119]. In another placebo-controlled study of testosterone undecanoate, older men with depressed mood, sexual dysfunction, and fatigue had a significant decrease in fatigue and improvement in mood and sexual function [120]. Although these studies reported improvements in mood with testosterone treatment, there were several studies that did not. A small study reported no improvement in mood in elderly men treated with intramuscular (IM) testosterone [121]. In two randomized, placebo-controlled trials of IM testosterone in men with major depression, testosterone was associated with a significant decrease in depressive symptoms, but there were no differences between the placebo and the treated group [122, 123] and no association between change in depressive symptoms and testosterone levels [122].

Testosterone Treatment in Subthreshold Depression

Two placebo-controlled studies found that testosterone improved mood in hypogonadal men with less severe depressive disorders [124, 125]. In a 6-week double-blind placebo-controlled clinical trial in middle-aged men with dysthymic disorder and low-normal testosterone levels, IM testosterone was associated with a significant decrease in depressive symptoms [124, 125]. In a 12-week double-blind placebo-controlled study of men with subthreshold depression and low testosterone levels, 7.5 g of testosterone gel was associated with decreased depression and a greater remission of depressive symptoms. Finally, in the recent Testosterone Trials in older hypogonadal men ($n = 772$) with a mean age of 72, testosterone treatment was associated with a significant decrease in depressive symptoms in men who had mild-moderate depressive symptoms as measured by the PHQ-9, a well-validated measure of depressive symptoms [126]. This baseline level of depressive symptoms is consistent with subthreshold depression. Testosterone treatment was also associated with improved positive mood and decreased negative mood as measured by the Positive and Negative Affect Schedule (PANAS) [127, 128]. The positive results of testosterone treatment in these studies suggest that testosterone may be effective in treatment of older hypogonadal men with subthreshold depression or dysthymia.

Testosterone Augmentation

Two studies reported that testosterone augmentation in men with antidepressant-refractory depression was effective in decreasing depressive symptoms [129, 130]. In a recent meta-analysis of augmentation strategies for refractory depression, testosterone augmentation in hypogonadal men was felt to be "clinically effective in high evidence studies" [131]. An augmentation study using testosterone to treat SSRI-associated sexual dysfunction showed positive benefit with testosterone in improving sexual function [132]. Although some augmentation studies for refractory depression were positive, there have been several negative studies of testosterone augmentation [133–135]. However, these studies were limited due to short treatment period of 6 weeks [133, 134], a low testosterone dose (5 g gel) [133, 135], inclusion of eugonadal men [134], and a small sample size with a high dropout rate of 30% [135].

Meta-Analyses of Testosterone Treatment and Mood

Four meta-analyses [136–139] examined the effect of testosterone on mood symptoms, but only two of these meta-analyses required that studies selected for inclusion utilized validated depression rating scales [136, 137].

Zarrouf et al. (2009)

In a meta-analysis of seven placebo-controlled studies of 354 hypogonadal and eugonadal men, testosterone was associated with a marked decrease in depressive symptoms. Men who had a greater improvement in depressive symptoms were those who were hypogonadal, HIV+, or treated with testosterone gel [136].

Amanatkar et al. (2014)

In a meta-analysis of 16 studies of 944 hypogonadal and eugonadal men, lasting at least 6 weeks, testosterone treatment was significantly associated with improved mood. Men who were more likely to respond to testosterone were hypogonadal, younger than 60 years, and had mild subthreshold depressive symptoms or had testosterone augmentation for antidepressant-refractory depression. Men who were less likely to respond to testosterone were men who were eugonadal or had a major depressive disorder [137].

Elliott et al. (2017)

In a network meta-analysis of 12 studies of 852 men, testosterone was compared to placebo or active control, to another testosterone formulation, and to the same testosterone formulation but at a different dose. The studies lasted a minimum of 12 weeks and included both eugonadal and hypogonadal men. Limits were that most studies did not examine follow-up testosterone levels. As a class effect, testosterone treatment was associated with improved quality of life and erectile function and a significant decrease in depression. However, no specific testosterone formulation was associated with decreased depression [138].

Ponce et al. (2018)

In a meta-analysis of four studies of 1779 hypogonadal men that lasted at least 12 weeks, testosterone treatment was not associated with an improvement in mood, but was associated with small increases in libido, erectile function, and sexual satisfaction [139].

In conclusion, the results of testosterone treatment trials on mood have been conflicting, which may be related to differences in baseline gonadal status; depression severity and chronicity; medical comorbidities; testosterone dose, formulation, and duration; androgen receptor polymorphisms; and whether testosterone replacement results in physiologic testosterone levels [64, 140, 141]. Three of four meta-analyses reported improved mood with testosterone replacement, and two meta-analyses reported that improvements in sexual libido and sexual function were found more consistently than improvements in mood [138, 139].

The predictors of improved mood from the meta-analyses included hypogonadal status, age less than 60 years, HIV+, and less severe depressive symptoms. An open-label registry study found similar predictors of response to testosterone to include age less than 60 years, low total testosterone levels <250 ng/dL (<8.68 nmol/l), HIV+, and concurrent use of antidepressants or opioids [142].

Summary

Prevalent mental health conditions differ greatly between men and women, and these differences may be related to the effects of androgens. Testosterone and its metabolites have numerous effects on brain structure and function including neurogenesis, neurotransmitters, and cerebral perfusion and metabolism. Testosterone levels decrease with aging and medical morbidity, and most studies have found that low testosterone levels are associated with prevalent depressive symptoms and with a risk for incident depressive illness. However, despite the results that low testosterone is associated with depressive illness, clinical trials of testosterone treatment in depression have been conflicting. The results may be inconsistent due to differences in patient populations, testosterone dose and duration, and study methodology. In addition, it appears that some subgroups of men may be more responsive to testosterone treatment. Men who appear to be more responsive to testosterone are hypogonadal men, younger than age 60, and with less severe, subthreshold depressive illness. Due to conflicting results from prior studies, testosterone cannot be recommended as routine treatment for men with depressive illness, particularly for men with major depression. However, in men with hypogonadism, potential beneficial mood effects could be considered when assessing the overall benefits and risks of testosterone treatment. Further studies are needed to better characterize the effects of testosterone on mood and to clarify subgroups of men who may be more responsive to it [143, 144].

Acknowledgments This study was supported by grant R01 AG042934-01 from the National Institutes of Health – National Institute on Aging and by the VA Office of Research and Development, Seattle, Washington. The author has no conflicts of interest to declare. This work was supported with resources and the use of facilities at the VA Puget Sound Health Care System. The contents do not represent the views of the US Department of Veterans Affairs or the US Government.

References

1. Werling DM. The role of sex-differential biology in risk for autism spectrum disorder. Biol Sex Differ. 2016;7:58.
2. Kessler RC, Chiu WT, Demler O, et al. Prevalence, severity, and comorbidity of 12-month DSM-IV disorders in the National Comorbidity Survey Replication. Arch Gen Psychiatry. 2005;62:617–27.

3. Kessler RC, Berglund P, Demler O, et al. Lifetime prevalence and age-of-onset distributions of DSM-IV disorders in the National Comorbidity Survey Replication. Arch Gen Psychiatry. 2005;62:593–602.
4. SAMSA. Addressing the specific behavioral health needs of men. Treatment Improvement Protocol (TIP) series 56. In: Substance abuse and mental health services administration. HHS Publication No.(SMA) 13-4736. Rockville: Substance Abuse and Mental Health Services Administration; 2013. p. 1–124.
5. Ferri SL, Abel T, Brodkin ES. Sex differences in autism spectrum disorder: a review. Curr Psychiatry Rep. 2018;20:9.
6. Schaafsma SM, Pfaff DW. Etiologies underlying sex differences in autism spectrum disorders. Front Neuroendocrinol. 2014;35:255–71.
7. Auyeung B, Baron-Cohen S, Ashwin E, et al. Fetal testosterone and autistic traits. Br J Psychol. 2009;100:1–22.
8. James WH. Further evidence that some male-based neurodevelopmental disorders are associated with high intrauterine testosterone concentrations. Dev Med Child Neurol. 2008;50:15–8.
9. Baron-Cohen S, Lombardo MV, Auyeung B, et al. Why are autism spectrum conditions more prevalent in males? PLoS Biol. 2011;9:e1001081.
10. McHugh RK, Votaw VR, Sugarman DE, Greenfield SF. Sex and gender differences in substance use disorders. Clin Psychol Rev. 2017;66:12–23.
11. Kolodny A, Courtwright DT, Hwang CS, et al. The prescription opioid and heroin crisis: a public health approach to an epidemic of addiction. Annu Rev Public Health. 2015;36:559–74.
12. Huecker MR, Gossman WG. Opioid, addiction. Treasure Island: StatPearls; 2018.
13. Le Roux C, Tang Y, Drexler K. Alcohol and opioid use disorder in older adults: neglected and treatable illnesses. Curr Psychiatry Rep. 2016;18:87.
14. Manchikanti L, Kaye AM, Kaye AD. Current state of opioid therapy and abuse. Curr Pain Headache Rep. 2016;20:34.
15. Sharma B, Bruner A, Barnett G, Fishman M. Opioid Use Disorders. Child Adolesc Psychiatr Clin N Am. 2016;25:473–87.
16. Wilkerson RG, Kim HK, Windsor TA, Mareiniss DP. The opioid epidemic in the United States. Emerg Med Clin North Am. 2016;34:e1–e23.
17. Nicholls L, Bragaw L, Ruetsch C. Opioid dependence treatment and guidelines. J Manag Care Pharm. 2010;16:S14–21.
18. Fullerton CA, Kim M, Thomas CP, et al. Medication-assisted treatment with methadone: assessing the evidence. Psychiatr Serv. 2014;65:146–57.
19. Notley C, Blyth A, Maskrey V, et al. The experience of long-term opiate maintenance treatment and reported barriers to recovery: a qualitative systematic review. Eur Addict Res. 2013;19:287–98.
20. Thomas CP, Fullerton CA, Kim M, et al. Medication-assisted treatment with buprenorphine: assessing the evidence. Psychiatr Serv. 2014;65:158–70.
21. Bawor M, Bami H, Dennis BB, et al. Testosterone suppression in opioid users: a systematic review and meta-analysis. Drug Alcohol Depend. 2015;149:1–9.
22. Ali K, Raphael J, Khan S, et al. The effects of opioids on the endocrine system: an overview. Postgrad Med J. 2016;92:677–81.
23. Basaria S, Travison TG, Alford D, et al. Effects of testosterone replacement in men with opioid-induced androgen deficiency: a randomized controlled trial. Pain. 2015;156:280–8.
24. Bhasin S, Brito JP, Cunningham GR, et al. Testosterone therapy in men with hypogonadism: an endocrine society clinical practice guideline. J Clin Endocrinol Metab. 2018;103:1715–44.
25. Lemieux AM, Saman DM, Lutfiyya MN. Men and suicide in primary care. Disease-a-month. 2014;60:155–61.
26. McDowell AK, Lineberry TW, Bostwick JM. Practical suicide-risk management for the busy primary care physician. Mayo Clin Proc. 2011;86:792–800.
27. Raue PJ, Ghesquiere AR, Bruce ML. Suicide risk in primary care: identification and management in older adults. Curr Psychiatry Rep. 2014;16:466.

28. Ljusic D, Ravanic D, Filipovic Danic S, et al. Contemporary principles of suicide prevention. Med Pregl. 2016;69:367–71.
29. Szanto K, Kalmar S, Hendin H, et al. A suicide prevention program in a region with a very high suicide rate. Arch Gen Psychiatry. 2007;64:914–20.
30. Chu C, Klein KM, Buchman-Schmitt JM, et al. Routinized assessment of suicide risk in clinical practice: an empirically informed update. J Clin Psychol. 2015;71:1186–200.
31. Steele IH, Thrower N, Noroian P, Saleh FM. Understanding suicide across the lifespan: a United States perspective of suicide risk factors, assessment & management. J Forensic Sci. 2018;63:162–71.
32. Fiore V, Marci M, Poggi A, et al. The association between diabetes and depression: a very disabling condition. Endocrine. 2015;48:14–24.
33. Blazer D. Depression in late life: review and commentary. J Gerontol A Biol Sci Med Sci. 2003;58:249–65.
34. Burgel PR, Escamilla R, Perez T, et al. Impact of comorbidities on COPD-specific health-related quality of life. Respir Med. 2013;107:233–41.
35. Wang JT, Hoffman B, Blumenthal JA. Management of depression in patients with coronary heart disease: association, mechanisms, and treatment implications for depressed cardiac patients. Expert Opin Pharmacother. 2011;12:85–98.
36. Hall CA, Reynolds-Iii CF. Late-life depression in the primary care setting: challenges, collaborative care, and prevention. Maturitas. 2014;79:147–52.
37. Gureje O. Dysthymia in a cross-cultural perspective. Curr Opin Psychiatry. 2011;24:67–71.
38. Devanand DP. Dysthymic disorder in the elderly population. Int Psychogeriatr. 2014;26:39–48.
39. Rodriguez MR, Nuevo R, Chatterji S, Ayuso-Mateos JL. Definitions and factors associated with subthreshold depressive conditions: a systematic review. BMC Psychiatry. 2012;12:181.
40. Seidman SN, Araujo AB, Roose SP, et al. Low testosterone levels in elderly men with dysthymic disorder. Am J Psychiatry. 2002;159:456–9.
41. Delhez M, Hansenne M, Legros JJ. Andropause and psychopathology: minor symptoms rather than pathological ones. Psychoneuroendocrinology. 2003;28:863–74.
42. Blazer D. Depression and the older man. Med Clin North Am. 1999;83:1305–16.
43. Callahan CM, Wolinsky FD, Stump TE, et al. Mortality, symptoms, and functional impairment in late-life depression. J Gen Intern Med. 1998;13:746–52.
44. Meeks TW, Vahia IV, Lavretsky H, et al. A tune in "a minor" can "b major": a review of epidemiology, illness course, and public health implications of subthreshold depression in older adults. J Affect Disord. 2011;129:126–42.
45. Hybels C, Blazer D, Pieper C. Toward a threshold for subthreshold depression: an analysis of correlates of depression by severity of symptoms using data from an elderly community sample. Gerontologist. 2001;41:357–65.
46. Wagner HR, Burns BJ, Broadhead WE, et al. Minor depression in family practice: functional morbidity, co-morbidity, service utilization and outcomes. Psychol Med. 2000;30:1377–90.
47. Affleck W, Carmichael V, Whitley R. Men's mental health: social determinants and implications for services. Can J Psychiat. 2018;63:581–9.
48. Addis ME, Mahalik JR. Men, masculinity, and the contexts of help seeking. Am Psychol. 2003;58:5–14.
49. Case A, Paxson C. Sex differences in morbidity and mortality. Demography. 2005;42:189–214.
50. Brownhill S, Wilhelm K, Barclay L, Schmied V. 'Big build': hidden depression in men. Aust N Z J Psychiatry. 2005;39:921–31.
51. Seedat S, Scott KM, Angermeyer MC, et al. Cross-national associations between gender and mental disorders in the World Health Organization world mental health surveys. Arch Gen Psychiatry. 2009;66:785–95.
52. Filova B, Ostatnikova D, Celec P, Hodosy J. The effect of testosterone on the formation of brain structures. Cells Tissues Organs. 2013;197:169–77.
53. Cooke B, Hegstrom CD, Villeneuve LS, Breedlove SM. Sexual differentiation of the vertebrate brain: principles and mechanisms. Front Neuroendocrinol. 1998;19:323–62.

54. McHenry J, Carrier N, Hull E, Kabbaj M. Sex differences in anxiety and depression: role of testosterone. Front Neuroendocrinol. 2014;35:42–57.
55. Puralewski R, Vasilakis G, Seney ML. Sex-related factors influence expression of mood-related genes in the basolateral amygdala differentially depending on age and stress exposure. Biol Sex Differ. 2016;7:50.
56. Ebinger M, Sievers C, Ivan D, et al. Is there a neuroendocrinological rationale for testosterone as a therapeutic option in depression? J Psychopharmacol. 2009;23:841–53.
57. Parducz A, Hajszan T, Maclusky NJ, et al. Synaptic remodeling induced by gonadal hormones: neuronal plasticity as a mediator of neuroendocrine and behavioral responses to steroids. Neuroscience. 2006;138:977–85.
58. MacLusky NJ, Hajszan T, Prange-Kiel J, Leranth C. Androgen modulation of hippocampal synaptic plasticity. Neuroscience. 2006;138:957–65.
59. Carrier N, Kabbaj M. Testosterone and imipramine have antidepressant effects in socially isolated male but not female rats. Horm Behav. 2012;61:678–85.
60. Frye CA, Koonce CJ, Edinger KL, et al. Androgens with activity at estrogen receptor beta have anxiolytic and cognitive-enhancing effects in male rats and mice. Horm Behav. 2008;54:726–34.
61. Robichaud M, Debonnel G. Oestrogen and testosterone modulate the firing activity of dorsal raphe nucleus serotonergic neurones in both male and female rats. J Neuroendocrinol. 2005;17:179–85.
62. de Souza Silva MA, Mattern C, Topic B, et al. Dopaminergic and serotonergic activity in neostriatum and nucleus accumbens enhanced by intranasal administration of testosterone. Eur Neuropsychopharmacol. 2009;19:53–63.
63. Kranz GS, Wadsak W, Kaufmann U, et al. High-dose testosterone treatment increases serotonin transporter binding in transgender people. Biol Psychiatry. 2015;78:525–33.
64. Khera M. Patients with testosterone deficit syndrome and depression. Arch Esp Urol. 2013;66:729–36.
65. Kranz GS, Hahn A, Kaufmann U, et al. Effects of testosterone treatment on hypothalamic neuroplasticity in female-to-male transgender individuals. Brain Struct Funct. 2018;223:321–8.
66. Azad N, Pitale S, Barnes WE, Friedman N. Testosterone treatment enhances regional brain perfusion in hypogonadal men. J Clin Endocrinol Metab. 2003;88:3064–8.
67. Zitzmann M. Testosterone and the brain. Aging Male. 2006;9:195–9.
68. Derntl B, Windischberger C, Robinson S, et al. Amygdala activity to fear and anger in healthy young males is associated with testosterone. Psychoneuroendocrinology. 2009;34:687–93.
69. Pasquali R. The hypothalamic-pituitary-adrenal axis and sex hormones in chronic stress and obesity: pathophysiological and clinical aspects. Ann N Y Acad Sci. 2012;1264:20–35.
70. Schneider HJ, Sievers C, Klotsche J, et al. Prevalence of low male testosterone levels in primary care in Germany: cross-sectional results from the DETECT study. Clin Endocrinol. 2009;70:446–54.
71. Araujo AB, Esche GR, Kupelian V, et al. Prevalence of symptomatic androgen deficiency in men. J Clin Endocrinol Metab. 2007;92:4241–7.
72. Bhasin S, Pencina M, Jasuja GK, et al. Reference ranges for testosterone in men generated using liquid chromatography tandem mass spectrometry in a community-based sample of healthy nonobese young men in the Framingham Heart Study and applied to three geographically distinct cohorts. J Clin Endocrinol Metab. 2011;96:2430–9.
73. Huhtaniemi IT. Andropause--lessons from the European Male Ageing Study. Ann Endocrinol (Paris). 2014;75:128–31.
74. Travison TG, Araujo AB, Kupelian V, et al. The relative contributions of aging, health, and lifestyle factors to serum testosterone decline in men. J Clin Endocrinol Metab. 2007;92:549–55.
75. Yeap BB, Alfonso H, Chubb SA, et al. Reference ranges and determinants of testosterone, dihydrotestosterone, and estradiol levels measured using liquid chromatography-tandem mass spectrometry in a population-based cohort of older men. J Clin Endocrinol Metab. 2012;97:4030–9.

76. Sartorius G, Spasevska S, Idan A, et al. Serum testosterone, dihydrotestosterone and estradiol concentrations in older men self-reporting very good health: the healthy man study. Clin Endocrinol. 2012;77:755–63.
77. Travison TG, Shackelton R, Araujo AB, et al. The natural history of symptomatic androgen deficiency in men: onset, progression, and spontaneous remission. J Am Geriatr Soc. 2008;56:831–9.
78. Almeida OP, Yeap BB, Hankey GJ, et al. Low free testosterone concentration as a potentially treatable cause of depressive symptoms in older men. Arch Gen Psychiatry. 2008;65:283–9.
79. Giltay EJ, van der Mast RC, Lauwen E, et al. Plasma testosterone and the course of major depressive disorder in older men and women. Am J Geriatr Psychiatry. 2017;25:425–37.
80. Joshi D, van Schoor NM, de Ronde W, et al. Low free testosterone levels are associated with prevalence and incidence of depressive symptoms in older men. Clin Endocrinol. 2010;72:232–40.
81. Barrett-Connor E, Muhlen DV, Kritz-Silverstein D. Bioavailable testosterone and depressed mood in older men: the Rancho Bernardo Study. J Clin Endocrinol Metab. 1999;84:573–7.
82. Kratzik CW, Schatzl G, Lackner JE, et al. Mood changes, body mass index and bioavailable testosterone in healthy men: results of the Androx Vienna Municipality Study. BJU Int. 2007;100:614–8.
83. Morsink LF, Vogelzangs N, Nicklas BJ, et al. Associations between sex steroid hormone levels and depressive symptoms in elderly men and women: results from the Health ABC study. Psychoneuroendocrinology. 2007;32:874–83.
84. Westley CJ, Amdur RL, Irwig MS. High rates of depression and depressive symptoms among men referred for borderline testosterone levels. J Sex Med. 2015;12:1753–60.
85. Berglund LH, Prytz HS, Perski A, Svartberg J. Testosterone levels and psychological health status in men from a general population: the Tromso study. Aging Male. 2011;14:37–41.
86. Shores MM, Sloan KL, Matsumoto AM, et al. Increased incidence of diagnosed depressive illness in hypogonadal older men. Arch Gen Psychiatry. 2004;61:162–7.
87. Shores MM, Moceri VM, Sloan KL, et al. Low testosterone levels predict incident depressive illness in older men: effects of age and medical morbidity. J Clin Psychiatry. 2005;66:7–14.
88. Ford AH, Yeap BB, Flicker L, et al. Prospective longitudinal study of testosterone and incident depression in older men: The Health In Men Study. Psychoneuroendocrinology. 2016;64:57–65.
89. Kische H, Pieper L, Venz J, et al. Longitudinal change instead of baseline testosterone predicts depressive symptoms. Psychoneuroendocrinology. 2018;89:7–12.
90. Kische H, Gross S, Wallaschofski H, et al. Associations of androgens with depressive symptoms and cognitive status in the general population. PLoS One. 2017;12:e0177272.
91. Alexander GM, Swerdloff RS, Wang C, et al. Androgen-behavior correlations in hypogonadal men and eugonadal men. II. Cognitive abilities. Horm Behav. 1998;33:85–94.
92. Burris AS, Banks SM, Carter CS, et al. A long-term, prospective study of the physiologic and behavioral effects of hormone replacement in untreated hypogonadal men. J Androl. 1992;13:297–304.
93. Wang C, Alexander G, Berman N, et al. Testosterone replacement therapy improves mood in hypogonadal men--a clinical research center study. J Clin Endocrinol Metab. 1996;81:3578–83.
94. Schmidt PJ, Berlin KL, Danaceau MA, et al. The effects of pharmacologically induced hypogonadism on mood in healthy men. Arch Gen Psychiatry. 2004;61:997–1004. https://doi.org/10.1001/archpsyc.61.10.997.
95. Zitzmann M, Faber S, Nieschlag E. Association of specific symptoms and metabolic risks with serum testosterone in older men. J Clin Endocrinol Metab. 2006;91:4335–43.
96. Zitzmann M. The role of the CAG repeat androgen receptor polymorphism in andrology. Front Horm Res. 2009;37:52–61.
97. Harkonen K, Huhtaniemi I, Makinen J, et al. The polymorphic androgen receptor gene CAG repeat, pituitary-testicular function and andropausal symptoms in ageing men. Int J Androl. 2003;26:187–94.

98. Schneider G, Nienhaus K, Gromoll J, et al. Depressive symptoms in men aged 50 years and older and their relationship to genetic androgen receptor polymorphism and sex hormone levels in three different samples. Am J Geriatr Psychiatry. 2011;19:274–83.

99. Colangelo LA, Sharp L, Kopp P, et al. Total testosterone, androgen receptor polymorphism, and depressive symptoms in young black and white men: the CARDIA Male Hormone Study. Psychoneuroendocrinology. 2007;32:951–8.

100. Schneider G, Zitzmann M, Gromoll J, et al. The relation between sex hormone levels, the androgen receptor CAGn-polymorphism and depression and mortality in older men in a community study. Psychoneuroendocrinology. 2013;38:2083–90.

101. T'Sjoen GG, De Vos S, Goemaere S, et al. Sex steroid level, androgen receptor polymorphism, and depressive symptoms in healthy elderly men. J Am Geriatr Soc. 2005;53:636–42.

102. Seidman SN, Araujo AB, Roose SP, McKinlay JB. Testosterone level, androgen receptor polymorphism, and depressive symptoms in middle-aged men. Biol Psychiatry. 2001;50:371–6.

103. McIntyre RS, Mancini D, Eisfeld BS, et al. Calculated bioavailable testosterone levels and depression in middle-aged men. Psychoneuroendocrinology. 2006;31:1029–35.

104. Rupprecht R. Neuroactive steroids: mechanisms of action and neuropsychopharmacological properties. Psychoneuroendocrinology. 2003;28:139–68.

105. Rupprecht R, Rupprecht C, Rupprecht M, et al. Different reactivity of the hypothalamo-pituitary-gonadal-axis in depression and normal controls. Pharmacopsychiatry. 1988;21:438–9.

106. Steiger A, von Bardeleben U, Wiedemann K, Holsboer F. Sleep EEG and nocturnal secretion of testosterone and cortisol in patients with major endogenous depression during acute phase and after remission. J Psychiatr Res. 1991;25:169–77.

107. Unden F, Ljunggren JG, Beck-Friis J, et al. Hypothalamic-pituitary-gonadal axis in major depressive disorders. Acta Psychiatr Scand. 1988;78:138–46.

108. Rubin RT, Poland RE, Lesser IM. Neuroendocrine aspects of primary endogenous depression VIII. Pituitary-gonadal axis activity in male patients and matched control subjects. Psychoneuroendocrinology. 1989;14:217–29.

109. Levitt A, Joffee R. Total and free testosterone in depressed men. Acta Psychiatr Scand. 1988;77:346–8.

110. Pope HG Jr, Kouri EM, Hudson JI. Effects of supraphysiologic doses of testosterone on mood and aggression in normal men: a randomized controlled trial. Arch Gen Psychiatry. 2000;57:133–40; discussion 155–136.

111. Piacentino D, Kotzalidis GD, Del Casale A, et al. Anabolic-androgenic steroid use and psychopathology in athletes. A systematic review. Curr Neuropharmacol. 2015;13:101–21.

112. Talih F, Fattal O, Malone D Jr. Anabolic steroid abuse: psychiatric and physical costs. Cleve Clin J Med. 2007;74:341–4, 346, 349–352.

113. Orengo C, Kunik ME, Molinari V, et al. Do testosterone levels relate to aggression in elderly men with dementia? J Neuropsychiatry Clin Neurosci. 2002;14:161–6.

114. O'Connor DB, Archer J, Hair WM, Wu FC. Exogenous testosterone, aggression, and mood in eugonadal and hypogonadal men. Physiol Behav. 2002;75:557–66.

115. O'Connor DB, Archer J, Wu FC. Effects of testosterone on mood, aggression, and sexual behavior in young men: a double-blind, placebo-controlled, cross-over study. J Clin Endocrinol Metab. 2004;89:2837–45.

116. Grinspoon S, Corcoran C, Stanley T, et al. Effects of hypogonadism and testosterone administration on depression indices in HIV-infected men. J Clin Endocrinol Metab. 2000;85:60–5.

117. Rabkin JG, Wagner GJ, Rabkin R. A double-blind, placebo-controlled trial of testosterone therapy for HIV-positive men with hypogonadal symptoms. Arch Gen Psychiatry. 2000;57:141–7; discussion 155–146.

118. Rabkin JG, Wagner GJ, McElhiney MC, et al. Testosterone versus fluoxetine for depression and fatigue in HIV/AIDS: a placebo-controlled trial. J Clin Psychopharmacol. 2004;24:379–85.

119. Giltay EJ, Tishova YA, Mskhalaya GJ, et al. Effects of testosterone supplementation on depressive symptoms and sexual dysfunction in hypogonadal men with the metabolic syndrome. J Sex Med. 2010;7:2572–82.
120. Cavallini G, Caracciolo S, Vitali G, et al. Carnitine versus androgen administration in the treatment of sexual dysfunction, depressed mood, and fatigue associated with male aging. Urology. 2004;63:641–6.
121. Sih R, Morley JE, Kaiser FE, et al. Testosterone replacement in older hypogonadal men: a 12 month randomized controlled trial. J Clin Endocrinol Metabol. 1997;82:1661–7.
122. Seidman S, Spatz E, Rizzo C, Roose S. Testosterone replacement therapy for hypogonadal men with major depressive disorder: a randomized, placebo-controlled clinical trial. J Clin Psychiatry. 2001;12:406–12.
123. Seidman SN, Roose SP. The sexual effects of testosterone replacement in depressed men: randomized, placebo-controlled clinical trial. J Sex Marital Ther. 2006;32:267–73.
124. Shores MM, Kivlahan DR, Sadak TI, et al. A randomized, double-blind, placebo-controlled study of testosterone treatment in hypogonadal older men with subthreshold depression (dysthymia or minor depression). J Clin Psychiatry. 2009;70:1009–16.
125. Seidman SN, Orr G, Raviv G, et al. Effects of testosterone replacement in middle-aged men with dysthymia: a randomized, placebo-controlled clinical trial. J Clin Psychopharmacol. 2009;29:216–21.
126. Kroenke K, Spitzer RL, Williams JB. The PHQ-15: validity of a new measure for evaluating the severity of somatic symptoms. Psychosom Med. 2002;64:258–66.
127. Snyder PJ, Bhasin S, Cunningham GR, et al. Effects of testosterone treatment in older men. N Engl J Med. 2016;374:611–24.
128. Watson D, Clark LA, Tellegen A. Development and validation of brief measures of positive and negative affect: the PANAS scales. J Pers Soc Psychol. 1988;54:1063–70.
129. Pope HJ, Cohane G, Kanayama G, et al. Testosterone gel supplementation for men with refractory depression: a randomized, placebo-controlled trial. Am J Psychiatry. 2003;160:105–11.
130. Seidman SN, Rabkin JG. Testosterone replacement therapy for hypogonadal men with SSRI-refractory depression. J Affect Disord. 1998;48:157–61.
131. Kleeblatt J, Betzler F, Kilarski LL, et al. Efficacy of off-label augmentation in unipolar depression: a systematic review of the evidence. Eur Neuropsychopharmacol. 2017;27:423–41.
132. Amiaz R, Pope HG Jr, Mahne T, et al. Testosterone gel replacement improves sexual function in depressed men taking serotonergic antidepressants: a randomized, placebo-controlled clinical trial. J Sex Marital Ther. 2011;37:243–54.
133. Pope HG Jr, Amiaz R, Brennan BP, et al. Parallel-group placebo-controlled trial of testosterone gel in men with major depressive disorder displaying an incomplete response to standard antidepressant treatment. J Clin Psychopharmacol. 2010;30:126–34.
134. Seidman SN, Miyazaki M, Roose SP. Intramuscular testosterone supplementation to selective serotonin reuptake inhibitor in treatment-resistant depressed men: randomized placebo-controlled clinical trial. J Clin Psychopharmacol. 2005;25:584–8.
135. Orengo CA, Fullerton L, Kunik ME. Safety and efficacy of testosterone gel 1% augmentation in depressed men with partial response to antidepressant therapy. J Geriatr Psychiatry Neurol. 2005;18:20–4.
136. Zarrouf FA, Artz S, Griffith J, et al. Testosterone and depression: systematic review and meta-analysis. J Psychiatr Pract. 2009;15:289–305.
137. Amanatkar HR, Chibnall JT, Seo BW, et al. Impact of exogenous testosterone on mood: a systematic review and meta-analysis of randomized placebo-controlled trials. Ann Clin Psychiatry. 2014;26:19–32.
138. Elliott J, Kelly SE, Millar AC, et al. Testosterone therapy in hypogonadal men: a systematic review and network meta-analysis. BMJ Open. 2017;7:e015284.
139. Ponce OJ, Spencer-Bonilla G, Alvarez-Villalobos N, et al. The efficacy and adverse events of testosterone replacement therapy in hypogonadal men: a systematic review and meta-analysis of randomized, placebo-controlled trials. J Clin Endocrinol Metab. 2018.

140. Amore M, Scarlatti F, Quarta AL, Tagariello P. Partial androgen deficiency, depression and testosterone treatment in aging men. Aging Clin Exp Res. 2009;21:1–8.
141. Amiaz R, Seidman SN. Testosterone and depression in men. Curr Opin Endocrinol Diabetes Obes. 2008;15:278–83.
142. Khera M, Bhattacharya RK, Blick G, et al. The effect of testosterone supplementation on depression symptoms in hypogonadal men from the Testim Registry in the US (TRiUS). Aging Male. 2012;15:14–21.
143. Buvat J, Maggi M, Guay A, Torres LO. Testosterone deficiency in men: systematic review and standard operating procedures for diagnosis and treatment. J Sex Med. 2013;10:245–84.
144. Yeap BB. Hormonal changes and their impact on cognition and mental health of ageing men. Maturitas. 2014;79:227–35.

Chapter 13
Billing and Coding for Infertility Services

Paul R. Shin

The financial reimbursement for fertility-related services ranges from the simple and straightforward to the byzantine. Uncertainty of insurance coverage coupled with the diligence required for proper revenue collection makes for a landmine-ridden financial landscape.

The preface to any financial advice or discussion applies here as well. There are tremendous differences regionally as to how billing and collecting issues are handled. A minority of states mandates insurance coverage for infertility-related services. Many do not. Insurances vary by locale and region as to what is required for appropriate filing and reimbursements of claims. Individual employers may also opt into fertility coverage either through conventional insurance plans (Blue Cross, Aetna, etc.) or through fertility-focused financial programs (Progyny).

Add to that the financial pressures most physicians are under to maximize revenue and the sum total is, frankly, a very messy financial environment to navigate.

Disclaimer: This chapter is merely a guideline for efficient and effective billing regarding fertility-based care of the male patient. The advice contained herein is garnered through successes and failures, through time and experience. It should, by no means, serve as a concrete "how-to" manual. Regional differences in medical practice patterns and insurances mandate that the individual physician and practice remain accountable.

P. R. Shin (✉)
Reproductive Urology, Shady Grove Fertility and Reproductive Science Center, Rockville, MD, USA
e-mail: paul.shin@sgfertility.com

© Springer Nature Switzerland AG 2021   249
J. P. Alukal et al. (eds.), *Design and Implementation of the Modern Men's Health Center*, https://doi.org/10.1007/978-3-030-54482-9_13

Personnel

One cannot begin any financial discussion without first understanding the importance of a good financial and clinical team. A good analogy for financial team success can be drawn from the restaurant world – think of service from a "front of the house" (front desk staff) and "back of the house" (financial and administrative support) perspective.

The initial point of contact with any provider's office is the "front desk" staff that the patient will contact to make the initial appointment. Having pleasant, good-natured, and even-tempered representatives sets the right tone. Accurate collection of information at this initial point of contact cannot be understated. Logistical and insurance information must be accurately collated and entered into the practice management software. Financial discussions of any substance should not be made at this juncture. Determining whether or not a referral is required for the visit and co-pay collection should be the extent of financial discussions at this early stage.

The true work of determining coverage falls to a dedicated financial counselor or team. Verification of benefits, communication with patients, working disputed claims, providing supporting documentation, and ultimately collection of revenue are all tasks that the provider's financial team must be facile and efficient with.

The final piece of the administrative puzzle is solid administrative support to maximize scheduling efficiency and verify all financial matters are clarified and communicated with the patient prior to rendering of services. Clear communication within the provider team is also paramount to presenting a unified and consistent message to the patient.

Pre-authorizations vs Predeterminations

The confusion around pre-authorizations, particularly for surgical procedures, can be summed in one neat and tidy phrase, often included in some version on every explanation of benefits (EOB). "Pre-authorization is not a guarantee of payment." This phrase accounts for much of the confusion regarding billing, collecting, and working claims for fertility-related procedural reimbursement.

One key point to clarify is the difference between pre-authorization and pre-determination.

Pre-authorization refers to the process by which a provider obtains authorization and approval to perform a procedure from an insurer. This is a requirement set forth by insurers. In a somewhat confusing turn of phrase, though, pre-authorization is not a guarantee of reimbursement, but failure to obtain pre-authorization may result in non-reimbursement with no recourse other than to write off the loss. This process normally takes up to 30 days but in practice is usually fairly quick and routine.

Predetermination is a more involved, lengthy, and discrete process. Predetermination involves a medical review to determine the necessity of the procedure. By going through the predetermination process, providers usually get a concrete determination of coverage prior to rendering service. Predetermination also has the advantage of addressing any questionable areas regarding coverage under a patient's policy. This is particularly useful in the setting of infertility. The main drawback, however, is that predeterminations may take up to 90 days to finalize. When caring for couples grappling with infertility, this delay can represent a significant amount of time.

Fertility Coverage or Not?

Government-issued healthcare such as Medicaid and Medicare do not provide coverage for fertility services. Additionally, many smaller "stop-gap" insurers also provide little-to-no fertility benefits. These types of insurance programs are generally limited to coverage for catastrophic medical issues while someone is either between jobs or taking extended leave without work.

Employer-based health insurance can run the gamut of coverage levels, so a simple place to begin is with the mandated states. At the time of the authorship of this piece, 15 states require health insurers to cover the diagnosis and treatment of infertility. These states are Arkansas, California, Connecticut, Hawaii, Illinois, Louisiana, Maryland, Massachusetts, Montana, New Jersey, New York, Ohio, Rhode Island, Texas, and West Virginia. Because much of the United States relies on employer-based health insurance, a key point to remember is that any business based in these states will likely provide some coverage for fertility medical services.

In the majority of states, though, fertility coverage is not mandated. This vetting process usually begins with some form of contact with the patient's insurer. More of these types of verifications can be done online through insurer-based portals, but calling the insurer directly is arguably the most straightforward way to ascertain a patient's benefits.

Once benefits are verified, clear communication of these benefits to the patient is crucial to maintain a good relationship.

Certain health conditions manifest as infertility. Testicular cancers, varicocele, endocrinopathies, and genetic issues like Klinefelter's Syndrome are all significant medical conditions that can present as infertility. Thus, insurances often will provide some level of diagnostic coverage.

An in-person evaluation, exam, ultrasound, serum hormonal and genetic bloodwork, and semen testing are often included under the "Diagnosis Only" type of insurance that many states and employers offer. The primary importance of any male fertility evaluation is to first diagnose any significant medical condition that is contributing to infertility. Secondarily, treatment of male factor fertility is cost-effective and less burdensome to the female partner. In many cases, even diagnostic biopsy of the testis is often a covered service.

This trend toward diagnostic coverage, though, does not routinely apply to coverage for infertility treatment. Once significant medical conditions germane to the male patient are ruled out, therapy for infertility is often uncovered. This includes sperm retrieval procedures, vasal reconstruction, microdissection, and the costs associated with cryopreservation of gametes.

Coding and Billing 101

Patients who are without fertility coverage or uninsured are self-pay (fee for service). This is a relatively straightforward concept – they pay what the provider charges. It is always sound financial practice to make sure these types of financials are tidied up PRIOR to the rendering of any care. Although we would all like to see altruism shine through, once people have gone through treatment, irrespective of success or failure, their inclination to pay often decreases.

Determination of coverage for therapeutic fertility interventions is the single most important aspect of efficient billing and coding. If a patient has therapeutic fertility coverage, then, by virtue of the provider's contract with the insurer, services must be rendered and billed accordingly to the insurer with acceptance of whatever payment is rendered. This also excludes any possibility of balance billing once the charges and revenues are settled.

Men presenting for counseling and treatment for post-vasectomy options are also fairly straightforward. Most commercial insurers will have a "sterilization exclusion" clause that effectively renders post-vasectomy men as uncovered for any therapeutic fertility intervention. Both sperm retrievals and vasal reconstructive procedures are generally out-of-pocket expenses for the patient.

Medicare and Medicaid patients will also generally be without fertility coverage. There is a definite trend toward older paternal age, and male patients in their 60s and 70s may sometimes want to have children. A quick word about Medicare participation – there are three types of Medicare providers – participating, non-participating, and opt-out.

Evaluation and Management (E&M) Codes – These are a collection of 5-digit Current Procedural Terminology (CPT) codes that start with the number 9. There have been three traditional types of initial patient visits – new patient visits, consultation requests, and second opinions. New patient visits were self-referred patients. Consultations were requested by a referring provider, and second opinions were also patient generated. Many insurers in the mid-Atlantic area have essentially discontinued payment for the set of codes for consultation and second opinion. Our practice is to simply bill each new patient encounter as exactly that.

Infertility as a medical issue is physically quite focused, but the counseling and planning can be very complex. For this reason, new patient encounters are often billed on time spent with the patient rather than scope of exam or review of systems. Electronic medical records can still be helpful in this regard, as detailed records regarding the history, review of systems, and the physical exam can be documented. A brief statement in the note should also be included to document the time spent delivering care and counseling as regards decision-making.

In most circumstances, the initial patient consultation and subsequent testing will be covered under the "diagnostic" rubric of a patient's policy. On occasion, E&M claims will bounce back or be denied. This initial denial stems from the need to provide documentation – clinical notes and justification for testing to diagnose infertility. The importance of having a diligent member of the medical team whose responsibility is to identify these denied claims and provide the necessary clinical information cannot be understated.

When an insurance claim is denied or contested, the revenue loss to the practice is not only a financial burden but a temporal one as well. The simple principle of dollar-cost averaging dictates that a dollar today is worth more than a dollar tomorrow. Timely documentation also helps immensely with the turnaround for contested claims.

Procedural (CPT) codes – Distinct CPT codes exist for most male fertility related procedures. Varicocelectomy, vasectomy, vasovasostomy, and diagnostic biopsy of the testis and epididymis have designated CPT code numbers. Obtaining pre-procedure authorization for these procedures is fairly straightforward and easy to do. Keep in mind that vasal reconstruction is often excluded from coverage because of elective sterilization exclusions.

Unfortunately, some of the most commonly performed male fertility procedures are lacking a specific CPT code. These include sperm retrieval procedures (PESA, TESE, MESA, and microdissection), which are performed with a certain therapeutic intent. Therefore, determining a patient's level of fertility coverage at the outset of their treatment is key to maintaining a clear line of communication, thus preventing frustration on both the patients and provider's behalf.

The use of the diagnostic codes for testis and epididymal biopsy for sperm retrieval may, in some cases, constitute fraud, as those procedures have only a diagnostic intent.

The CPT code 55899 is a "catch-all" nonspecific surgery code for urologic procedures not accurately described by conventionally available codes. One important aspect of using this code is to understand that it is not a fertility-specific code. It simply refers to a procedure for which a CPT code does not exist. Contacting an insurer for pre-authorization using this code, even when coupled with a fertility-related ICD-10 code often results in authorization. As covered previously though, authorization in no way guarantees payment.

The use of the 55899 code will essentially require that supporting documentation is sent to the insurer prior to reimbursement. It is therefore crucial to understand the level of a patient's therapeutic fertility coverage prior to submission of this code. In our practice, if a patient has no therapeutic fertility benefits, he is automatically considered a self-pay patient. Patients often will ask for procedures to be submitted to insurance first to see "what comes out the other side." Doing this jeopardizes one's revenue. In the time necessary to sort through these claims, an entire treatment cycle can progress and patients can achieve their end goal of becoming pregnant. At this point, altruism and honoring debts owed often take a backseat to the end goal achieved.

Another frequently performed procedure for men with compromised fertility is a varicocele repair. When billing for varicocele repair, because it has a defined CPT code and ICD-10 code, authorizations and payments are generally straightforward. A useful tip is the addition of both a surgical microscope CPT code as well as a Doppler ultrasound code, as both of these technologies are commonly employed in microsurgical varicocelectomy.

Effective use of modifiers is another effective way to enhance revenue. Modifiers for bilateral procedures, distinctly separate procedures, and procedures done on the same day as a counseling visit can improve the yield from a provider's work.

Negotiating with Insurance

As a male reproductive specialist, the unique set of skills also opens a window of opportunity to negotiate with insurers directly to increase reimbursement for specific procedures. These "carveout" types of arrangements are specific in nature and apply only to a handful of procedures in which the provider demonstrates an added level of expertise. For procedures that are commonly performed there is some revenue advantage to the effort it takes to make this happen with insurers.

Take Home Points
- Clarification of a patient's fertility benefits is a crucial first step.
- Effective, timely, and consistent communication and messaging.
- Appropriate use of both pre-authorization and pre-determination when appropriate.
- Data analysis of revenue can lend insight into gaps and revenue problems as well as openings to negotiate better rates with insurers.
- Maintaining a diligent staff to work claims and contested submissions is important for efficient billing and collecting.

Chapter 14
The Role for Nurse Practitioners and Physician Assistants in Men's Health

Susanne A. Quallich

Introduction

Many of the authors in this book have attested to the reality that there is not a recognized "men's health" provider, nor does the literature suggest who might best fill this role. This opens the field up to any providers who have a wish to focus on the care of men, but this desire is limited by the lack of curricula offerings for medical, nursing, and physician assistant students alike. Providers are forced to learn specific information on their own or at continuing education activities; this does offer specific advantages, however, as the present focus on men's health may be somewhat free of institutional bias as a result.

A men's health clinic (MHC) can serve a variety of purposes in community and as such needs to acknowledge the specific *local* population it is intended to serve, despite the potential for a larger watershed referral area. This starts with the definition of the local community, whether it be predominantly rural, inner city, designed to meet the needs of elderly men, or designed to appeal to an LGBTQ community. The idea and realization of a men's health clinic lags considerably behind the well-established women's health clinics that are offered at many high-ranking academic medical centers [1].

Background

While there are ample examples in the literature of nurse practitioners and physician assistants (APP) specializing in particular domains of medical care (e.g., diabetes management, emergency medicine, cardiology), there is very little that can be drawn

S. A. Quallich (✉)
University of Michigan/Michigan Medicine, Department of Urology, Ann Arbor, MI, USA
e-mail: quallich@umich.eud

© Springer Nature Switzerland AG 2021
J. P. Alukal et al. (eds.), *Design and Implementation of the Modern Men's Health Center*, https://doi.org/10.1007/978-3-030-54482-9_14

from the literature regarding the role of the APP specifically in men's health clinics. This is owing in part to the fact that there is no single specialty that claims the domain of men's health, creating a situation in which providers of all types may specialize in men's health- from urology clinics, internal medicine clinics, family practice clinics, mental health, and cardiology clinics. However, urology providers often fill this role by default, especially as men with sexual health and reproductive complaints may bypass primary care completely and self-refer to urology providers because they feel that primary care is ill-equipped to identify and manage their specific concerns.

From the perspective of urology, there is some data that can be used to extrapolate a valuable role for APPs in a specialty men's health clinic. Langston et al. [2] reported that APPs in urology were predominantly involved in ambulatory clinics and usually worked independently. These authors further reported that survey participants ($n = 296$) reported most of their time spent in managing general urology concerns and reported various percentages of time-performing procedures that were unique to the care of men. This included transrectal ultrasound (6%), LHRH antagonist insertion (28%), hydrocele aspiration (13%), penile injection teaching (43%), transrectal ultrasound-guided prostate biopsy (6%), Xiaflex injections (3%), circumcision (2%), and vasectomy (1%). Furthermore, respondents reported predominantly practicing in an urban, institutional setting with communities large enough that could sustain a specialty men's health clinic.

Langston et al. [3] also reviewed Medicare Physician Supplier Procedure Summary Master Files to extract procedures that were performed by APPs, to further characterize their role in urology clinics. These authors reported a steady increase in the number of cystoscopies performed by APPs from 1999 through 2010. Rates of other male-specific urologic procedures, such as in penile injection, also showed a slower but steady increase from 1999 to 2013.

Taylor and Hotaling [4] offer an exemplar that describes the role of APPs in a specifically designed men's health clinic that was established at the University of Utah in 2013. These authors offer their experience with the success of adding APPs to this clinic environment. Adding APPs to a men's health clinic results in decreased wait times, promotes integration with other medical disciplines, and addresses specific concerns of men that have emerged as a result of direct-to-consumer advertising around issues such as testosterone replacement. This MHC arrangement also has the advantage of offering men the option to coordinate further care through the men's health clinic, resulting in the fewest number of total visits and a prudent use of healthcare resources. Taylor and Hotaling go on to propose that APPs improve a clinic's visit capacity and can be very productive members of the care team when standardized care pathways are in place. These authors go on to report that APP-performed procedures in this MHC at the University of Utah clinic include cystoscopy, testosterone pellet implantation, plaque injection for Peyronie's disease, and penile injection for erectile dysfunction.

Academic medical centers have only recently begun to add specific men's health clinics to their list of specialties. Choy et al. [1] evaluated the availability of men's health clinics versus women's health clinics in academic medical centers. These authors highlighted a clear disparity in the number of men's health clinics that were available when compared with the availability of specific women's health clinics. They also reported that men's health clinics were staffed by multidisciplinary providers that included internal medicine, family practice, cardiology, endocrinology, and urology. For those clinics that advertise services, the services tended to be urology-specific and included treatment for hypogonadism, erectile dysfunction, benign prostatic hyperplasia, and male infertility.

Men's Clinics: Developing a Role for the APP

It is clear that APPs can be trained to do most procedures, even those that are considered complex procedures, with a program of formal or on-the-job training with a physician or more experienced APP. But the issue remains in defining what the best role is for APPs in a specialized men's health clinic. More and more specialties are using APPs to improve access and offer a method for continuity of care [2, 3, 5–9], and this APP role is particularly effective with geriatric patients [10, 11]. This may be of particular interest as the US population continues to age, as there is a clear intersection for urology and geriatric care [12]. Stange [13] reported that the actual provider providing care might be less vial than the *environment* in which that care is provided, suggesting that a clinical environment designed with the needs of a particular population in mind (such as men) may have more success than a clinic designed to appeal to all patients.

Developing a men's health clinic, or furthering the capacity for men's health clinic, must keep in mind some of the issues that have kept men from pursuing primary care in the past. These issues, such as the local geographic definition of masculinity, are well detailed and other sources and beyond the scope of this chapter. But the local definition and cultural forces that define health are key determinants in the use of preventive health services by male populations. Establishing the needs of an individual man should begin with an investigation of how he personally defines health: is it the ability to work, maintain roles as father and spouse, or exercise at a marathon-athlete level? Men who present with a urology or sexual function concern after an absence from routine care should be viewed as needing a "gateway visit" that reintroduces men to routine care needs. As recommended by Miner et al. [14], this reintroduction visit can include (in addition to blood pressure measurements and waist circumference)

- Serum glucose vs glycosylated hemoglobin (HgbA1c)
- Serum creatinine
- Albumin/creatinine ratio
- Fasting lipids
- Assessment of cardiovascular risk
- Measurement of total testosterone
- Coronary artery calcium (CAC) score as an additional measure of cardiovascular risk

Additional evaluation could include (based on age and risk) PSA screening, referral for screening colonoscopy, screening for osteoporosis, referral for mental health concerns, and social work referrals for socioeconomic challenges. Initiating and interpreting all of these studies and referrals falls well within the APP scope of practice.

One perspective on developing the role of the APP in a MHC could be a focus on patient follow-up and coordination of care with other specialists that may also be a designated part of the MHC). This would allow a lengthier and complete results discussion with the APP, in turn allowing the physician to focus his/her schedule on more complex new patients to the clinic, concentrating on management of those men that require specialty-specific follow-up. This structure could promote billing at the highest rate possible and create a broader-based education and coordination role for the APP that takes advantage of their training curricula and education.

The role of the APP in a MHC can also be determined by a broader perspective, one that aligns with the needs of the community and the definitions of health and wellness that are prevalent. This can capitalize on the components of the NP/PA curricula that emphasize a primary care or family/internal medicine perspective. The additional of APPs to men's health clinics can obviously increase access, but it is also a value-added move (especially in a MHC that is more urology-focused) that can capitalize on more holistic or complete assessment of men, a perspective that can be vital with men who do not have or choose not to have a regular primary care provider. This makes the MHC a place that promotes both quality and value from an interdisciplinary perspective, recognizing that the "best" provider for specific visits at a MHC may not be a urologist or other physician, but an APP. Nurse practitioners and physician assistants excel in the management of chronic conditions that require episodic *medical* management, in this may be the context in which they are most valuable in a men's health clinic. They may become the primary MHC providers who provide management of conditions such as erectile dysfunction and sexual function concerns, BPH, hypertension, and obesity management. This perspective on health care management also aligns with the concept that healthcare is preventive care, and must come from a management-across-the-lifespan perspective rather than from an episodic, single contact perspective that only addresses acute illness.

APPs may be the providers that are well-suited for community outreach programs that emphasize the need for routine care, and educate men in an environment where they may be more comfortable. This offers the opportunity to investigate facets of the male community that may have high-risk behaviors; this can be sexual behaviors, inactivity, diet issues, or alcohol and drug use issues that may not be a readily obvious in a formal clinic environment. This would offer many opportunities to integrate the recognized social determinants of men's health into community interventions. This would include acknowledgments of patients who suffer from poverty, lack of healthcare savvy, geography and access issues, incarceration, unemployment or underemployment, and insurance challenges. Furthermore, the identification of these particular issues has implications for disease management and treatment adherence, as well as overall physical health.

Lastly, a key role for APPs in the men's health clinic will be to function as instructors and preceptors for students from all healthcare disciplines, as way to introduce them to the nuances that are involved in the care of men, cultivating next generation of nurse practitioners and physician assistants who may be interested in moving into this particular specialty focus.

Conclusions

The value of APPs in any clinical environment has been well-established, both anecdotally and with support in the literature. Including APPs in a focused men's health clinic is a natural progression of the increasing presence of APPs in specialty clinical environments. Focusing on men's health is a vital component to impact the health of families and communities in overall society, and nurse practitioners and physician assistants can play a vital role in health promotion for men.

References

1. Choy J, Kashanian JA, Sharma V, Masson P, Dupree J, Le B, Brannigan RE. The men's health center: disparities in gender specific health services among the top 50 "best hospitals" in America. Asian J Urol. 2015;2(3):170–4.
2. Langston JP, Orcutt VL, Smith AB, Schultz H, Hornberger B, Deal AB, et al. Advanced practice providers in US urology: a national survey of demographics and clinical roles. Urol Pract. 2017;4(5):418–24.
3. Langston JP, Duszak R Jr, Orcutt VL, Schultz H, Hornberger B, Jenkins LC, et al. The expanding role of advanced practice providers in urologic procedural care. Urology. 2017;106:70–5.
4. Taylor K, Hotaling J. A men's health clinic exemplar: experience at the University of Utah. In: Quallich SA, editor. Manual of men's health: a practice guide for APRNs and PAs. New York: Springer Publishing Company; 2018.
5. Chaney AJ, Harnois DM, Musto KR, Nguyen JH. Role development of nurse practitioners and physician assistants in liver transplantation. Prog Transplant. 2016;26(1):75–81.
6. Colvin L, Cartwright A, Collop N, Freeman N, McLeon D, Weaver T, Rogers A. Advanced practice registered nurses and physician assistants in sleep centers and clinics: a survey of current roles and educational background. J Clin Sleep Med. 2014;10(5):581–7.
7. Day CS, Boden SD, Knott PT, O'rourke NC, Yang BW. Musculoskeletal workforce needs: are physician assistants and nurse practitioners the solution? AOA critical issues. JBJS. 2016;98(11):e46.
8. Hooker RS, Brock DM, Cook ML. Characteristics of nurse practitioners and physician assistants in the United States. J Am Assoc Nurse Pract. 2016;28(1):39–46.
9. Morgan P, Himmerick KA, Leach B, Dieter P, Everett C. Scarcity of primary care positions may divert physician assistants into specialty practice. Med Care Res Rev. 2017;74(1):109–22.
10. Morilla-Herrera JC, Garcia-Mayor S, Martín-Santos FJ, Uttumchandani SK, Campos ÁL, Bautista JC, Morales-Asencio JM. A systematic review of the effectiveness and roles of advanced practice nursing in older people. Int J Nurs Stud. 2016;53:290–307.
11. Reuben DB, Ganz DA, Roth CP, McCreath HE, Ramirez KD, Wenger NS. Effect of nurse practitioner comanagement on the care of geriatric conditions. J Am Geriatr Soc. 2013;61(6):857–67.

12. Quallich SA. Geriatric urology and the role of the nurse practitioner. Urol Nurs. 2017;37(3):114–8.
13. Stange K. How does provider supply and regulation influence health care markets? Evidence from nurse practitioners and physician assistants. J Health Econ. 2014;33:1–27.
14. Miner MM, Heidelbaugh J, Paulos M, Seftel AD, Jameson J, Kaplan SA. The intersection of medicine and urology: an emerging paradigm of sexual function, cardiometabolic risk, bone health, and men's health centers. Med Clin. 2018;102(2):399–415.

Chapter 15
Future Directions in Men's Health Technology

Mike Pell

The Fundamental Problem

The last thing most men want to do is talk about their personal health issues. Why? Stubbornness, embarrassment, pride, stupidity. Pick any or all. And it doesn't seem to matter who's asking either – a trusted friend, wife, partner, children, even close family. It's just not discussed, and that's the problem. Even as sensitive women's health issues such as ovarian and breast cancer are openly talked about and rallied around, men's health issues still remain taboo to discuss for much of Western society.

The fact that men generally don't want to talk about these things (even with the people closest to us) means we are not getting out in front of potentially serious issues. Even after signs that something is wrong, we typically wait until there seems to be little choice but to engage with professionals. This prideful type of behavior, as we all know, often leads to situations where help comes too late in the process.

Not all men act this way, of course. Some do proactively use Google searches, medical websites, and self-diagnosis apps in an attempt to learn just enough about the situation to know what to do next. The trouble with this type of self-diagnosis is they can still miss something by avoiding talking with a medical professional.

Billions of web searches and thousands of medical-related websites have been serving the function of providing "expert" advice for decades. We have successfully published and crowd-sourced the world's combined opinions on men's health into a

---

DISCLAIMER – As neither a doctor nor researcher, the perspective and assertions set forth here by the author are his own, and do not necessarily reflect those of his employer or associated organizations. The following discussion and design is highly informed by decades of creating usable and impactful technological solutions for millions of people, but is not a proven and validated solution endorsed for wide deployment in the medical space.

M. Pell (✉)
Envisioneer, Woodinville, WA, USA

© Springer Nature Switzerland AG 2021
J. P. Alukal et al. (eds.), *Design and Implementation of the Modern Men's Health Center*, https://doi.org/10.1007/978-3-030-54482-9_15

confusing mountain of information. It's incredibly useful when you hit upon the right source and context, and frustratingly confusing when you can't discern fact from opinion, or protocol from advice.

So, what are we to do? How do we heal ourselves when all we're willing to do is randomly poke through a miles long search result list hoping for clarity? It turns out this situation is precisely where a particular combination of technologies has a useful part to play.

The Role of Technology in Men's Health

What became clear after many discussions with current patients and observations from professionals is that what men need most during these stressful and upsetting times is not a generic web search or medical app, but rather a trusted professional to talk with, who could tell us exactly what to do next in unequivocal terms, leaving out any unnecessary jargon or clinical descriptions.

Our insight and the guiding principle for this exploration is that despite our natural aversion to discussing these topics, most men actually do prefer talking with a person directly rather than sifting through an electronic pile of information to guide them to the next step in their diagnosis or treatment. Having some clarity around that condition started us down a path of exploration that calls for a fundamental shift in how we approach this problem of habitual avoidance.

The shift involves moving men away from interacting with web searches and knowledge bases to a more personal conversational interface to access the information and next steps we need to move ahead.

Our approach is two pronged – (1) leverage some promising new technology to mimic discreet conversations you'd have with a trusted professional and (2) involve the person's support system in the solution.

First, we do recognize very acutely that you cannot just substitute technology, however sophisticated, for an expert physician's experience, technique, and instinct in a completely reliable way. People are still indispensable. Despite the daily advances in tech like artificial intelligence and machine learning, it is very difficult to replicate the intangibles of human instinct. Our personal interactions are often very subtle and nuanced. We can however codify the collective knowledge and insights of experts into a conversational form that can be used to guide next steps and decisions.

Second, since men are reluctant to seek medical advice or treatment until it's almost too late, we need to put part of this effort into other people's hands. We can't count on men themselves changing their behavior or attitudes overnight, but we can try to have their friends and family advocate an easy path forward. At least for this initial experiment, we'll leave it to our loved ones to talk some sense into us by leveraging some clever technology.

Combined, these two aspects provide a promising alternative to today's habitual avoidance and self-diagnosis. They essentially yield a digital guide and support system to move forward, modeled on interactions with a real-life men's health medical professional.

Your Personal Guide to Men's Health

In some medical departments, clinics, and practices around the world, there is a person or a small set of people who direct patients, family members, and friends to the right person to talk with or next step in their journey. These people are often called *patient coordinators* or *patient navigators*. Their main purpose is to move people through the medical system with the ultimate goal of successful resolution. In no way do they pretend to be a physician, surgeon, or other medical professional. They are very clear about their role.

Using that type of real-world men's health professional as our primary model, we are experimenting with providing that function to medical organizations in the form of digital assistant when a person is not available. Being mindful of the failures and limitations with this type of solution, our goal is to fill the gap with a first-line responder for people who are hesitant to reach out to a real person initially, for whatever reason.

> Part skillful navigator of health systems, part personal confidant, part scheduler, part super-connector, this thoughtfully crafted *digital navigator* gives men, and the people who make up their support system, a way to quickly take action to move them to the next step in their journey, whatever that may be.

The most common situations where a patient navigator proves helpful involve hugely stressful medical events such as a life-threatening diagnosis for yourself or a loved one. In these cases, do you really want a faceless, mechanical construct telling you what all this means and what to do next? Not usually. Our nature is to seek out other people to advise us quickly with their expertise. Our confidence in their advice is drawn from our interaction.

Enter technology as a friendly, neutral, and non-judgmental assistant in getting to the bottom of men's health issues.

Common Scenarios

Here are some examples of situations we're targeting for this use of technology to help open up discussions and enable people to take direct action, which in many cases would lead to talking with a professional.

1. *What could be wrong?*

   This is a bit too embarrassing to discuss with my wife or friends, but I have been feeling some real discomfort from time to time when urinating. Doesn't happen all the time, but when it does, it's pretty uncomfortable. I have dealt with worse pain before, but not like this. I can live with it for now, but it does seem like it's getting worse.

   Wonder if I should search the web to see what it could possibly be. Could be anything. Ugh. Where do I start? How do I know if this is it, or not? Thinking I may have to talk to someone about this. Really can't stand that though. Wish there was a way to do this without going into the office.

2. *Understanding a diagnosis*

   After a routine annual physical, you're shocked to hear that your doctor suspects you have prostate cancer. It never occurred to you that occasional pain while urinating was being caused by a growing cancer. As you try to understand what all this means sitting in your doctor's office, an unsettling feeling of confusion and detachment quickly set in, making it almost impossible to listen and understand what the doctor is saying.

   It is not until you arrive home, sit for some time, and try to recall the conversation that you realize much of what was said is just a blur. Wanting to be better informed before talking with your family, you start typing words into the Google search box hoping it will somehow give you an idea of what to do next. Nothing doing. I wish there was an app or better tool that would let me figure this out.

3. *What should we do next?*

   After being told second-hand that your husband has prostate cancer, you immediately shift into problem-solving mode. What is that disease exactly? Do we need a second opinion? Is it fatal or treatable? What's the very next thing we should do? There are a million questions to ask. Without direct access to the doctor who provided the diagnosis, it's natural to start searching the web for answers.

   The problem of course is you don't know exactly what terms to type in, and which search result link to click when it returns over a million. Who is reliable? Which of these are ads? After an hour of trying to figure out what to do next, you realize that just calling the doctor is really the next step. I want to be educated before I call the doctor's office directly. Wish there was someone I could talk with or something on their website to help me figure out how this process works.

All of these scenarios can be experienced by the same person, or an entire group of concerned people. Perhaps even worse is when this is happening to a family member or friend who isn't near enough to care for personally. It's in these times that we need a trusted source of information and next steps. We need a better solution.

Key Aspects

The previous scenarios illustrated some of the important drivers behind our foundational design decisions and overall direction for the digital patient navigator.

1. The first and most important reason for this digital system to exist is to *guide people toward a next action that involves a real medical professional*, not just provide information that is easily misinterpreted or ignored.
2. Designing the system to *learn what the most useful responses to patient and family inquiries are* provides an invaluable feedback mechanism and turning capability. Without resorting to traditional patient surveys, we can observe and adapt to subsequent actions to provide real value for people choosing to use this approach to fact gathering and decision making.
3. Scaling this solution out addresses the *scarcity of real patient navigators* is the next big reason to invest in this type of technology solution. Given their importance and value to people, you'd think these patient navigators would be found everywhere. But sadly, they are rare today. Why? Not every medical organization can find someone skilled enough to do this, nor can strapped programs afford to pay the salary of this type of person.

Experience Design

In thinking about how to address the challenge of providing better direction and guidance, our model for the patient experience is simple – having a conversation with a trusted medical professional. Similar with family and friends – our goal is to give you easy access to the kind of answers and facts your loved one may not be able to relay properly or just doesn't know the answer to.

To achieve that desired level of trust for patients and their families throughout this experience, we would optimally need to provide a real person, not a website or app. And that's precisely the issue. There are not enough medical departments and clinics with these real patient navigators to guide people through the process. Given that, we need to assemble technology that models that personal type of conversation as closely as we can.

Designing a conversational digital medical assistant that enables people to access critically important information during stressful times is very difficult to get right. In these stressful situations, our collective patience is short and nerves frayed. Each interaction needs to be modeled as closely as possible to a real conversation so that the participant is afforded all the same choices and can observe the same type of hinting a human would exhibit.

Humans are very attuned to awkward exchanges, stilted speech, or canned responses. Not to mention that being factual and clear has never been more important. Adhering to highly ethical standards of information disclosure and citation cannot be compromised or discounted.

Advanced Technologies

In order for us to achieve the level of trust we are aiming for, there are several new technologies and approaches we'll need to employ in our system design. These can be mix and match among providers or all found within one vendor. The specific implementations are not important at first; the fact that we are taking a leap forward from the typical static website is key.

Artificial Intelligence (AI) is a very broad area of technologies and thinking that we'll leverage. Often associated with malevolent villains in science fiction movies and stories, AI is terribly miscast. True it's a technology that enables machines to approximate human intelligence, but its role in computing is the opposite of its movie persona. It is actually very useful as a worker bee, doing the things that people are not good at, such as spotting microtrends in huge data sets, monitoring events at scale, and learning how to identify things in the same way humans do.

AI is clearly an integral part of our lives already, hardly noticed by most due to its behind-the-scenes role in today's common scenarios. When your phone does something that seems incredibly useful without you asking it to – that's AI. When your Amazon Echo plays your favorite song without you explicitly telling it to, that's AI. When Windows reminds you that 2 days ago you promised Sam you'd send that report, that's AI. We'll use some very particular aspects of AI in our conversational patient navigator design described below.

Machine Learning (ML) is a subfield of AI that deals with systems that learn over time (which is very important to our project). The critical part of ML for this application is that without being explicitly programmed to do so, these advanced software systems are trained to recognize and learn by examining and analyzing many large data sets. From that analysis, a model is trained, similar to how we learn by observing and testing the world around us as we grow up. Being able to recognize an object, pattern, or behavior is extremely useful when building systems to deal with conversations. Though ML, we can spot trends in how people ask questions that may lead to early identification of issues or a helpful diagnosis.

Reinforcement Learning is an approach within AI systems to find the optimal behavior or path in a particular situation, which is beneficial to the person using the system. We do this by using systems to observe the real-world behavior of people over time to see what they choose or pass on, do or don't, revisit or ignore. Inherent to this approach is the notion of people somehow being rewarded for good choices through an enhanced experience. For example, if enough people use our digital navigator to get advice on a particular aspect of men's health such as bladder cancer, the system can recommend a particular set of responses that appear to have satisfied previous queries properly. No other responses need be offered to those types of inquiries in the future to optimize the experience.

Bots or Chatbots are AI-powered software agents that enable a conversational interface to provide answers to frequently asked questions. These bots are often used for doing repetitive and predictable responses for customer service questions on websites. The key aspect of bots is their ability to learn how to better answer questions over time based on getting more information from previous sessions. The interaction model is a person asks the bot a question via a website, phone app, or digital assistant. The response will be based on a model and database that the bot is tied to for its domain knowledge.

All combined, these new technologies fill out the framework of a conversational service designed to lead patients and their families to the next step along their journey in men's health issue diagnosis and treatment.

Example Interactions

Here's what some typical patient interactions with this type of conversational system would be like.

1. *What could be wrong?*
   After enduring a few weeks of increasingly painful urinations, George decides it's finally time to figure out what could be wrong, but is too embarrassed to discuss it with his wife, kids, or even his doctor (mostly for fear of having a lot of useless and expensive tests). Not wanting to talk about this, his first thought is to just start typing search terms into Google and see what it returns, which he does, only to find it has both confused him and scared him. How am I to know which of these descriptions to trust given so many sound similar? His frustration grows to the point of wanting to go back to ignoring the problem.

   After talking with a friend at lunch the next day, he decides to try a different approach. By going to his doctor's website, he can use a new tool that focuses on figuring out what's wrong by asking a series of questions based on your initial questions. That sounds much better than talking directly with his doctor or staff, so he tries it out. The results were very different than he thought.

   Instead of getting a ton of possibilities of what could be wrong, the system asked a few questions back and forth, and then focused down on one area in particular – prostate cancer. His expectation was not having the system tell him exactly what's wrong and what to do about it, but rather provide some strong guidance. And he got it – yet instead of speculation, he learned more about the probable causes and was strongly encouraged to connect with a professional who can help him get the proper diagnosis and treatment. Not wanting to ignore the symptoms any longer, he took the advice of the professionals via the site and did schedule an appointment.

2. Understanding a diagnosis
   Shortly after being told by her husband that his doctor suspects he has a form of prostate cancer, Meixia gets right to work. She was mad that he waited so long to find out what was wrong and tell her, but that's not the issue now – she needs to figure out what to do next. He didn't even know exactly what the diagnosis was – just a vague description is all he can remember.

She starts by Googling "bladder cancer" and is immediately overwhelmed by the amount of information available. But none of the top responses or pages are telling her what it means for his future. What are the next immediate steps to take? What kind of a journey are they about to undertake? A million questions arise from just the first few pages clicked on. There must be a better way to educate herself before talking with the doctor. And there is.

By going to the men's health clinic's website, she sees a download link for a new smartphone app to help her navigate men's health issues. After installing it, a friendly looking person's picture who says they'd be happy to answer questions. Little did she know that it felt just like talking with a person, not some robot. In almost no time, she was able to understand what her husband couldn't explain very well. And she was presented with an easy-to-follow roadmap for potential next steps along the journey of proper diagnosis and treatment.

Relieved by what she was able to learn by talking with the digital patient navigator, she leapt into action by getting her husband and older children involved in a plan to get to the bottom of the problem and tackle it head on together.

3. *What should we do next?*

After learning about his father's prostate cancer diagnosis, Alok is floored. He never thought his dad would have a problem like this – he's been the model of health his whole life. Tough as nails. Devastating to think he could lose him so quickly. But, then he realizes there's very little he actually knows about this disease.

His mom told him to go to the doctor's website to access an incredible tool to learn more about it. But instead, he asks Alexa through his *Amazon Echo* what prostate cancer is. She is able to give him a short and general description, but not enough info to calm his fears. Asking for a deeper explanation, Alexa is able to reference a new service that can have a conversation about men's health issues.

In the privacy of his home, through his own Amazon Echo, he is able to have a back and forth conversation with this new men's health service to get some of his most pressing questions answered surprisingly well. The nature of the disease, common symptoms, treatments, and mortality statistics. The ease of getting information in this way is encouraging him to continue digging.

After 10 minutes, it's time to confront the issue head on, armed with better information. He calls his dad to make sure there's an appointment with the doctor that his family can also attend. Of course, he didn't set up a follow-up visit to deal with his treatment options. So, he gets off the phone, and asks Alexa to request an appointment with the doctor's office for the next week so they can get to the bottom of all this together.

By now, you can see the pattern of how these technological aides to learning more about men's health issues can open up dialogue and discussion not only between patients and professionals, but also with their families and friends.

System Design

This conversational system could be designed with any number of technologies we discussed previously applied to the problem, but for this example we'll focus on some well-known techniques, technologies, products, and services for the key system components.

There are typically three parts (layers or tiers as they are known in tech circles) to the design of a system like this. The *presentation layer* or user experience is how we interact with the system, the *application layer*, or business logic portion controls the exchange of information between the person and the technologies. And finally, the *data layer* or backend is the faceless portion that does the processing, storage, and heavy lifting for the system. Together, these sections form a seamless experience for the patient and their support network.

Presentation Layer

In essence, the user interface or presentation layer of a technology system is how we communicate and interact with it. For most situations, this would take the physical form of a website, app, or digital assistant of some kind.

These interfaces are implemented in a variety of forms that cater to a person's devices and their preferred method of input. The key to designing a great "front end" is enabling enough choice within expected input methods that we have effectively removed any barrier to use. If the person can find and use it on their iPad, Android phone, Google Home, or Microsoft Surface Book, we have provided enough access for it to be considered accessible.

For a website, we'd enable the expected mouse and keyboard input, touch perhaps on a phone or tablet, and voice or other specialized methods that fall into the accessibility category.

For a digital assistant, a voice-only interface (like found in Amazon's Alexa) has become fairly standard. Same with our navigation systems within automobiles.

The presentation layer is typically constructed from HTML and Javascript technologies for web-based offerings, and a variety of languages and tech for the voice-based services.

The key aspects of the presentation layer are flexibility, speed, and forgiveness.

Application Layer

Understanding what a person is asking for and getting it for them is the role of the application layer of a system like this. We often overlook this important function because it's almost completely invisible to most of us. When we ask for something, it just magically appears. The sequence of events, logic involved, and interchange of information are all contained within this layer. That's why this layer is often referred to as the business logic of a system.

This layer is typically kept separate from the presentation layer to allow for multiple types of input experiences that can leverage a single implementation of logic and accessor functions for the information and data needed by the system. Think of it as a self-contained service running in the cloud that can be accessed by many different types of front ends such as websites, apps, and devices.

Application layers are typically implemented as online services that are hosted on Microsoft Azure, Amazon Web Services, or Google Cloud Platform. These services are faceless, meaning they are meant to be a piece of middleware that is accessed by various front ends through and Application Programming Interface (API). This allows reuse and scalability.

The key aspects of the application layer are reusability and efficiency.

Data Layer

The "backend" of a system is where all of the information and data is stored and collected. If we ask questions about something, the answer will be retrieved from here. It's also where new information is stored as the system is used over time. This portion is composed of a continuously updated database, which is full artifacts important to the overall mission of system, such as textual responses, videos, photos, and records.

These collections of data can be massive and continue to grow over time. Often, the data layer pulls information from multiple sources, not all physically housed in the same place. Being able to source data from multiple locations makes the design more flexible and robust. Being able to keep this critical information secure and private is also a very important consideration when designing the implementation of the data layer.

The data layer is built out of large-scale databases and data warehouses hosted in Microsoft Azure and Amazon Web Services, employing SQL and other database technologies.

The key aspects of the data layer are integrity, security, and privacy.

Next Steps

Given the breadth of this solution space, our only way forward is to break the problem down into manageable steps and components.

The obvious first step is to create a website and mobile app that inspires a high degree of trust in patients through its simple language, direct approach, and detailed information. These experiences would embody a warm but professional look and feel that inspires confidence.

Next would come employing an AI system to convey the knowledge base to patients and their families in a conversational manner. In order to do that successfully, we'd have to train the AI model using our largest and most up-to-date knowledge bases and articles, along with testing the common scenarios found within normal conversations about men's health topics.

And finally, we'd experiment with voice-only or conversation first devices to try and get this service into the homes of people who are more comfortable dealing with questions and answers in that way.

By building out and testing our initial assumptions and hypothesis at each stage, we can make meaningful progress in this pursuit of better outcomes.

Conclusion

The first steps toward a human-like patient navigator are already behind us, but the journey ahead is long and challenging. The key is to keep experimenting and trying new approaches to keep it as humane as possible.

Our best work must be done in the realm of converting digital inquiries into in person conversations with Men's Health professionals – because in the end, people are the only thing that will solve both our medical and interpersonal issues.

Index

© Springer Nature Switzerland AG 2021
J. P. Alukal et al. (eds.), *Design and Implementation of the Modern Men's
Health Center*, https://doi.org/10.1007/978-3-030-54482-9